The
Fat Pedagogy
Reader

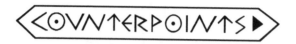

Studies in the Postmodern Theory of Education

Shirley R. Steinberg
General Editor

Vol. 467

The Counterpoints series is part of the Peter Lang Education list.
Every volume is peer reviewed and meets
the highest quality standards for content and production.

PETER LANG
New York • Bern • Frankfurt • Berlin
Brussels • Vienna • Oxford • Warsaw

The
Fat Pedagogy
Reader

CHALLENGING WEIGHT-BASED OPPRESSION
THROUGH CRITICAL EDUCATION

Edited by Erin Cameron & Constance Russell

PETER LANG
New York • Bern • Frankfurt • Berlin
Brussels • Vienna • Oxford • Warsaw

Library of Congress Cataloging-in-Publication Data

Names: Cameron, Erin, editor of compilation. | Russell, Constance, editor of compilation.
Title: The fat pedagogy reader: challenging weight-based oppression
through critical education / edited by Erin Cameron, Constance Russell.
Description: New York: Peter Lang, 2016.
Series: Counterpoints: studies in the postmodern theory
of education; vol. 467 | ISSN 1058-1634
Includes bibliographical references and index.
Identifiers: LCCN 2015042700 | ISBN 978-1-4331-2568-3 (hardcover: alk. paper)
ISBN 978-1-4331-2567-6 (paperback: alk. paper) | ISBN 978-1-4539-1784-8 (e-book)
Subjects: LCSH: Discrimination in education. | Discrimination against overweight persons.
Classification: LCC LC212.F38 2016 | DDC 379.2/6—dc23
LC record available at http://lccn.loc.gov/2015042700

Bibliographic information published by **Die Deutsche Nationalbibliothek**.
Die Deutsche Nationalbibliothek lists this publication in the "Deutsche
Nationalbibliografie"; detailed bibliographic data are available
on the Internet at http://dnb.d-nb.de/.

Contents

Part Four: Expanding Fat Pedagogies

Acknowledgments

First, the two of us want to express our heartfelt gratitude to all of the chapter authors. Simply put, without your contributions this book would not exist. We have learned much from you and look forward to future conversations and, perhaps, future collaborations.

We are very grateful to series editor Shirley Steinberg, who first encouraged us to develop a book on fat pedagogy. We also want to thank the team at the New York office of Peter Lang who helped turn this book into reality, particularly managing editor Chris Myers, Phyllis Korper, editorial assistant Stephen Mazur, and production director Bernie Shade.

Kathleen Knowling kindly gave us permission to reprint her evocative art on the cover, which we very much appreciate. Thank you to Natalie Beausoleil for introducing us to Kathleen and for letting us borrow this piece of art that hangs proudly in her home.

The advertisement in Chapter 21 is reprinted with permission of Propaganda Advertising, Romania.

Individually, we each have many other people to thank as well.

Connie. To begin, Tema Sarick first introduced me to fat acceptance; while it may have taken years for the fat acceptance Tema modeled in her own inimitable way to stick and, alas, it still comes unstuck fairly easily even now, I remain grateful. Conversations with a number of friends, family members, colleagues, and students have been invaluable to me on this journey of learning and un-learning as has the cheerleading and the more quiet yet still rock solid support of others. So, a great big fat thank you to Jean Aguilar-Valdez, Anne Bell, Paul Berger, Mary Breunig, Jocelyn Burkhart, Joan Chambers, Lori Chambers, Lauren Corman, James Czank, Glynis Digby, Justin Dillon, Leesa Fawcett, Natalie Gerum, Annette Gough, Sue Hamel, Joe Heimlich, Kristen Hardy, Richard Kahn, Morgan Kensington, Gail Kuhl, Alex Lawson, Teresa Lloro-Bidart, Greg Lowan-Trudeau, Janice Mason, Ledah McKellar, Hannah McNinch, Marcia McKenzie, Rachel Mishenene, Helle

Möller, Blair Niblett, Jan Oakley, Leigh Potvin, Alan Reid, Emily Root, Donna Russell, Ken Russell, Pauline Sameshima, Lex Scully, Marilyn Silverman, Keri Semenko, Teresa Socha, Bob Stevenson, Christina van Barneveld, Peter van der Veen, Pam Wakewich, Gerald Walton, Hilary Whitehouse, Karen Williams, and the late Brent Cuthbertson. I particularly want to thank Erin Cameron for pushing me to finally start writing about fat pedagogy after so many years of talking about it, and also for insisting that we edit this book together; I have learned much from you and from the process of working on our various projects. Finally, I very much appreciate the unwavering support of my husband, Mike Hosszu; I feel very fortunate to have him in my corner.

Erin. I have described elsewhere my encounters with weight-based oppression in the settings of sport, physical education, and teacher education. Despite these unsettling encounters, it wasn't until pursuing doctoral studies that I found critical "obesity" and fat scholarship—it felt like coming home. It put into context the discomfort I had felt for years as I witnessed constant weight-based oppression in sport and gymnasium settings. In my first year of doctoral studies, it was reading Geneviève Rail's article "Canadian Youth's Discursive Constructions of Health in the Context of Obesity Discourse" and interacting with her when she was a guest scholar at Lakehead University that cemented my academic interest in this field. It was thus fitting that four years later Geneviève served as the external reviewer for my dissertation defense. I have many other people to thank for nurturing and supporting my interest in this growing field. I would first like to thank the 26 individuals who participated in my dissertation research, who shared with me their pedagogical approaches, challenges, and successes as accomplished scholars and teachers working in the fields of critical obesity studies, critical weight studies, critical geographies of body size, Health at Every Size, and fat studies. Their humility, generosity, and genuine interest in my study was a gift and inspired, in many ways, my interest in working on this book. I'd also like to thank my doctoral committee who offered valuable insights and input into my thinking about fat pedagogy, namely, Teresa Socha (supervisor), Joe Barrett, Connie Russell, Gerald Walton (committee members), Lori Chambers (internal examiner), and as mentioned, Geneviève Rail (external examiner). In particular, I'd like to thank Connie, whose excitement and interest in anything fat was inspiring and indeed instrumental in fueling my own interests in the field. As a new scholar dealing with imposter syndrome, Connie's guidance through co-editing this book has been much appreciated. I am also indebted to many individuals for their support, friendship, and humanity as I delved into critical scholarship deconstructing notions of health, wellness, and fatness. A big thank you to Paul Berger, James Czank, Juan-Miguel Fernandez-Balboa, Joannie Halas, Michelle Kilborn, David Kirk, Kathy-Kortes-Miller, Jody Mitchell, Helle Möller, Jan Oakley, Alexa Scully, Earle Seigler, Ellen Singleton, Kelly Skinner, Mirella Stroink, Richard Tinning, and Pam Wakewich. I'd also like to thank the Social Sciences and Humanities Research Council of Canada for funding my doctoral research and showing me that scholarship related to critical obesity and fat studies can, and hopefully will someday, be mainstream! Lastly, I am indebted to my extended family and to my husband, Jeffrey, and two young children, Carter and Yannik. This is as much your journey as mine. I am particularly thankful to my mom, Heather Dean, who as an academic in the health sciences has provided unwavering support and offered invaluable insights into my thinking, research, and work.

Preface

How did I know, from my first days in kindergarten, that I was fat and didn't count the way other children did?

I was round-faced, slightly larger than my peers. I recall no overt statements, but by age 4, not quite 4, I knew that I was, indelibly, an outsider.

Was it the hint of disapproval in their voices when family members picked me up and pronounced the usual line, "My, you're getting big"? Was it the other children who knew each other from preschool and showed me I had no place in their pecking order? Was it my teachers whose attention fell on me differently, especially as they oversaw snack time and exercise routines? Did my beautiful, brilliant, fat mother convey this knowledge to me via her unspoken concern that I might face precisely these attitudes and this treatment? However, I found out—I learned she was right. Nothing about me could mitigate my bottom-rung position on the weight hierarchy. It never occurred to me to try to lose weight because I couldn't imagine anything I could do that would be enough to offset an exclusion that felt so thorough. (A feeling of futility for which I'm now deeply grateful. I've lived mostly free from the weight-loss industry's self-hate rituals.) In grammar school, my teachers reprimanded the students who teased or bullied me if they found out about it, saying my tormentors were wrong to torment me. But they never said that the kids were wrong about *me*. They never said I was fine as I was. I suspect the idea would have been as unthinkable to them as it had become to me.

Other than being fat and being a girl living under patriarchy, I carried all sorts of privilege and the luck of being good at school. Sexism and anti-fat attitudes altered my understanding of every interaction and while that combination offered me particular insights, fat people who face racism, homophobia, transphobia, ableism, and classism become expert in how these oppressions magnify, and are magnified by, weight bigotry.

The high school teacher who single-handedly turned me into a writer went hungry nibbling raw vegetables during her lunch hour and tailored her own clothes to hide the parts of her body that deviated in minor ways from her received idea of an acceptable figure. Years later, when I had come out as a fat person and created the print zine *FAT!SO?*—using everything she taught me—I sent her a copy but never heard a word. A fellow student who visited her around that time told me that when my name came up in their conversation, she had one word for my fat activism: "disgusting."

I came to fat identity through feminism. In college, I took feminist theory courses outside my required coursework. I was hoping to ease a pain I wasn't able to name. When I read the work of Julia Kristeva and Kim Chernin and others, it was obvious to me that "the body" they were so concerned about was not my fat body. I finally found words to describe my experience in my mid-20s when I read the groundbreaking 1983 anthology *Shadow on a Tightrope: Writings by Women on Fat Oppression*, edited by Lisa Schoenfielder and Barb Wieser.

During my zine years, I learned about three young people who committed suicide after weight-based bullying left them hopeless: Brian Head, Samuel Graham, and Kelly Yeomans. Brian had faced years of bullying for his weight when he brought a gun to high school one day. He stood up to his bully but ended by shooting himself that day, saying, "I'm sick of it."[1] Samuel undertook to lose weight the summer before he entered middle school, but feared it wasn't enough to prevent bullies from targeting him. He hung himself from a tree the night before school started.[2] Kelly's bullies escalated from attacking her at school to repeatedly throwing food at her house and yelling taunts. She took an overdose at age 13.[3]

Because of these tragic deaths, I felt I had to do more than publish a zine. These three young people were not the only ones in pain. Despite my fear of public speaking, I couldn't remain silent, so I started giving talks about weight-based oppression and fat liberation. I hoped to do whatever I could to address the cruelty and suffering. For my first talk, a teacher friend invited me to speak to students in his middle school health education class. If I had to locate a time in my life when I felt most vulnerable to anti-fat attack and ostracism, it could easily have been my own seventh-grade health education class.

Now that I've given hundreds of talks in all sorts of settings, I know that people of all sizes suffer directly from weight-based oppression and are eager for better ways to navigate it. At the heart of each talk is an exercise that I call "Speed Anthropology." For 5 or 10 minutes, I ask people to be anthropologists and come up with the concepts that our culture associates with fat and thin. I write down their findings, divided by a line that later comes to represent the weight-based social hierarchy. I hope to use what people already know (but may not *know* they know) to raise their consciousness of weight oppression as a real and pervasive system that affects us all and that does serious harm. I hope to inspire people's outrage and tap into their self-interest to fight this system. I invite people to join me in rejecting weight-based oppression in ways that are fun and satisfying for them.

A necessary part of fat liberation is reclaiming ideas about health, eating, and physical activity from the anti-fat attitudes that have come to pervade them. As this anthology demonstrates, that project will take a long time and a lot of effort. It is a necessary endeavor if we are to address the fundamental question of whether fat people can be at home in our bodies and welcome in a society made up of a weight-diverse population, or whether we are a target to be eradicated. Embedded in all of the ostensibly salubrious efforts to reduce or prevent so-called obesity is an inherently eugenics-y worldview. I tell the stories of Brian, Samuel, and

Kelly because this anti-fat worldview is a particular threat to children and young people. It has certainly been a threat to me all of my life. I see its impact on people in the fat community and general society every day.

This preface serves as a latter-years version of a plea for help, safety, and personhood from my 4-year-old self standing in the doorway of that kindergarten classroom. Fat pedagogy—and more important a politicized fat pedagogy—is so very necessary. It can mean life or death.

~Marilyn Wann, author of *FAT!SO?* and creator of Yay! Scales

Notes

1   http://web.archive.org/web/20090403041656/http://www.esquire.com/ESQ1002-OCT_TERRIBLEBOY_rev
2   http://articles.chicagotribune.com/1996–08-27/news/9608270254_1_hanged-new-school-boy, http://articles.sun-sentinel.com/1996–09-01/news/9608310354_1_sunrise-middle-school-fat-jokes-religious-boy
3   http://news.bbc.co.uk/2/hi/uk_news/148765.stm

Introduction

Erin Cameron and Constance Russell

Why *The Fat Pedagogy Reader?*

Over the past decade, concerns about a global "obesity epidemic" have flourished (World Health Organization, 1998), appearing in media (Saguy & Almeling, 2008), popular culture (Kwan & Graves, 2013), and in speeches by health leaders who have made claims such as "obesity" being "more threatening than weapons of mass destruction" (Carmona, 2003, para. 66). Public health messages around physical activity, fitness, and nutrition permeate society and validate fat-phobic behaviors and practices. This "obesity" discourse dominates and serves to reproduce a framework of thinking, talking, and action in which thinness is privileged and in which a "size matters" message fuels narratives about fat people's irresponsibility and lack of willpower (see Gard & Wright, 2005; Lupton, 2013; Wann, 2009). Consider as well the photos of "headless fatties" that typically accompany news articles. In her analysis of this phenomenon, Charlotte Cooper (2007) notes how "the body becomes symbolic: we are there but we have no voice, not even a mouth in a head, no brain, no thoughts or opinions. Instead we are reduced and dehumanized as symbols of cultural fear" (para. 3). Such depictions, alongside images of people Photoshopped to unrealistic proportions, serve to inform society about whose bodies count as "normal." As Susan Bordo (1993) states, "This is perpetual pedagogy, how to interpret your body 101. These images are teaching us how to see … [and] training our perceptions in what's a defect and what is normal" (p. xvii).

A growing body of research provides alternative perspectives on "obesity" and fatness. Within this literature, scholars dispute scientific rationalizations of "obesity"; draw attention to the cultural, historical, political, and social contexts of "obesity" and fatness; and highlight how obesity discourse perpetuates harmful and oppressive assumptions, behaviors, and actions. New inter-disciplinary fields that problematize "obesity" have emerged, including critical obesity studies, critical weight studies, critical geographies of body size, and fat studies (Colls & Evans, 2009; Cooper, 2010). While these fields differ somewhat in focus, theoretical grounding, and meth-odologies, they are "united in their refusal to simply reproduce/legitimate/endorse biomedical narratives that would have us 'tackle' this putative problem" (Monaghan, Colls, & Evans, 2013, p. 251).

There also is a small but growing literature on how formal education (elementary, second-ary, and tertiary) acts as a powerful site for the (re)production of dominant obesity discourse, fat phobia, and weight-based oppression; scholars have critically examined curriculum, peda-gogy, policy, school culture, and the physical environment (e.g., Azzarito, 2007; Cameron, 2015a; Cameron et al., 2014; Evans, Rich, Davies, & Allwood, 2008; Farrell, 2013; Gard, 2008; Gard & Pluim, 2014; Guthman, 2009; Hetrick & Attig, 2009; Koppleman, 2009; Leahy, 2009; Petherick & Beausoleil, 2015; Powell & Fitzpatrick, 2013; Pringle & Pringle, 2012; Quennerstedt, Burrows, & Maivorsdotter, 2010; Rice, 2007; Rich, 2010; Russell, Cam-eron, Socha, & McNinch, 2013; Sykes, 2011; Sykes & McPhail, 2008; Weinstock & Krehbiel, 2009). Others have shared stories of teaching practices or their experiences of weight-based oppression or thin privilege in education settings (e.g., Boling, 2011; Brown, 2012; Cameron, 2015b; Escalera, 2009; Fisanick, 2006, 2007, 2014; Hopkins, 2011; Jones & Hughes-Deca-tur, 2012; Tirosh, 2006; Watkins & Concepcion, 2014; Watkins, Farrell, & Hugmeyer, 2012; Watkins & Hugmeyer, 2013).

In their book *Education, Disordered Eating and Obesity Discourse*, John Evans, Emma Rich, Brent Davies, and Rachel Allwood (2008) draw attention to how dominant obesity discourse is operationalized in educational contexts through a culture of body perfection and perfor-mance. They suggest that body pedagogies—"the conscious activities undertaken by people, organizations, or the state that are designed to enhance individuals' understanding of their own and others' corporeality" (p. 17)—reveal the "contributory" relationship between dominant obesity discourse in schools and harmful health consequences such as body dissatisfaction, disordered eating, excessive exercise, and depression. They also assert that we need to appreci-ate the complexity of the social conditions of students' embodied lives. Arguably, addressing the wider structures will require not just a politics of fat but also a politics of pedagogy, where teachers and scholars engage in reimagining an experience of education that is inclusive of size diversity.

Feminist and critical scholars working in education have advocated emancipatory and lib-eratory pedagogies, demonstrating that classrooms and other learning contexts are not separate from but instead extensions of a society fraught by hierarchies and structures of dominance (e.g., Darder, Baltodano, & Torres, 2009; hooks, 1995; Kincheloe, 2008; Sensoy & DiAngelo, 2011). To date, these scholars have focused on many social justice issues such as gender, race, class, sexuality, and ability, but few have focused on body size (Cameron et al., 2014). We as-sert that *all* educators need to pay attention to how classrooms and other learning contexts can turn bodies into political sites of privilege and oppression as well as the ways in which domi-nant obesity discourse and weight-based oppression, often expressed as fat phobia, fat hatred, and fat bullying, are being addressed within spaces and places of teaching and learning. While socially just pedagogies alone cannot redress the depth of inequity in educational institutions

(Apple, 2000), they certainly can play an important role in bringing attention, awareness, and recognition to specific areas of difference. With this in mind, this book is dedicated to exploring various ways in which educators are politically positioning critical perspectives of "obesity" and fatness in formal and informal educational settings, and thereby helping develop this emerging field of fat pedagogy. Given the growth in critical obesity and fat scholarship, the time does indeed appear ripe for *The Fat Pedagogy Reader*.

Before providing a brief overview of the book, we first want to describe four core concepts we used to frame it. While literature on disrupting dominant obesity discourse and addressing weight-based oppression has begun to enter the mainstream in some fields such as sociology and women's studies, it has not yet gained traction in many others, including education (Brown, 2012). Taking a few moments, then, to situate the book seems to be in order.

Building Upon *The Fat Studies Reader*

In the late 1960s, a social movement began to emerge that called for a radical shift in understandings of fatness. Like other social movements of the time such as the gay liberation movement, second wave feminism, and the civil rights movement, a focus on a specific oppression, in this case weight-based oppression, motivated much activism. This is not to say that these activists did not have other concerns nor were they unaware of intersecting identities, but rather that single-issue activism was mobilizing for many. Nonetheless, fat activism was largely influenced by second wave feminism (Farrell, 2011) and a common rallying idea was that "fat is a feminist issue" (Fikkan & Rothblum, 2012; Saguy, 2012).

In the beginning of the twenty-first century, the work of these early activists and a number of scholars began to coalesce into the field of fat studies (Wann, 2009). Given its roots in fat activism, fat studies scholars defined it as an inherently "radical field" (Wann, 2009, p. ix) that "critically examines societal attitudes about body weight and appearance, and that advocates equality for all people with respect to body size" (Rothblum, 2011, p. 173). In 2009, two pivotal academic texts were published in the field, *The Fat Studies Reader* (Rothblum & Solovay, 2009) and *Fat Studies in the UK* (Tomrley & Naylor, 2009) and helped to establish fat studies in the academy by highlighting the breadth and depth of work being done. In 2012, the first academic journal, *Fat Studies: An Interdisciplinary Journal of Body Weight and Society*, was launched.

As we conceptualized *The Fat Pedagogy Reader*, the two of us were particularly inspired by *The Fat Studies Reader*. It remains an exemplar in the field with its historical, social, political, and cultural examination of the nascent field of fat studies; as such, it has served as an invaluable resource for academics and activists alike. While we recognize that not all of the authors who have contributed to *The Fat Pedagogy Reader* define themselves as fat studies scholars nor describe their work as necessarily radical, we argue that any scholar or educator addressing the "problem" of how "obesity" and fatness are constructed or working to challenge weight-based oppression is, by nature of the contexts in which we are operating, doing critical work. We thus intentionally chose to use the term "fat pedagogy" for this book and we invite readers to pause, consider the everyday ways in which we learn and teach about fatness, and as Sondra Solovay and Esther Rothblum (2009) said in their introduction to *The Fat Studies Reader*, "Do something daring and bold" (p. 2) about weight-based oppression.

Fat Pedagogues Come in Many Shapes and Sizes

As scholars influenced by feminist, intersectional, poststructuralist, and environmental theories, the two of us believe that situating ourselves is an important academic undertaking. For example, Erin identifies as a thin, straight, able-bodied, white cisgender woman who is an Anglophone French-speaking Canadian, and Connie as a fat, straight, able-bodied, white, Anglophone Canadian, once lower- and now middle-class, cisgender woman. Like Carla Rice (2009), we believe that "such descriptions tend to encourage centering of researchers' embodied subjectivities" (p. 250). We recognize that the two of us come at this work with different lived and embodied experiences, as does each author who has contributed to this book. Whatever our shape or size, we have all been implicated in weight-based oppression and we each can play a role in challenging dominant obesity discourse and stopping fat hate. As Marilyn Wann (2009) points out in her foreword to the *Fat Studies Reader*:

> People all along the weight spectrum may experience fat oppression. … [A] young woman who weighs eighty-seven pounds because of her anorexia knows something about fat oppression. … A fat person who is expected to pay double for the privilege of sitting down during an airplane flight. … [I]f we imagine that the conflict is between fat and thin, weight prejudice continues. Instead, the conflict is between all of us against a system that would weigh our value as people. (p. xv)

Words Have Weight

Scholars and activists who identify with fat studies or fat acceptance purposely use the word "fat" and assert that doing so is a political action. Arguing that "fat" ought simply to act as a descriptor of size and shape, they strategically use the "f-word" (Wann, 1998) to counter the stigmatizing and privileging of particular body sizes and weights (Cooper, 2010). These scholars suggest that the deployment of biomedical weight categories such as "obesity" and "overweight" have served to normalize and privilege thin bodies and oppress fat ones (Anderson, 2012; Braziel & LeBesco, 2001; Rothblum & Solovay, 2009). They demonstrate how the use of biomedical weight categories continues to validate fat hate and fat phobia and has led to much harm, including unhealthy body preoccupations, weight-cycling, low self-esteem, and eating disorders (see Aphramor, 2005; Bacon & Aphramor, 2011).

This process of reclaiming a word is not unique to fat studies. It is a cultural and political strategy that has been used by other marginalized groups to reappropriate the power of disparaging words. However, not everyone agrees with or feels comfortable with this strategy. In this book, authors use various terms, demonstrating the theoretical and political breadth within the field. Regardless of what perspective one takes, it is impossible to ignore that words do carry important meaning and convey different things to different people. Sometimes fat is used to describe a food (e.g., fatty meat), something good (e.g., fat wallet), or something unlikely to happen (e.g., fat chance). Still, when directed at humans, in contemporary Western society fat generally has come to infer "reckless excess, prodigality, indulgence, lack of restraint, violation of order and space, transgression of boundary" (Braziel & LeBesco, 2001, p. 3). Attending to the power of language, most authors in *The Fat Pedagogy Reader* have put words like "obesity" and "overweight" in quotation marks unless referring to concepts like dominant obesity discourse or fields like critical obesity studies. Many, too, have chosen to reclaim that dreaded f-word in their writing.

An Important Social Justice Issue

There is growing awareness that current biomedical approaches to "obesity" are contributing to what has been coined a "shadow epidemic" (Daghofer, 2013, p. 6): as obesity concerns have escalated, so too have rates of weight bias, stigmatization, and discrimination. Research is continuing to demonstrate that weight bias, defined as negative weight-related attitudes, beliefs, assumptions, and judgments towards individuals, often results in false and negative stereotypes (Puhl & Heuer, 2009). It is on the rise, negatively impacting fat people's educational opportunities, employment opportunities, health care, health insurance coverage, income, physical and mental health, and social relations (Brownell, Puhl, Schwartz, & Rudd, 2005).

As noted earlier, weight-based oppression is rampant in educational settings. Consider the case of Geoffrey Miller, an evolutionary psychology professor who in 2013 came under fire for tweeting, "Dear obese PhD applicants: If you don't have the willpower to stop eating carbs, you won't have the willpower to do a dissertation. #truth" (Kingkade, 2013, para. 3). Miller's tweet caused instant outrage across the Internet and in academic circles. By shining a bright light on weight-based oppression, one of the unintended but positive consequences is that some universities are now offering weight bias sensitivity training (Inego, 2013). In a culture that "pathologizes, insults, and oppresses difference and fatness" (Aphramor, 2005, p. 334), there is a great need for educational theory, research, and practice to address weight-based oppression in a wide variety of educational settings.

Overview of Chapters

Bodies are integral in teaching and learning no matter the context or topic—we are constantly learning in, through, and about our bodies. *The Fat Pedagogy Reader* draws attention to the ways in which weight-based oppression, often expressed as fat phobia, fat hatred, and fat bullying, can be addressed within spaces and places of teaching and learning. The book not only calls attention to the need for a fat pedagogy, but also illustrates the diverse and powerful ways this international contingent of scholars, activists, and teachers are working to end weight-based oppression. They share their personal experiences, their pedagogical practices, their research findings, and their ideas for further developing the field of fat pedagogy. While we have grouped the chapters into four distinct parts (storying, practicing, researching, and expanding), there is much overlap and indeed some of the chapters engage in all four activities.

Part One: Storying Fat Pedagogies
As one way to ensure that the voices of those who have endured weight-based oppression remain at the forefront, the book kicks off with Ellen Abell's memoir of her time at a fat camp. Her chapter illustrates how stories can be a powerful medium for sharing counter-discourses that help reposition fatness as a form of rebellion against a dangerous culture of thinness. She calls for a "re-storying" of fatness and the war that has been waged against bodies and lives. Similarly, Tracy Royce shares her own experiences as a fat graduate student and the constant

weight-based oppression she encounters in the academy. Drawing on these experiences, she makes a compelling case for the urgent need for fat pedagogy and calls for heightening visibility of fat hate in spaces of teaching and learning. Victoria Kannen also grounds her chapter in her own experiences. As a young instructor teaching critical approaches to "obesity" and fatness, she was asked by a visibly distressed student, "How can you be teaching this?" Sharing the challenges she faced and the role her body plays in teaching this content, she illustrates well the idea that every*body* is implicated in weight-based oppression. So too do Linda Bacon, Caitlin O'Reilly, and Lucy Aphramor as they reflect on their thin privilege and what they can do with it in the academy. They argue that their role as thin allies is to actively and iteratively work to address weight-based oppression and ensure that the voices and experiences of fat people are central in that work.

Part Two: Practicing Fat Pedagogies

Many of the authors in the book share their own teaching strategies for disrupting dominant obesity discourse and addressing weight-based oppression. For example, Cat Pausé describes how and why she has found it very important to nurture safe spaces for learning in her teaching across the university; for her, creating a "fat positive" classroom is key. Teaching in a small liberal arts college, Amy Farrell shares how mindfulness, deep listening, and empathy for student learning have been central to her pedagogical approach, illustrating through examples and her students' own words the shifts she has witnessed. Esther Rothblum, building on her years of teaching courses in women's studies, psychology, and LGBT studies, has found it is critical to navigate the complicated assumptions and truths about health and weight that her students bring to class; in so doing, she works to disarm what she dubs "weapons of mass distraction." Pam Ward, Natalie Beausoleil, and Olga Heath also work to challenge assumptions about "obesity" in various disciplines within the health sciences and describe how they, individually and collectively, have used reflections, dialogue, and storying to do so. Teaching in a kinesiology faculty, Moss Norman and Leanne Petherick share similar goals and share tactics that have worked for them. They begin with activities that get students thinking *through* rather than *about* the body to create a more productive space for challenging them to reconsider "obesity truths" they have learned elsewhere. Arguably, to take such an approach, one needs to have a good handle on where one's students are likely coming from, and this is something that Lisette Burrows describes as being integral to her own attempts to disrupt "obesity" discourse. Also central for her is critically interrogating her own practices.

Part Three: Researching Fat Pedagogies

A number of chapters describe research on weight-based oppression in educational contexts or the efficacy of different pedagogical strategies. Kicking off this section, Hannah McNinch reports on a research study in which she interviewed six young women who had experienced fat bullying in elementary and secondary schools and who were then in the midst of a teacher education program. Analyzing their often quite painful stories, she concludes with specific recommendations for teacher education. Also concerned with teacher education, Richard Pringle and Darren Powell share the results of their research in two elementary schools on what and how children learn about fitness, fatness, bodies, and health. Their findings have directly impacted their own practices in teacher education as they work to disrupt weight bias in teachers. In her research, Lori Don Levan was also interested in the perspectives of children and youth.

She asked them to visually represent fat people and was disturbed by the results, so much so that it has influenced her own teaching at the college level. Jan Wright and Deana Leahy offer a critical analysis of a number of body image programs currently operating in Australian schools that, despite good intentions, end up reproducing rather than challenging normative notions of the body. They argue instead for taking a more socio-critical and truly educative approach to fat pedagogy. Angela Alberga and Shelly Russell-Mayhew also review programs and approaches to promoting children's physical activity, and found that weight bias can indeed limit children's participation. The next three chapters in this section switch gears somewhat to focus on research in higher education. Patti Lou Watkins describes a variety of strategies she uses in teaching fat studies as part of her institution's social justice curriculum. She shares both the challenges she has faced and the successes she has enjoyed, using the voices of her students to good effect. Using self-study to enable critical self-reflection, Erin Cameron recounts an experience teaching a graduate course in public health focused on obesity discourse. Taking the learner rather than the content as her starting point, she was able to effectively support students through their discomfort with challenging dominant obesity discourse. Also concerned with the education of public health professionals, Krishna Bhagat and Shannon Jette critically reflect on an educational intervention they tried with their kinesiology students. To help them assess its efficacy, they relied on analysis of student discussions, recording of the session, and a short student evaluation survey. In the final chapter in this section, Caitlin O'Reilly shares research that she conducted on an online professional development tool focused on reducing weight bias in health care professionals, pointing to both the challenges and possibilities of interdisciplinary and interprofessional collaboration.

Part Four: Expanding Fat Pedagogies
The final part of this book offers critiques of fat pedagogy as well as ideas for expanding our horizons and pushing the field further. Heather Brown argues for the need to develop a theoretical framework to support fat pedagogy practices in higher education settings. Her analysis of the fat studies literature leads her to propose four key components for such a framework. Constance Russell and Keri Semenko focus on the pedagogical potential they see in intersectional analyses that grapple with the complex interplay of various oppressions. Particularly concerned with how sexism, sizeism, and speciesism intersect, they describe their pedagogical efforts to fatten humane, environmental, and social justice education. Breanne Fahs also argues that fat pedagogy must continue to push itself to make the most of its radical potential. Sharing examples from three different courses she teaches, she points to the possibilities of engaging with intellectual allies of fat studies such as queer studies, disability studies, gender studies, and freak studies. In a chapter that takes fat pedagogy beyond formal education settings, Emma Rich argues for taking up a public pedagogical approach. She offers a number of compelling examples from the arts, social media, community health, and various sites of activism, particularly given that "obesity" construction does not only happen within educational settings. Michael Gard offers an honest and thoughtful chapter that challenges all of us to grapple with the moral, political, and intellectual complexities of fat pedagogy. He urges us all to be more self-critical and consider more fully the role of science in fat pedagogy and the tension between education and advocacy. Finally, to wrap up the book, the two of us conclude with "a fat pedagogy manifesto" that we hope sparks reflection, discussion, and action.

Celebrating New Beginnings

We have been delighted by the support *The Fat Pedagogy* Reader has already received. In particular, fat studies and critical obesity scholars as well as fat activists have told us that they are eager to read it. This project did not start out with such enthusiasm, however. In fact, this book is a direct result of an encounter with resistance. The two of us had been developing a proposal for a symposium focused on fat pedagogy to submit to the American Educational Research Association annual conference and we were pondering what division or "special interest group" would be the best fit. We sent email inquiries to a few different groups, making clear the connections we saw between fat pedagogy and the focus of the respective group. To our surprise and dismay, all responded coldly. Frustrated, Connie shared the experience in a Facebook discussion group, strategic connections were made, and the symposium eventually found a home. Shirley Steinberg, who was part of that Facebook group, was excited by the concept and suggested that we put together a book on the topic. Thrilled, we accepted and, well, here we are. In a culture where weight-based oppression is rampant, including in educational settings, we are excited to see a book on fat pedagogy in print. We hope that it does indeed contribute to creating the conditions for all bodies to flourish.

References

Anderson, J. (2012). Whose voice counts? A critical examination of discourses surrounding the Body Mass Index. *Fat Studies, 1*(2), 195–207.

Aphramor, L. (2005). Is a weight-centered health framework salutogenic? Some thoughts on unhinging certain dietary ideologies. *Social Theory & Health, 3*(4), 315–340.

Apple, M. (2000). The shock of the real: Critical pedagogies and rightist reconstructions. In P. P. Trifonas (Ed.), *Revolutionary pedagogies* (pp. 225–250). New York, NY: Routledge.

Azzarito, L. (2007). "Shape up America!": Understanding fatness as a curriculum project. *Journal of the American Association for the Advancement of Curriculum Studies, 3*, 1–25.

Bacon, L., & Aphramor, L. (2011). Weight science: Evaluating the evidence for a paradigm shift. *Nutritional Journal, 10*(9), 1–13.

Boling, P. (2011). On learning to teach fat feminism. *Feminist Teacher, 21*(2), 110–123.

Bordo, S. (1993). *Unbearable weight: Feminism, Western culture and the body.* Los Angeles, CA: University of California Press.

Braziel, J. E., & LeBesco, K. (2001). *Bodies out of bounds: Fatness and transgression.* Los Angeles, CA: University of California Press.

Brown, H. (2012). *Fashioning a self from which to thrive: Negotiating size privilege as a fat woman learner at a small liberal arts college in the Midwest* (Doctoral dissertation). Northern Illinois University, DeKalb, IL.

Brownell, K., Puhl, R., Schwartz, M., & Rudd, L. (2005). *Weight bias: Nature, consequences, and remedies.* New York, NY: Guilford Press.

Cameron, E. (2015a). Toward a fat pedagogy: A study of pedagogical approaches aimed at challenging obesity discourse in post-secondary education. *Fat Studies, 4*(1), 28–45.

Cameron, E. (2015b). Teaching resources for post-secondary educators who challenge dominant obesity discourse. *Fat Studies, 4*(2), 212–226.

Cameron, E., Oakley, J., Walton, G., Russell, C., Chambers, L., & Socha, T. (2014). Moving beyond the injustices of the schooled healthy body. In I. Bogotch & C. Shields (Eds.), *International handbook of educational leadership and social (in)justice* (pp. 687–704). New York, NY: Springer.

Carmona, R. (2003, March 11). *Reducing racial and cultural disparities in health care: What actions now?* Keynote speech for National Healthcare Congress Summit, Washington, DC. Retrieved from http://www.surgeongeneral.gov/news/speeches

Colls, R., & Evans, B. (2009). Questioning obesity politics. *Antipode, 41*(5), 1011–1020.

Cooper, C. (2007, January). Headless fatties. Retrieved from http://charlottecooper.net/publishing/digital/headless-fatties-01–07

Cooper, C. (2010). Fat studies: Mapping the field. *Sociology Compass, 4*(12), 1020–1034.

Daghofer, D. (2013). *From weight to well-being: Time for shift in paradigms? A discussion paper on the inter-relationships among obesity, overweight, weight bias, and mental well-being.* Retrieved from http://www.phsa.ca/population-public-health-site/Documents/W2WBTechnicalReport_20130208FINAL.pdf

Darder, A., Baltodano, M. P., & Torres, R. D. (2009). *The critical pedagogy reader* (2nd ed.). New York, NY: Routledge.

Escalera, E. A. (2009). Stigma threat and the fat professor: Reducing student prejudice in the classroom. In E. Rothblum & S. Solovay (Eds.), *The fat studies reader* (pp. 205–212). New York, NY: New York University Press.

Evans, J., Rich, E., Davies, B., & Allwood, R. (2008). *Education, disordered eating and obesity discourse: Fat fabrications.* New York, NY: Routledge.

Farrell, A. E. (2011). *Fat shame: Stigma and the fat body in American culture.* New York, NY: New York University Press.

Farrell, A. E. (2013). Academia's anti-fat problem. *Bitch.* Retrieved from http://bitchmagazine.org/post/academias-anti-fat-problem

Fikkan, J. L., & Rothblum, E. D. (2012). Is fat a feminist issue? Exploring the gendered nature of weight bias. *Sex Roles, 66*(9/10), 575–592.

Fisanick, C. (2006). Evaluating the absent presence: The professor's body at tenure and promotion. *Review of Education, Pedagogy, and Cultural Studies, 28,* 325–338.

Fisanick, C. (2007). "They are weighted with authority": Fat female professors in academic and popular cultures. *Feminist Teacher, 17*(3), 237–255.

Fisanick, C. (2014). Fat professors feel compelled to overperform. *Chronicle of Higher Education.* Retrieved from https://chroniclevitae.com/news/425-christina-fisanick-fat-professors-feel-compelled-to-overperform#sthash.EQn4lThq.dpuf

Gard, M. (2008). Producing little decision makers and goal setters in the age of the obesity crisis. *Quest, 60*(4), 488–502.

Gard, M., & Pluim, C. (2014). *Schools and public health: Past, present and future.* Lanham, MD: Lexington.

Gard, M., & Wright, J. (2005). *The obesity epidemic.* London, England: Routledge.

Guthman, J. (2009). Teaching the politics of obesity: Insights into neoliberal embodiment and contemporary biopolitics. *Antipode, 4*(5), 1110–1133.

Hetrick, A., & Attig, D. (2009). Sitting pretty: Fat bodies, classroom desks, and academic excess. In E. Rothblum & S. Solovay (Eds.), *The fat studies reader* (pp. 197–204). New York, NY: New York University Press.

hooks, b. (1995). *Teaching to transgress: Education as the progress of freedom.* New York, NY: Routledge.

Hopkins, P. (2011). Teaching and learning guide for: Critical geographies of body size. *Geography Compass, 5*(2), 106–111.

Inego, L. (2013, August 7). #Penalty. *Inside Higher Ed.* Retrieved from https://www.insidehighered.com/news/2013/08/07/fat-shaming-professor-faces-censure-university

Jones, S., & Hughes-Decatur, H. (2012). Speaking of bodies in justice-oriented feminist teacher education. *Journal of Teacher Education, 63,* 51–61.

Kincheloe, J. L. (2008). *Critical pedagogy primer.* New York, NY: Peter Lang.

Kingkade, T. (2013, July 2). Geoffrey Miller claims mocking obese people on Twitter was research: University disagrees. *The Huffington Post.* Retrieved from www.huffingtonpost.com

Koppelman, S. (2009). Fat stories in the classroom: What and how are they teaching about us? In E. Rothblum & S. Solovay (Eds.), *The fat studies reader* (pp. 197–204). New York, NY: New York University Press.

Kwan, S., & Graves, J. (2013). *Framing fat: Competing constructions in contemporary culture.* New Brunswick, NJ: Rutgers University Press.

Leahy, D. (2009). Disgusting pedagogies. In J. Wright & V. Harwood (Eds.), *Biopolitics and the obesity epidemic: Governing bodies* (pp. 172–182). London, England: Routledge.

Lupton, D. (2013). *Fat.* New York, NY: Routledge.

Monaghan, L., Colls, R., & Evans, B. (2013). Obesity discourse and fat politics: Research, critique and interventions. *Critical Public Health, 23*(3), 249–262.

Petherick, L., & Beausoleil, N. (2015). Female elementary teachers' biopedagogical practices: How health discourse circulates in Newfoundland elementary schools. *Canadian Journal of Education, 38*(1), 1–29.

Powell, D., & Fitzpatrick, K. (2013). "Getting fit basically just means, like, nonfat": Children's lessons in fitness and fatness. *Sport, Education and Society, 20*(4), 463–484.

Pringle, R., & Pringle, D. (2012). Competing obesity discourses and critical challenges for physical educators. *Sport, Education and Society, 17*(2), 143–162.

Puhl, R., & Heuer, C. (2009). The stigma of obesity: A review and update. *Obesity, 17*(5), 941–964.

Quennerstedt, M., Burrows, L., & Maivorsdotter, L. (2010). From teaching young people to be healthy to learning health. *Utbilning & Demokrati, 19*(2), 97–112.

Rice, C. (2007). Becoming "the fat girl": Acquisition of an unfit identity. *Women's Studies International Forum, 30*, 158–174.

Rice, C. (2009). Imagining the other? Ethical challenges of researching and writing women's embodied lives. *Feminism & Psychology, 19*(2), 245–266.

Rich, E. (2010). Obesity assemblages and surveillance in schools. *International Journal of Qualitative Studies in Education, 23*(7), 803–821.

Rothblum, E. D. (2011). Fat studies. In J. Cawley (Ed.), *The Oxford handbook of the social science of obesity* (pp. 173–183). New York, NY: Oxford University Press.

Rothblum, E. D., & Solovay, S. (Eds.). (2009). *The fat studies reader.* New York, NY: New York University Press.

Russell, C., Cameron, E., Socha, T., & McNinch, H. (2013). "Fatties cause global warming": Fat pedagogy and environmental education. *Canadian Journal of Environmental Education, 18*, 27–45.

Saguy, A. (2012). Why fat is a feminist issue. *Sex Roles, 66*(9/10), 600–607.

Saguy, A. C., & Almeling, R. (2008). Fat in the fire? Science, the news media, and the "obesity epidemic." *Sociological Forum, 23*(1), 53–83.

Sensoy, Ö., & DiAngelo, R. (2011). *Is everyone really equal? An introduction to key concepts in social justice education.* New York, NY: Teachers College Press.

Solovay, S., & Rothblum, E. (2009). Introduction. In E. Rothblum & S. Solovay (Eds.), *The fat studies reader* (pp. 1–7). New York, NY: New York University Press.

Sykes, H. (2011). *Queer bodies: Sexualities, genders and fatness in physical education.* New York, NY: Peter Lang.

Sykes, H., & McPhail, D. (2008). Unbearable lessons: Contesting fat phobia in physical education. *Sociology of Sport, 25*(1), 66–96.

Tirosh, Y. (2006). Weighty speech: Addressing body size in the classroom. *Review of Education, Pedagogy, and Cultural Studies, 28*(3–4), 267–279.

Tomrley, C., & Naylor, A. K. (2009). *Fat studies in the UK.* York, England: Raw Nerve Books.

Wann, M. (1998). *FAT!SO?* New York, NY: Ten Speed Press.

Wann, M. (2009). Foreword: Fat studies: An invitation to revolution. In E. Rothblum & S. Solovay (Eds.), *The fat studies reader* (pp. ix–xxv). New York, NY: New York University Press.

Watkins, P. L., & Concepcion, R. Y. (2014). Teaching Health At Every Size to health care professionals and students. In E. Glovsky (Ed.), *Wellness not weight: Motivational interviewing and Health At Every Size* (pp. 159–169). San Diego, CA: Cognella.

Watkins, P. L., Farrell, A., & Hugmeyer, A. (2012). Teaching fat studies: From conception to reception. *Fat Studies, 1*(2), 180–194.

Watkins, P. L., & Hugmeyer, D. (2013). Teaching about eating disorders from a fat studies perspective. *Transformations: The Journal of Inclusive Scholarship and Pedagogy, 23*(2), 177–188.

Weinstock, J., & Krehbiel, M. (2009). Fat youth as common targets for bullying. In E. Rothblum & S. Solovay (Eds.), *The fat studies reader* (pp. 120–126). New York, NY: New York University Press.

World Health Organization. (1998). *Obesity: Preventing and managing the global epidemic.* Report of a WHO consultation on obesity. Geneva, Switzerland: World Health Organization.

PART ONE

Storying Fat Pedagogy

ONE

Picking the Bones

Ellen S. Abell

I am 55 and have a lifetime of experience with the discrimination this book aims to identify and reduce. I am a counselor, life coach, professor of psychology and gender studies, amateur comedian, and survivor of seven years of fat camp.

Three years ago, a close friend of mine from fat camp died. She was 51. Of the original gang of six of us who'd been friends since we met at camp, Kim was the fourth to die prematurely. The presumption is she died of "obesity." When you weigh 450 pounds and they have trouble getting your body out of the house where you lived, they don't even do an autopsy. Fat is a killer, after all.

A month after Kim died, after Andi, Gail, and Tommie all died before her, I elected to have lap band surgery. Weight started to drop, seemingly without trying. At age 52, I was becoming what I'd longed to be for as long as I could remember: thin. This compelling transformation marked the recognition of my dual life—a fat person now living inside of a thin body. One body, two worlds.

I want to tell you about my life and what it was like to be the "fat girl," although rarely was the word "fat" ever used. I was simply "big-boned." I also want to introduce you to some of my "big-boned" friends who, despite the stereotypes, were beautiful, hard-working, sensitive, and sexy young women.

The Power of Stories

According to Jane Halonen (1995), memoirs typically have an emotional impact on readers, which can facilitate thinking, build insight, and increase motivation. Using narratives as a pedagogical tool to assist others to better understand the lives and challenges often experienced by fat people can be a powerful and productive way to bring these stories and characters alive. It also invites readers to reflect upon the narrow ways in which dominant stories can be extremely limiting (White & Epston, 1990). The dominant narratives surrounding fatness in our culture make claims about fat people's laziness, lack of self-worth, and poor discipline, requiring educators committed to fat pedagogy to contradict such claims by offering alternative perspectives and counter-stories that are more accurate and humane.

Psychologist Jerome Bruner (1990) suggests there are always feelings and key experiences left out of dominant stories. One way to challenge the skewed dominant narratives about fat people is to look to authors who introduce fat characters that undermine these negative images while presenting counter-stories that present these characters as self-determined, sexually attractive, and multidimensional. Doing so is likely to encourage a deeper and more realistic view of fat people while increasing the reader's ability to relate to, rather than distance herself from, these characters.

My Story

My mother and I are opposites. She is Barbie; I'm more like Ken. She is beautiful, thin, skating through life on her good looks. Her life has been about attracting and pleasing men. Through these men, she wrangled the dream house, the fancy cars, the expensive wardrobe, and the accouterments befitting a celebrity. Despite the lines on her face that betray her, her age is top-secret intel to which very few have security clearance.

Mom's the woman who followed all the perfectly prescribed rules including marriage, children, and beauty obsession while fighting the aging process like a true gladiator. I'm the anti-Barbie. I hate wearing makeup, and have short, curly, brunette hair; I feel adamantly that high heels should be outlawed, and my boobs are far from perky. Did I also mention that I date women? In fact, I recently married one. And if that's not enough to chase Ken away, I was also fat for most of my life. I am not the sort of woman who fits most men's definition of a trophy wife.

I've had my share of lovers but my primary relationship has always been with food. I was obsessed with it since nursery school, when my mother warned me that if I ate two treats in one day, I'd end up fat as a teenager, unable to wear a bikini to the beach. I took her advice to heart, choosing at nursery school snack time "vanilla" milk instead of chocolate. Chocolate was the enemy of girls who wanted to be liked by boys, i.e., girls who wanted to be thin. I always loved sweets. Buttercream icing was my favorite. Any time cake was served I'd strip the icing off the top with my finger, then off the sides, until there was only the cake left, which I'd throw into the trash. But oh, that sweet, sugary icing … that was pure heaven. And ice cream. Vanilla, of course, and thick, creamy milkshakes. I'd take great risks sneaking these foods into my room when no one was looking. If we were out of ice cream, I'd find the next best thing: sugary jams, cocoa powder, even chewing gum would do. My private life was filled with sweet indulgence, but in public I was the perfect dieter, eating only that of which my mother would approve.

The fall of 1974 was when my passionate love affair with food began to take over my life. Over the next 40 years food became my friend, my mistress, and my therapy. The intimacy I shared with vanilla ice cream, Butterfingers, and M&M's was deep. I was hooked and there was no breakup in sight. Desire took over my life. I wanted to be loved, I wanted to be thin, I wanted to be happy, but most of all, I wanted to eat. Often. And in secret. I'd wait until everyone in the house was asleep so I could sneak into the kitchen and eat whatever I'd denied myself throughout the day. I wouldn't eat at school out of sheer embarrassment that people would actually see the fat girl eating. After school, I'd go directly to swim practice, having not eaten since the night before. We'd swim for two, sometimes three, long, hard, calorie-burning hours. Sprints, relays, distance, and I could barely keep up. I was weak from hunger, yet too ashamed to let anyone see me eat.

For the two of us, my mother made dry chicken or tuna with salad and broccoli, while my father, brother, and sister enjoyed pizza, lasagna, and burgers. They had brownies for dessert, piled high with whipped cream. They had pasta and cheesecake. I was never allowed pasta, never allowed sweets. The longer I was deprived of these delicacies, the more my fascination with them grew. It was all out of proportion, the feeling I could drum up for a cookie I wanted but could not have. The cookie, the brownie, and the donut took on celestial qualities. These items were not mere food anymore; they were benefits of a life I'd not gained entrance to. When our family went out to dinner, I would sit next to my sister who was encouraged to get "whatever you want" while I had to order from one tiny section of the menu—with choices limited to scoops of cottage cheese, pallid canned pears, anemic iceberg lettuce, or clear chicken broth. While I forked into my cottage cheese, a flavor I detest to this day, my sister would have juicy hamburgers with thick shakes and greasy fries that she'd smear with ketchup. I would've given up my allowance for one of those fries.

The thing about desire is that it is all consuming. It knows no bounds. It wants what it wants and patience is not its virtue. There's only one way to tame desire and that is by giving in to its every demand. Desire had taken me prisoner and I was serving a life sentence.

During the summer of 1975, my mother's friend Jane saw an ad in the New York Times Magazine section. "Camp Clover for overweight girls. Results guaranteed." The camp was in the Catskill Mountains; we lived in Poughkeepsie, only 75 minutes away. From their excitement when they told me about Camp Clover, it was clear that my mother and Jane were very concerned about my 180-pound body. Jane had recently joined Weight Watchers, and went quickly from a size 18 to a size 10. My mother had always been thin.

The whole thing was very rushed and had the feel of an emergency. Calls were made, and we learned that the second session was just starting; I could join up midstream. My mother signed me up for the remaining 4 weeks and the day after Jane had seen the ad, I was packed and delivered. When we arrived, my mom accompanied me to the office where we met the owners, one of whom was fat herself. I found this funny. My mother asked how much weight I would lose in 4 weeks. The owner, who told me to call her Aunt Ruth, carefully looked me up and down and then informed my mother that I was "big boned," so she could only expect me to lose about 10 pounds in a month. My mother seemed satisfied.

When my mother drove away Aunt Ruth called a counselor, who was also fat, to take me to my room. I would be rooming with the 13-year-old girls because there were no available rooms with the girls my own age of 15 or 16. The room that would be my home for the next 4 weeks had yellow linoleum floors, red-checkered curtains, and three identical twin beds. My bed was the one with no linens, on the far right, pushed up against the cold, white wall. The lodge, as this building was called, reeked of mildew. The hallway with red, industrial-type carpeting was in desperate need of vacuuming. The other campers were at their required activities. I could hear them in the distance laughing and splashing around. Others were playing what sounded like a competitive game of volleyball. As I began to unpack, my mind raced with fears. Who were these people? How had I been dropped off at a place I knew nothing about? What if these people were mean? Crazy? Or worse?

Everyone else knew one another because they had all been together for the first session. I was one of the only ones to arrive for the second half of the summer. It was like starting at a new school *after all the cliques had already been established. The one key difference? All these girls were fat. Or someone thought they were.*

Like any community, fat camp had its royals and its peasants. The popular girls, like royals anywhere, got what they wanted and were powerful among the campers and counselors. The peasantry was humble and managed the best they could. It wasn't hard to determine who was who. The royals were often the loudest in the dining hall and in the lodge and typically were also the best athletes. They were the leaders during all the activities, and the younger girls, you could tell, aspired to become them. When I arrived on my first day, I was not a royal. That was a title I would have to earn.

Camp Clover was a far cry from my former camp. Chipinaw was five stars by anyone's standards, with rolling hills, a private lake, beautiful tennis courts, and first-class cuisine. The campers were rich kids, mostly from Long Island—they were beautiful, athletic, creative, and talented dancers, singers, and actors. I was an outsider there.

Camp Clover was ordinary. No rolling hills, no private lake. Just a tiny, algae-ridden pool. We were fed the bare minimum and required to exercise all day. Who wouldn't lose weight under those conditions? It was torture.

I sat between Lil' and Kim in the dining hall. I laugh even referring to this place as a "dining" hall, considering the lack of actual dining that occurred there. There were no smells of cookies or brownies baking, no pancakes and bacon and eggs in the mornings. No Saturday night cookouts with burgers and weenies and s'mores for dessert. Foods you associate with camp we definitely didn't have.

It was chicken night. Our favorite. It was one of the only times some of the campers actually left food on their plates. Not because they didn't like chicken. Some of them just didn't clean all their bones, which meant that the rest of us could take the bones from their otherwise empty plates and eat the chicken skin or marrow that remained. These scraps of flesh always went to the popular girls.

I doubt if any of us got the irony as we were cleaning the flesh from the chicken bones how we were also desperate to eliminate the flesh from our own bodies. To be boney, like "normal" girls were. Desirable girls, loved by their mothers, and boys.

Saturday mornings we were weighed—the most important 20 seconds of the week. Getting on the scale in front of the head counselor and her assistant was humiliating, but it was the moment we'd waited for all week long. Who'd lost weight and how much? The night before the big weigh-in we did whatever it took to see the scale go down. We were offered and enthusiastically accepted laxatives, doled out like candy by the camp nurse. Some of us were so desperate that we removed anything and everything we could think of to make the scale our friend. We tweezed eyebrows, squeezed zits, shaved legs, and cut toenails. One girl cut her hair.

I was especially neurotic. Most of the girls would find any excuse to get out of doing slimnastics or swimming, but in the evenings when all the other campers were playing cards or socializing on the lodge porch, I could be found outside my room doing 100 jumping jacks or killer sit-ups. I feared going home without having lost an acceptable amount of weight. How would I face my friends and family unless I came home a smaller, better version of myself? I would be crushed, and my mother— how would she ever face Jane?

"Hey Ja-cock," Lil' yelled. She was referring to the light blue Camp Jeckoce (pronounced ja-co-see) T-shirt I was wearing. I was standing on the porch of the main house where our counselors were handing out our morning snack, a piece of fruit the size of a raisin. But we were happy to be eating anything.

I recognized Lil' as the precocious 12-year-old who moved through camp as if she owned the place, flashing her sweet smile at everyone she saw. I was 15, and amazed by her youthful self-confidence and sheer chutzpah. Her blue cut-offs and her white, sweat-stained T-shirt matched her knee-high jock socks and blue and white Adidas high tops. She sported a Dorothy Hamill haircut, still damp from her morning swim.

"It's pronounced Ja-co-see," I said. Lil' just smiled and went to get her plum.

If a casting agent made a movie of Camp Clover, they would have cast a young Ashley Judd to play Lil'. She was pretty. She had been at camp the first 4 weeks and knew everyone, and everyone knew her. She was a natural athlete and charismatic leader. Someone once nicknamed her the "gentle giant" because of her charm and wit. She was at home at camp. Even happy. I envied her.

Lil' and I became friends, in the way a 12-year-old and 15-year-old can be friends. I was sort of a big sister to her. When she got in trouble with the counselors, they sent for me to set her straight, to talk some sense into her.

As the youngest of three children, I'd never been anyone's big sister. My brother was two and a half years older than I, and my sister was in between us. My mother had three children in less than three years, which I figured was why she was always so tired and mad.

Camp had a way of making even the least likely friendships develop. Andi was three years older, and Lil' three years younger, but at camp age didn't dictate connection; fat did. We were all there for the same reason, and while we were at camp, we wore swimsuits and shorts without getting the jeers we garnered on the outside.

We were a gang of six. All royals. Andi was the leader. She was from the Bronx and she was tough. To prove it, she'd put her lit cigarettes out on her calloused bare feet. She had one sister who she hated yet she always wore a T-shirt from the play My Sister Eileen. *Andi was Italian, and proud of it. She always had a cigarette in her hand and a pic in her Afro. Andi planned to become thin and wealthy one day, and move far away from her family and her moderate upbringing in the Bronx. She also wanted straight hair. She wanted to be everything she wasn't.*

Tommie was a counselor, and 10 years older than most of us. She had a way of making everyone laugh with her impressions of rock stars and actors, especially Billy Idol and Elvis, exaggerating the way they both elevated the side of their lips when they sang. She cracked us up. She smoked long brown cigarettes called Nat Shermans that made her look old and cool. She was Puerto Rican with gorgeous long red hair and freckles that covered her face and body. We called her Tommie Tennis because she was so good on the court. When she wasn't being our camp counselor, she was in New York City with her mother. Her parents never married so she grew up with her father's family in Ohio until she was old enough to decide that she wanted to move to Manhattan to live with her mother. She was 25 years old before she discovered that the mother she imagined her whole life was much better than the real life version.

Andi and Tommie were both quick-witted. Andi in a cutting, harsh way; Tommie in a clever, dry way. I loved their humor. We all did. Whenever we weren't at activities, we'd all meet on the lodge porch, collapse into the old, cracked Adirondack chairs, and share the stories of our lives while relighting the rest of our half-smoked cigarettes. I smoked Merit Ultra Light 100s. I figured they couldn't be too bad for me if they were "light." We'd take turns telling one another about our lives, our families, and the friends who were waiting for us to return home. Sometimes we read each other the letters we got at mail call, and at other times we traded clothes as we each grew out of and into various sizes. One evening, Tommie began telling us about her mother and how she told everyone she was Puerto Rican even though she was actually from the Dominican Republic. With a heavy Spanish accent, pretending to be her mother, Tommie stood up, brushed her hair from her face, and delivered the impression: "Darling," she imitated, "I came to New York to take a bite out of the Big Apple. I thought I would become a famous movie star, like Lana Turner or Ava Gardner, but instead, I wash other people's hair at Estée Lauder. If only I could lose this damn accent, I'd surely get my big break!" We all laughed as she continued the rendition of her mom, pretending to apply lipstick and give her hair some height. No matter how funny we found this, when Tommie finished her performance and we applauded, she seemed sad.

Gail was from a "blended" family in Trenton, New Jersey. That's what they started to call families back then when not everyone in the house was related by blood. She was 2 years old when her mother died and Gail wore the scars of a motherless child. She felt alone and abandoned and compensated by developing and nurturing intense fantasy relationships with actors. She especially loved Robbie Benson. Gail aspired to be an actor herself, go to drama school in New York City, and meet all the people she'd read about in People magazine. What she lacked in physical beauty, she made up for with her dynamic personality. Gail saw the world as a large play composed of a huge cast of characters. She loved to cast people in imaginary movie roles. She cast me as a manager of a McDonald's. I never understood why. She once told Tommie she would cast her as the bitchy next-door neighbor in a television sitcom. Tommie never forgot that, and always held it against Gail. Tommie could really hold a grudge.

Then there was Kim—the charmer. Kim was from West Orange, New Jersey, the only child of a hard-working single mother who had escaped a violent relationship. With her long, brown hair, big, brown eyes, and delicate, feminine features, Kim was the epitome of a beautiful girl. And she was beloved. Everyone's favorite, everyone's best friend. Kim could charm the food out of our hungry mouths.

My final weigh-in that first summer reflected a 12-pound loss over 4 weeks. It was the start I needed. At home, I imagined, I could continue the diet, lose more weight, and be thin, back to who I was before, as my mother said, "I blew up like a balloon."

On our last morning at camp, I wasn't the only one who was nervous. Every girl had a mother who was some version of my own—mothers whose love we'd not entirely earned because of the physical space we occupied in the world. Mothers who paid lots of money to ship us off for the summer where someone else could harass us about calories and fat, and be the one to deny us snacks. Our mothers were tired of being the calorie police.

The cars of our mothers started coming through the camp's gates at around the same time, all except my mother's. I watched all my friends leave one by one. "KIM!!! Your mom is here!" And she would go off to be seen by her mother. The mothers would embrace their daughters while carefully sizing them up. Had the mother's money been invested wisely? Was the difference noticeable? Was the weight loss something that could be maintained once the girl was brought home? Was fat a permanent plague?

I cried as each of my friends piled into their family cars. Would I see them again? Would we remain close once we all returned to the "real world"? Would we stay in touch? Meet for a reunion? None of us talked about returning to camp next summer, because returning could only mean one thing: you got fat again.

While waiting for my mother I sat with some of the counselors who weren't allowed to leave until the last camper was gone. But mostly I just sat with my thoughts. What would it be like back home? Would I be able to keep myself thin? How soon could I have ice cream?

The sun was at high noon when I finally saw my mother's black Cadillac drive through the gate. I flashed back to the last time I'd seen her, 4 weeks ago, and could almost feel the sweat that had rolled down my forehead that day as I'd scanned the sparse grounds, the shoddy buildings, and the girls: some fat, others less so. I'd been so nervous then, sent to a place where I knew no one, where people like me apparently had to go to become normal. But since that day, I had sung countless songs by the campfire, smoked cigarettes on the lodge porch, ate untold scoops of cottage cheese with cinnamon and Sweet'N Low, shared secrets, and earned my place among the royals. I belonged here. As I walked over to my mother's car in my white carpenter jeans and black, cap-sleeve T-shirt, she got out of the car wearing a big smile. She was beautiful, as always. Her blonde hair, fitted jeans, red silk top, and those ridiculously large sunglasses made me tear up with joy. My mom was finally here and by the look of it, she liked what she saw.

We hugged. She eyed me up and down. She was pleased. Relieved. "You look normal again. I'm so happy." She made me turn around and model my new figure. She placed her hand on my bottom, measuring how much less of it there was since the last time she'd seen me. "You lost your tush," she said. I was relieved my friends weren't here to witness this part of our reunion.

I said my final good-byes, hugging the few counselors who were gathered on the lodge porch waiting for their rides. Everyone was wearing "street clothes" today. No sweat pants or shabby cut-off shorts. We were all dressed for judgment day. My mother was eyeing Laurie, a counselor I really liked, but I'm sure all my mother saw was her large body.

"How much weight did you lose?" my mother asked, calling unnecessary attention to herself. My face was turning red. My face often turned red when my mother spoke to other people.

"Thirty-four pounds," Laurie replied.

"Good for you," my mother said. And then, "Keep it up. You have a very nice face."

I rushed to the car, hoping to shorten the amount of time my mom had to further embarrass me. I threw my duffel bag into the backseat and got in the front. Mom fussed with the adjustment of the rearview mirror, even though she'd been the last one to drive the car. She was always fussing with something, nothing was ever to her satisfaction. She was quiet and so was I. We had an hour and a half drive ahead of us. It was after noon, and the last meal served at camp had been breakfast—one hardboiled egg and 6 oz. of juice. I was back in the land of food, restaurants, grocery stores, things I'd not seen in weeks, and as we drove in silence, desire grew big inside me.

"Mom," I said. "Can we stop for lunch? I'd love a milkshake." Weeks of deprivation builds courage. Or was it desperation? I braced myself for her reply.

"Is that all you can think about?" she said. And then, "Shame on you!" In that moment, my carpenter pants suddenly seemed tight, digging into me at the hip-hugger waistband. Then she went on, something about good money and so on, and she was not going to let me ruin this.

I settled into my seat, looked out my window, anywhere but at her angry face. Then she stepped on the accelerator, bringing the Caddy from 0 to 55 mph in an instant, determined to get as far away as possible from the land of the fat people, Camp Clover, that land where I belonged.

If it hadn't been forbidden, I would've lit up a Merit, rolled down my window, and tapped the ash onto the racing road below me while looking at the lush green summer world, thinking about Andi, Tommie, Lil', and the rest. Instead I clicked on the radio, found a station my mom wouldn't hate, and let the music fill the huge gap between us, all the way home.

Using Memoirs in Fat Pedagogy

Sharon Hollander (2001) identifies several advantages of the pedagogical use of memoirs, including bridging gaps and allowing writers to introduce themselves and their lived experiences directly to the reader. Paul Gray (1997) suggests that some memoirs can serve as an opportunity to open up a new world to readers. Educators who use memoirs can ask students to reflect on various questions designed to elevate their insight and to foster compassion among readers. For example, based on the memoir presented previously, educators might ask students to reflect on the gendered nature of thinness and why Camp Clover was exclusively for girls.

We might also ask students to write their own memoirs about their relationship to food, body image, problems with eating, hunger, cravings, or about culture's role in creating beauty standards. The use of autobiography has a long tradition in feminist studies and pedagogy (e.g., Smith & Watson, 1998) and I argue it would work well in fat pedagogy, too.

Fat pedagogy must explore why some women and girls are choosing starvation and death as an alternative to becoming fat. Rather than placing the blame on individual girls and women for suffering from "disordered" eating, why not introduce counter-stories that take a stand against oppression and injustice? How might "overeating" or "undereating" be seen as a form of rebellion against sexism and fat oppression? Let's help our students re-story fat people as s/heroes fighting a battle against a dangerous culture of thinness. It's high time for us to put forth new narratives about fatness before more people become casualties of the cultural war that has been waged against our bodies, and our lives.

References

Bruner, J. S. (1990). *Acts of meaning: Four lectures on mind & culture*. Cambridge, MA: Harvard University Press.

Gray, P. (1997, April 21). Real-life misery. Read all about it! *Time*, 106.

Halonen, J. S. (1995). Demystifying critical thinking: *Teaching of Psychology, 22*(1), 75–81.

Hollander, S. A. (2001). Taking it personally: The role of memoirs in teacher education. *Electronic Journal for Inclusive Education, 1*(5).

Smith, S., & Watson, J. (1998). *Women, autobiography, theory: A reader*. Madison, WI: University of Wisconsin Press.

White, M., & Epston, D. (1990). *Narrative means to therapeutic ends*. New York, NY: Norton.

TWO

Fat Invisibility, Fat Hate: Towards a Progressive Pedagogy of Size

Tracy Royce

I wedge myself into my seat, tops of my thighs mashed painfully against the bottom of the desk. *Who are these things designed for anyway?* This classroom's desks are especially cramped, even more punitive than those in the other lecture halls in which I've served as a teaching assistant.[1]

The day's medical sociology lecture begins with the professor's straightforward assertion that patients' social location impacts the quality of the medical services they receive. The prof easily rattles off the usual examples of social categories that impact the provision of health care: race, class, and gender. I lean forward—uncomfortably—as she hesitates, then adds "age" to the list. Our eyes connect. Surely she'll see me, overflowing my Lilliputian desk, and think to mention body size or weight. Perhaps recalling my research interests, she sputters, "sexuality … ." Taking a deep breath, I puff out my cheeks like a blowfish and hold my rounded arms out at my side, mimicking an oversized beach ball. Only then does she finally utter, "weight." I exhale, relieved, yet literally and figuratively deflated. I have had to resort to broad pantomime to get the professor to see what is obvious to people who live inside bodies like mine: the consequentiality of body size.[2]

Same university, different day. My soon-to-graduate friend is warning me about the barbs of the academic job market, sharing a story another job-seeking friend has relayed:

Grad student to mentor: Now that I'm applying for academic jobs, do you have any advice?

Mentor to grad student: Yeah. Lose some weight.

One of the painful paradoxes of fatness is the simultaneous invisibility and hyper-visibility of large bodies. Fat people are frequently the targets of prejudice, discrimination, and even overt hatred, both inside and outside of educational settings (Puhl & Brownell, 2001).[3] Yet, our otherwise conspicuous bodies nonetheless have a way of receding into the background when it comes to curricular design and critical analysis. I've observed that academic colleagues who routinely display great sensitivity and analytic nuance when interrogating race, gender, and/or sexuality can be embarrassingly clumsy with regards to body size. Some conflate thinness with fitness and fatness with ill health. Others carelessly invoke the "O words," "obese" and "overweight," without the accompanying scare quotes or elaborate disclaimers they typically use to preface discussion of other contested terms (and oblivious to the fact that my eyebrows have shot up towards the ceiling). Still others comment on colleagues' weight or bodies in ways that per-petuate the toxicity of diet culture. And at the beginning of most academic terms, when the professor I'm assisting asks me to review the course syllabus, I scour the list of topics and read-ings, thinking, "Here is the syllabus. I am not on it."

Why Teach About Body Size?

An examination of body size and fatness (in particular, mainstream society's response to fatness) is especially worthwhile within sociology and other academic disciplines that critically investi-gate social life and teach students to consider the intersection of history and biography (Mills, 1959). Much of the "work" of teaching undergraduate students to think sociologically comes from challenging students' investment in "the myth of meritocracy" (McNamee & Miller, 2004), which exaggerates the rewards of hard work while obscuring the structural constraints that hamper success and reproduce inequality for people in historically oppressed social catego-ries. Ignoring the context in which inequality flourishes can foster victim-blaming: *Why can't these people just work harder to improve their own circumstances?* Good sociology courses provide students with the information and critical tools to challenge this all-too-human tendency to-wards believing that we exist in a "just world" (Lerner, 1980) in which effort is rewarded fairly and adverse circumstances constitute "just" punishment for lack of effort or wrongdoing.

Granted, undergraduates, many of whom are facing crushing student debt as a result of recent economic and policy trends, have a vested interest in meritocratic thinking. Many make significant sacrifices to attend college and therefore need to believe that the work they pour into their academic studies will eventually be rewarded, not only with "good grades" but also with fulfilling careers upon graduation. And, those former students who have achieved that most coveted of prizes within academia, a position as a tenured professor, sometimes skew to-wards meritocratic thinking as well (Grollman, 2014). Faced with the daunting task of training new scholars to compete for increasingly scarce full-time positions, many mentors fall back on old chestnuts like "there will always be jobs for good people," despite mounting evidence to the contrary (Iber, 2014; Weissmann, 2013).

Meritocratic thinking is especially problematic in that it fosters anti-fat attitudes (Crandall & Reser, 2005) and discourse: weight loss is simply a matter of "calories in, calories out," right? And if that is so, it stands to reason that fatness can only occur as a result of people's freely chosen actions: when people are gluttonous (too many calories in) and/or slothful (not enough calories out). Patricia Boling (2011) counters this popular discourse:

> This focus on individual redemption and change reflects a powerful tendency in contemporary American culture to understand people's problems or situations as fundamentally their own

responsibility or fault, and open to choice, control, and change provided they are sufficiently disciplined and put enough effort into transforming themselves. (p. 111)

Further, such an underinformed overinvestment in the power of individual effort ignores many factors that influence weight, including the role of stress, genetics, the effects of diseases, disorders, side effects of medications, hormones, the body's built-in biological regulatory systems, as well as the natural diversity of bodies (Bacon, 2010). Perhaps even more important to sociologists, a focus on meritocratic thinking also ignores the very real social mechanisms that perpetuate inequality for people of size, which include prejudice and discrimination, the medicalization of fatness as a disease, and the moral panic surrounding the so-called obesity crisis, not to mention the profit motives of a multibillion-dollar diet industry (Boero, 2012; Campos, Saguy, Ernsberger, Oliver, & Gaesser, 2006; Farrell, 2011; Saguy, 2013).

So, given that professors and students alike may fall prey to (or even regularly indulge in) meritocratic thinking, it's far from surprising when colleges and universities provide a less-than-hospitable climate for fat students. Undergraduate women at my university have confided that at times undergraduate men have perched in cafes along pedestrian thoroughfares in our local campus town and proceeded to comment upon the perceived attractiveness of female passersby and held up numbered cards as if they were sanctioned competition judges. More famously, in 2013, University of New Mexico evolutionary psychology professor Geoffrey Miller tweeted: "Dear obese PhD applicants: if you don't have the willpower to stop eating carbs, you won't have the willpower to do a dissertation #truth" (Farrell, 2013, para. 1). Miller later deleted the tweet, issuing an apology and claiming that the tweet was part of a social media experiment. While the social media response to Miller was both swift and condemnatory, Miller's attitudes are far from unique in educational settings. Research indicates that fat students face numerous interpersonal and institutional barriers within the education system, including peer rejection, harsh evaluations from instructors, lower college acceptance rates, harassment, and sometimes even dismissal (Puhl & Brownell, 2001). Rebecca Puhl and Kelly Brownell (2001) conclude, "Weight stigmatization can be more overt at higher levels of education" (p. 796).

Because fat invisibility and fat hatred are related problems not only in society at large, but also within the academy, both should be confronted directly in the classroom through progressive curricular design. Professors who are able to exercise control over their own course curricula have the opportunity to choose between thoughtlessly reproducing the biases and educational inequalities detailed earlier, or instead confronting and disrupting them. The latter can be achieved by heightening the visibility of the fat experience, and in particular by including modules examining fat hatred and responses to it.

Towards Heightened Visibility: Fat People Matter

Some Words on Language

In order to increase something's visibility, one needs to name it. As fat pride activist and author Marilyn Wann (2009) states, "Word choice is a good place to begin to examine assumptions" (p. xxi). While there is much heterogeneity among people who variously identify with ideologies, groups, and movements associated with fat pride, body size diversity, size acceptance, fat liberation, and fat power, most agree that the "O words" (p. xii), "overweight" and "obese," are objectionable and stigmatizing. As Wann beautifully explains:

> "Overweight" is inherently anti-fat. It implies an extreme goal: instead of a bell curve distribution of human weights, it calls for a lone, towering, unlikely bar graph with everyone occupying the same (thin) weights. If a word like "overweight" is acceptable and even preferable, then weight prejudice becomes accepted and preferred. ... [Further,] calling fat people "obese" medicalizes human diversity. (pp. xii–xiii)

Moreover, as Wann notes, medicalizing diversity leads to offensive and deleterious efforts to "cure" fat people of their difference.

Together, these "O words" work to establish larger bodies as unacceptably non-normative and in need of remediation. Where context demands their use (such as in discussion of the so-called obesity epidemic), scare quotes indicate some critical distance from mainstream anti-fat discourse. Instead of these stigmatizing "O words," the editors of *The Fat Studies Reader* (Solovay & Rothblum, 2009), alongside too many others to list, simply use "fat" as a value-neutral descriptor of people with large bodies. "Fat" has the advantage of being straightforward and unembarrassed. People who use "fat" prefer not to hide behind euphemisms, because there is no reason to hide except to preserve the comfort of the intolerant. The word "fat" continues to be levied as an insult, even against people in power such as Senator Kirsten Gillibrand (2014), whose memoir reveals acutely anti-fat comments from male colleagues. Nonetheless, professors can help implement positive cultural change by helping to alter the context in which the word is used. Academia is infamous for its jargon; why not confound its critics by adopting that simple, three-letter adjective that the most progressive voices within communities of size use to describe themselves?

The Contemporary Context of Fatness
In addition to a willingness to include sensitively worded discussions and readings pertaining to fat people, professors can further heighten fat visibility by elucidating the contemporary context in which fat people live their lives. This includes making explicit some of the structural constraints that impact fat people. As the anecdote that opens this chapter illustrates, body size doesn't always readily spring to mind when academics consider the aspects of identity that influence how people are treated; race, class, and gender tend to take center stage. In a classic essay on multiracial feminism, Maxine Baca Zinn and Bonnie Thornton Dill (1996) respond to critics of the feminist theoretical move towards an analysis of difference:

> Our perspectives take their bearings from social relations. Race and class differences are crucial, we argue, not as individual characteristics *(such as being fat)* but insofar as they are primary organizing principles of a society which locates and positions groups within that society's opportunity structures. (pp. 322–323, emphasis added)

Today, few critically oriented academics would dispute the relevance of race, class, or gender, but that doesn't mean that an exploration of intersectional identities needs to end there. Granted, the influential essay from which the previous excerpt was drawn was published nearly two decades ago; nonetheless, the dearth of progressive course content related to body size in today's college courses suggests that its sentiments still prevail. Outside of the dedicated work of fat studies scholars, fatness appears to have been largely relegated to the realm of the personal.

Yet empirical research suggests that body size *is* in fact an "organizing principle ... which locates and positions groups within that society's opportunity structures" (Zinn & Dill, 1996, pp. 322–323). Fatness (or rather prejudicial attitudes and discriminatory policies that penalize fat people) can serve as a barrier to hiring and receiving equitable wages and benefits (Fikkan & Rothblum, 2005; Puhl & Brownell, 2001), and as previously noted, gaining admission to college (Puhl & Brownell, 2001). Fat people report discrimination from potential landlords, denial of access to public transportation, inferior customer service, and a variety of types of unwelcome scrutiny and harassment from strangers (Sobal, 2005).

But no informed discussion of how fat individuals relate to society at large would be complete without at least a brief but critical examination of the so-called national and global obesity epidemic. The National Institutes of Health currently define two-thirds of the U.S. population as either "overweight" or "obese" (cf. Farrell, 2011). As public health agencies scramble to "cure" what has now been medicalized and designated as a disease, media alternately decry the "crisis," "epidemic," and/or "pandemic," along with the presumed moral laxity of fat people, particularly the poor and people of color (Campos et al., 2006).

Paul Campos, Abigail Saguy, Paul Ernsberger, Eric Oliver, and Glenn Gaesser (2006) identify four central claims of the proponents of the "war on obesity":

> that obesity is an epidemic; that overweight and obesity are major contributors to mortality; that higher than average adiposity is pathological and a primary direct cause of disease; and that significant long-term weight loss is both medically beneficial and a practical goal. (p. 55)

Although Campos et al. found these claims to be poorly supported by scientific evidence, they are nonetheless frequently repeated in the media and have become widely accepted conventional wisdom. This is bad enough in itself, but as Amy Farrell (2011) states, much of the reporting on the issue (or non-issue) takes on the flavor of "apocalyptic thinking":

> Such thinking not only clouds judgment, it also induces a moral panic about the "guilt" of the one who "causes" such a catastrophe, often leading to extraordinary and discriminatory actions on the basis of "health" and "well-being." (p. 9)

This situation has caused some to conclude that the true epidemic is the media frenzy surrounding "obesity" (Farrell, 2011; Wann, 2009) and the resulting stigmatization of fat people. Nonetheless, I've heard professors and students alike invoke "the obesity epidemic" without a hint of irony or criticism. Unfortunately, when professors fail to critically engage the structural forces that shape fat people's lives, they also forfeit an opportunity to challenge the discourses used to justify fat hatred.[4]

Calling It Like It Is: Fat Hatred

Language Revisited

Isn't "fat hatred" a little hyperbolic, a bit polemical? Wouldn't "fat phobia" be more fitting? Whereas I've adopted "fat phobia" in the past (e.g., Royce, 2009), more recently I've begun to use "fat hate" and "fat hatred" because it seems to more accurately represent the revulsion, loathing, mockery, and abuse that fat people sometimes experience at the hands of size bigots (Ansfield, 1998; Gailey & Prohaska, 2006; Prohaska & Gailey, 2010; Royce, 2009). Social psychologist Gregory Herek (2000) similarly advocates a transition away from the use of "homophobia" in favor of adopting the term "sexual prejudice." Herek contends that "homophobia" implies that anti-gay attitudes are motivated by irrational fear rather than negative attitudes towards gay, lesbian, and bisexual people. Although the term "fat phobia" has proved useful in reorienting attention away from blaming large bodies and towards holding size bigots accountable for their words and deeds, it likewise implies that anti-fat utterances and writings arise from fear, rather than emotions that are less easy to excuse. In addition to clarifying the visceral impact anti-fat words and ideologies can have on their intended targets, the term "fat hate" has the advantage of directly opposing in name that which it opposes in effect: fat pride.

(Un)Teaching Fat Hate: Fat Pig and "Hogging"

Given the infrequency with which size-related topics surface on course syllabi outside of courses in fat studies, it's probably unrealistic to expect professors of sociology, much less other disciplines, to design a stand alone module dedicated solely to "fat hate." Nonetheless, in addition to highlighting larger scale phenomena such as the moral panic surrounding the so-called "obesity epidemic," it's worth also including at least one reading or portion of a lecture that emphasizes interpersonal aspects of fat hatred. Here I'll provide descriptions of two examples, Neil LaBute's Fat Pig (2004) and Jeannine Gailey and Ariane Prohaska's examinations of the practice of "hogging" (2006, 2010).

Although playwright LaBute has at times been charged with sexism, misogyny, and misanthropy (Szalwinska, 2008), I understand most of his work as less of an endorsement of prejudice and hatred than an unflinching dissection of such. I find this to be particularly true of his play Fat Pig (2004), which traces the course of a romantic relationship between a thin male office drone, Tom, and a fat librarian, Helen. The play also depicts the scrutiny that Tom receives from two thin co-workers, Carter and Jeannie (the latter a former lover), as a result of their relationship. Helen is arguably LaBute's most sympathetically written character, but the story belongs to Tom, who is initially taken with Helen's frankness and humor (which, unlike that exhibited by most of LaBute's other characters, lacks cruelty). However, Tom remains ambivalent throughout much of the play: emotionally attached to Helen, but nonetheless ashamed of their association and how it reflects upon him.

What's striking about Fat Pig isn't so much the harsh words LaBute places in the mouths of some of his characters—at one point, Jeannie derides Tom's relationship with Helen: "I hope it's some mothering thing or whatever, because if it's not, it's just so off-the-charts gross that I don't know what to say. … She's really fat, Tom! A fat sow and you know it" (pp. 66–67, emphasis in original)—but that an established, acclaimed playwright created a play that explicitly centers on fat hatred and mainstream societal ideals of (thin) beauty. Protagonist Tom's fence-straddling between a rejection of those overly narrow ideals and a passive alignment with the fat-rejecting status quo may actually mirror the ambivalence some students feel as they process new ways of thinking about the significance of body size. Further, the play makes important connections among stigma, (hetero)masculinity, and the social constructedness of mainstream beauty ideals that conflate beauty and thinness.

Similarly worth exploring is the difficult-to-stomach practice of "hogging" (Gailey & Prohaska, 2006; Prohaska & Gailey, 2010). Gailey and Prohaska (2006) define "hogging" as "a practice in which men prey on overweight or unattractive women to satisfy their competitive and/or sexual urges" (p. 31). Fat victims of "hogging" may be the object of a bet or game, good for "laughs," or simply a sexual target of last resort after a night of drinking. Gailey and Prohaska (2006) also suggest that some of the men who participate in the practice may in fact be closeted fat admirers who sexually pursue fat women under the guise of "hogging" in order to avoid stigmatization for deliberately selecting fat female partners without a "good excuse" (such as drunkenness, a paucity of other options, or in order to ridicule fat women and use them for entertainment). In terms of the effects on the women involved, as well as the way men who engage in "hogging" represent them (often as animalistic and not fully human), hogging strikes me as the quintessential form of interpersonal fat hatred.

While "hogging" is not exclusively directed at fat women (also targeted are women who are otherwise deemed unattractive), the narratives of the male respondents in Gailey and Prohaska's (2006) research are dominated by vicious anti-fat, misogynistic rhetoric, and the men justify their mistreatment of the women by claiming that fat women's violation of gendered weight and beauty norms renders them abnormal. According to the authors, the men "indicated that these women are not really women at all, hence there is no victim because they deserve it" (p. 39). One man stated that a friend of his "homed in on fat girls" and "demanded oral sex" (p. 40), after which he would literally use his foot to *kick* them out of his car. Another man stated, "The next morning it was like waking up next to Jabba the Hut. Only in the sober reflection of daylight could I see how hideous and nasty-looking Sally really was" (p. 40). A particularly appalling excerpt describes how men who challenged a friend to have sex with a fat woman would "confirm" that he had followed through with his end of the wager, while collaborating in her abuse:

> A rodeo is when your buddy meets a girl and takes her back to his room to have sex and two or three guys are waiting in the closet, and [as] they're getting into it and right before she either appears as if she's going to get off or right before she's really getting into it, three guys jump out. One with a camera, one with a stopwatch, and one just there to yell, and they time how long the guy can hang onto the girl. That's what a rodeo is. (p. 46)

One can only imagine the horror felt by a woman who is thus humiliated during sexual intercourse. Presumably at the time of interruption by multiple yelling, photo-snapping men, she withdraws her consent to sex. Prohaska and Gailey (2010) liken this practice to gang rape. In sum: "hogging" constitutes a practice whereby male privilege and domination of women are reinforced through anti-fat mockery, coercion, and violence. Men bond through the act of dehumanizing and aggressing against fat women and then displace the responsibility for their acts onto their victims.

But why expose undergraduates to these horrors? First, at least some students are *already* exposed to them in their everyday lives; respondents who practiced "hogging" in Gailey and Prohaska's studies were college men. It's commonplace for professors to include sensitive material that undergraduates may feel is personally relevant, such as articles and lectures on hook-up culture and campus rape. A lecture addressing "hogging" has the advantage of making tangible the interpersonal effects of fat hatred, while tying in easily with pre-existing course modules on coercive/violent sexuality, violence against women, and/or hegemonic masculinity. Additionally, once students have been exposed to earlier course material that makes explicit the ways in which larger social forces shape the opportunities that fat people face in the aggregate, returning to the realm of interpersonal interaction allows students to engage fat hatred at a level at which they can immediately intervene. As previously mentioned, part of the task of teaching sociology, as well as other disciplines, lies in *unteaching* ignorant attitudes and beliefs absorbed from mainstream discourses. If fat hatred can be taught (at the societal level), calling it by name and engaging it in the classroom may just constitute a progressive step towards *unteaching* it.

Conclusion

I'll end with one final, brief anecdote drawn from my life outside academia. One day, as I approached the gas station counter after waiting in line for my turn to pay, a man breezed past me and engaged the attendant as though I wasn't even there. When I politely but firmly asserted my right to be served next, the man assumed a menacing physical posture and loudly called me "a fat fuckin' bitch." Shaken and more concerned for my immediate safety than with asserting my rights or confronting this man's anti-fat bigotry, I decided to patronize another gas station. Later, when I had gassed up and decompressed, I realized just how extraordinary this experience was. The rapidity with which I'd transformed from invisible and unworthy of acknowledgment to a target for this man's fat hatred gave me whiplash. And then I realized that this incident perfectly illustrated that being ignored and being hated are two sides of the same noxious coin.

Thankfully, I've never personally experienced anything quite this vitriolic within academic contexts. I'm more likely to end up annoyed at the oafish ignorance others typically display when discussing body size (briefly, sometimes reluctantly), when size or weight is even mentioned at all. More often the topic is simply overlooked. When opportunities to engage in well-informed, critical discussions of the experiences of people in oppressed social categories are systematically denied, academic colleagues and undergraduate students alike are robbed of an opportunity to confront and transform the prejudices they may have absorbed from society at large. When there's no critical discussion about issues such as fat stigma or the moral panic about "obesity" and the mounting public health war against fat bodies, it makes it that much easier for a professor to remain unchallenged when s/he comments on a colleague's body size. It makes it that much harder for a silently suffering student to assert herself or himself and request an accessible desk or chair (I know I didn't), much less find more radical ways of bringing classroom inaccessibility into focus (Hetrick & Attig, 2009). And within sociology, it impoverishes a discipline that touts social constructionism, but frequently fails to critically examine the structural constraints that contribute to inequality for fat people.

References

Ansfield, A. (1998). Rude remarks and right on rejoinders! *Radiance, 55*, 16–19.

Bacon, L. (2010). *Health At Every Size: The surprising truth about your weight.* Dallas, TX: BenBella.

Boero, N. (2012). *Killer fat: Media, medicine and morals in the American "obesity epidemic."* New Brunswick, NJ: Rutgers University Press.

Boling, P. (2011). On learning to teach fat feminism. *Feminist Teacher, 21*(2), 110–123.

Campos, P., Saguy, A., Ernsberger, P., Oliver, E., & Gaesser, G. (2006). The epidemiology of overweight and obesity: Public health crisis or moral panic? *International Journal of Epidemiology, 35*, 55–65.

Crandall, C. S., & Reser, A. H. (2005). Attributions and weight based prejudice. In K. D. Brownell, R. M. Puhl, M. B. Schwartz, & L. Rudd (Eds.), *Weight bias: Nature, consequences, and remedies* (pp. 83–96). New York, NY: Guilford Press.

Farrell, A. E. (2011). *Fat shame: Stigma and the fat body in American culture*. New York, NY: New York University Press.

Farrell, A. E. (2013). Academia's anti-fat problem. *Bitch*. Retrieved from http://bitchmagazine.org/post/academias-anti-fat-problem

Fikkan, J., & Rothblum, E. (2005). Weight bias in employment. In K. D. Brownell, R. Puhl, M. B. Schwartz, & L. Rudd (Eds.), *Weight bias: Nature, consequences, and remedies* (pp. 15–28). New York, NY: Guilford Press.

Fisanick, C. (2006). Evaluating the absent presence: The professor's body at tenure and promotion. *Review of Education, Pedagogy, and Cultural Studies, 28*, 325–338.

Fisanick, C. (2014). Fat professors feel compelled to overperform. *Chronicle of Higher Education*. Retrieved from https://chroniclevitae.com/news/425-christina-fisanick-fat-professors-feel-compelled-to-overperform#sthash.EQn4lThq.dpuf

Gailey, J. A., & Prohaska, A. (2006). "Knocking off a fat girl": An exploration of hogging, male sexuality, and neutralizations. *Deviant Behavior, 27*, 31–49.

Gillibrand, K. (2014). *Off the sidelines: Raise your voice, change the world*. New York, NY: Ballantine.

Grollman, E. A. (2014). *The myth of meritocracy in academia*. Retrieved from http://conditionallyaccepted.com/2014/04/17/meritocracy-in-academia/

Herek, G. M. (2000). The psychology of sexual prejudice. *Current Directions in Psychological Science, 9*, 19–22.

Hetrick, A., & Attig, D. (2009). Sitting pretty: Fat bodies, classroom desks, and academic excess. In E. Rothblum & S. Solovay (Eds.), *The fat studies reader* (pp. 197–204). New York, NY: New York University Press.

Iber, P. (2014). (Probably) refusing to quit. *Inside Higher Ed*. Retrieved from https://www.insidehighered.com/advice/2014/03/10/essay-about-inability-find-tenure-track-job-academe

LaBute, N. (2004). *Fat pig*. New York, NY: Faber & Faber.

Lerner, M. (1980). *The belief in a just world: A fundamental delusion*. New York, NY: Springer.

McNamee, S. J., & Miller, R. K., Jr. (2004). *The meritocracy myth*. Lanham, MD: Rowman & Littlefield.

Mills, C. W. (1959). *The sociological imagination*. London, England: Oxford University Press.

Prohaska, A., & Gailey, J. A. (2010). Achieving masculinity through sexual predation: The case of hogging. *Journal of Gender Studies, 19*(1), 13–25.

Puhl, R., & Brownell, K. (2001). Bias, discrimination, and obesity. *Obesity Research, 9*(12), 788–805.

Royce, T. (2009). The shape of abuse: Fat oppression as a form of violence against women. In E. Rothblum & S. Solovay (Eds.), *The fat studies reader* (pp. 151–157). New York, NY: New York University Press.

Saguy, A. C. (2013). *What's wrong with fat?* New York, NY: Oxford University Press.

Sobal, J. (2005). Social consequence of weight bias by partners, friends, and strangers. In K. D. Brownell, R. M. Puhl, M. B. Schwartz, & L. Rudd (Eds.), *Weight bias: Nature, consequences, and remedies* (pp. 150–164). New York, NY: Guilford Press.

Solovay, S., & Rothblum, E. (2009). Introduction. In E. Rothblum & S. Solovay (Eds.), *The fat studies reader* (pp. 1–7). New York, NY: New York University Press.

Szalwinska, M. (2008, June 2). Neil LaBute's sexist pig. *The Guardian*. Retrieved from http://www.theguardian.com/stage/theatreblog/2008/jun/02/neillabutessexistpig

Wann, M. (2009). Foreword: Fat studies: An invitation to revolution. In E. Rothblum & S. Solovay (Eds.), *The fat studies reader* (pp. ix–xxv). New York, NY: New York University Press.

Weissmann, J. (2013, February). The Ph.D. bust: America's awful market for young scientists—in 7 charts. *The Atlantic*. Retrieved from http://www.theatlantic.com/business/archive/2013/02/the-phd-bust-americas-awful-market-for-young-scientists-in-7-charts/273339/

Zinn, M. B., & Dill, B. T. (1996). Theorizing difference from multiracial feminism. *Feminist Studies, 22*(2), 321–331.

Notes

1   For an in-depth discussion of issues related to classroom accessibility and the "disciplinary effects of desks" see Hetrick and Attig (2009, p. 200).

2   I'd like to add that the individual described in this anecdote is actually someone who is receptive to critiques of mainstream, stigmatizing anti-fat discourses. This is all the more reason why her sluggishness to conjure up "weight" or "body size" is illustrative of the invisibility of body size as a legitimate category of inquiry.

3   Unfortunately, counter to dominant, idealized images of academe as transcending mainstream cultural concerns about appearance, the academy serves as "a mirror of our culture at large" (Fisanick, 2014, para. 7), where fat students and fat professors alike are vulnerable to anti-fat bias (Fisanick, 2006, 2014).

4   For recommendations on how professors can address these issues sensitively and reflexively despite inhabiting thin bodies, see Boling (2011).

THREE

"How Can You Be Teaching This?": Tears, Fears, and Fat

Victoria Kannen

"How can you be teaching this?" This question was posed to me one evening, just after I had fin-ished teaching a second-year "Introduction to Gender Systems" course in the fall of 2012. It was the fourth week of class and the lecture was "Appearance and the Body." At the outset of the class, I asked the students to consider, "Why do appearances matter to the study of identity? What can we learn from thinking about how we appear to one another? What are the limitations of 'appear-ing'?" As my courses focus heavily on using media representations in order to accessibly convey complex ideas, I had shown familiar yet disturbing images[1] on eating disorders (Greenfield, 2006) and from airbrushed cosmetic ads found in fashion magazines. To counter these images, I pre-sented a trailer for a 2011 short documentary directed by Margritte Kristjansson, *The Fat Body (In) Visible*. This clip enabled me to discuss fat activism and present an alternative to the self-loathing, body-shaming images of women's bodies that proliferate in the media. In the clip, a woman says, "[f]at acceptance is just accepting your body where it's at." The students in this particular course, of which there were nearly 120, were resoundingly silent following this clip, except when a few of the students acknowledged that they had never heard of fat activism or fat acceptance before, nor had they seen films that address body acceptance.

In order to give context to my teaching experience, a discussion of where I am and who I am is crucial. The location and population of the university that I teach in is a predominantly white, middle-class community in Ontario, Canada. As an able-bodied, cisgender, straight, femme, young, thin, tall, white woman whose research focus is on social privilege and higher education, I teach courses that require us to explore privilege as it manifests in and through theories, ideas, ourselves, and our classrooms. I have named the classrooms in which I teach "critical identity classrooms" (Kannen, 2012)—spaces where the pedagogical focus is on deconstructing the "normal" that is embedded within privileged identities and exposing students to concepts of appearance, gender, racialization, disability, and sexuality, for example. Understanding how social hierarchies shift *and* can also remain unchanged through the concepts of privilege, power, and oppression is fundamental to how I design these courses.

Sessional or contract instructors like me, who have a pedagogical focus on politicizing identities but who simultaneously do not have the same protections as tenure-track or tenured faculty, create decidedly contentious spaces in the university. In attempting to challenge the weight-based oppression found in media representations (and often found in the collective consciousness of the majority of students), I expected resistance in the classroom. But, as I mentioned earlier, I did not immediately encounter it. My expectations, however, did not prepare me for the dialogue that would immediately follow this particular lecture. I had remained in the lecture hall and was fielding some questions regarding an upcoming assignment, when I saw a young, thin, white woman standing off to the side with a concerned expression, staring at me. She waited until almost all of the students had left the lecture hall and asked if we could talk about the film clip that I showed. She then asked "the question" as tears began to well up in her eyes: "How can you be teaching this?"

In my memory of this encounter, I don't recall where the emphasis was placed in her statement. What I do remember is how I felt after she left the lecture hall. I had a few other students to chat with, and after they had left I sat in one of the empty seats and stared at the front of the room trying to process "the question" (and the conversation it resulted in). I very rarely receive questions on why I teach what I teach. Questions about the purpose of the lecture and the topics that I have chosen to include are something I don't remember having to account for previously. As I am still a fairly new instructor, this conversation was a first and it took me aback. It forced me to reflect on my process of teaching and the significance of teaching these critical ideas.

"The question" will serve as the guiding foundation for the rest of this chapter. Each component of this sentence presents unique analytical opportunities. By presenting the question in four ways, I focus my analysis on the teaching of body acceptance as a practice of critical education (How can you be *teaching* this?); the possibilities of introducing fat activism and body acceptance in the space of a critical identity classroom (*How* can you be teaching this?); the embodiment of an instructor with thin privilege teaching fat acceptance (How can *you* be teaching this?); and the objectification of women's bodies and fat-phobia in the classroom (How can you be teaching *this*?).

How Can You Be *Teaching* This?

Through my teaching, I try to be as accessible as possible with the theories of identity, privilege, oppression, and power that I present. Inspired by the work of Peggy McIntosh (1990), bell hooks (2000), Stuart Hall (1996, 2011), Rosemarie Garland-Thomson (1997, 2009), and others, I want my students to be exposed to critical ideals that confront social hierarchies such as race, gender, and disability in a way that is far removed from the "man-hating feminists" stereotype that many of them have come to mistakenly expect of classes that focus on gender. These ideas can be intimidating, personal, and fraught with conflict, so it is important for students to engage with them as "easily" as possible. In *Teaching Critical Thinking* (2010), bell hooks argues,

By the time most students enter college classrooms, they have come to dread thinking. Those students who do not dread thinking often come to classes assuming that thinking will not be necessary, that all they will need to do is consume information and regurgitate it at the appropriate moments. ... Fortunately, there are some classrooms in which individual professors aim to educate as the practice of freedom. In these settings, thinking, and most especially critical thinking, is what matters. (p. 8)

Entering into a second-year introductory course on gender, I expect that students have some assumptions about how the course will unfold, what kinds of topics on gender will be covered, and the resistance to feminist theories that I might encounter. As an instructor focused on embedding intersectionality within my teaching, I also see my job as presenting that which may be unexpected or non-traditional. For example, given that my focus is on teaching gender and privilege, the study of social privilege must extend beyond whiteness and masculinity. Using an intersectional framework (Crenshaw, 1994; Valentine, 2007), my teaching speaks to the ways in which our identities are found within systems of power and privilege. Our gender and race are not separate from each other, for example, but rather constantly affect and inform how we can understand those identities in our own lives. Teaching about privilege must include teaching about the problematic ways that "normal" seeps into our embodied expectations: thin privilege, straight privilege (heteronormativity), gender norms (being cisgender and knowing what that means), and able-bodiedness (being non-disabled) are experiences of privilege that need to be unpacked within introductory courses.[2]

In terms of mainstream scholarship, fat studies has experienced tremendous growth in the past five years (Watkins, Farrell, & Hugmeyer, 2012), but it is certainly not yet a mainstay in the academy as it is still seen as an "optional" inclusion in many gender studies curriculums. However, as Robyn Longhurst (2012) says, "[f]at studies has provided much critical insight into, and examination of, some of the social, cultural, political and ethical implications of the various meanings that have come to be associated with fat bodies" (p. 873). The ability to teach fat oppression *and* acceptance depends on moving beyond discussions of health (which I will return to shortly) and instead exploring the social values currently privileging certain sizes and shapes. As Longhurst (2005) argues,

Fatness and thinness are not binary terms but exist on a continuous spectrum. ... Even within a day people can *feel* different sizes and shapes depending on an array of factors such as clothing, feelings of well-being, the activity being undertaken, and interactions with people. ... Understanding fat in this way does not mean ignoring the materiality or fleshiness of bodies but recognizing that bodies are always situated in multiple psychoanalytic, discursive and material spaces. (pp. 249–250)

Teaching the fluidity of identities and bodies is not easy. In a 3-hour class, we also discuss concepts and theories of staring, social constructions of beauty, "normal" sizes and shapes, and what it means to be visible (see Dyer, 1997; Garland-Thomson, 1997, 2009; Watkins et al., 2012). A critical pedagogy of the body requires most students to be open to new possibilities for what their bodies may mean and the variety of social spaces they inhabit. This type of learning is a process; with any kind of process comes resistance, as evidenced in the following section.

How Can You Be Teaching This?

This question can feel like an accusation that seems to demand an apology or, at the very least, a justification for my teaching. Teaching the oppressions and privileges that bodies and identities experience should, at this historical moment, perhaps not require a justification, but that is not the reality I have experienced. This question seems to be one that is seeking broad answers to questions of social inequality that should have already been answered. Didn't the feminist movement take us past these kinds of gender-based oppressions? Don't we live in a diverse, tolerant society? How can you (still) be teaching this? As a scholar who relies heavily on the works of Michel Foucault (1980, 1986, 1990) in much of my research, I instead choose to read the question of "how" as a question of possibilities. How is fatness now possible as a pedagogical subject, specifically within gender studies? What conditions have made this pedagogy an important inclusion? How has body size and body acceptance become integral within my teaching in the face of medicalized resistance to fatness? While the answers to these questions require far more time and space than I am allowed here, I want to include them to show the depth of what was being asked of me. The question "How can you be teaching this?" is not only interesting for the multitude of answers that it offers but also for the amount of questions it inspires in return.

Instead of answering the student's question, I asked her a question in response. As I saw the tears beginning to stream down her face, I said, "Why do you think hearing women talking about how we should love our bodies—regardless of what size they are—is so upsetting to you?" As I teach courses that focus on gender, I am used to tears. Teaching about and for social justice invariably begins with histories and realities of oppression, discrimination, and marginalization. These subjects are ripe with personal discovery and reflection. Students crying, particularly with female professors, is now understood as fairly commonplace when teaching ideas that are so closely tied to our intimate lives (Varallo, 2008). These are difficult topics, ones that can lead to conflict, pain, and feelings of discomfort. I, naively, hadn't expected the subject of empowerment, body acceptance, and fat activism also to ignite tears.

The primary reason that I asked her this question was because I wanted her to reflect on her experience of hearing other women talk positively about their bodies and how that positivity was so difficult for her to connect with. The expectations of femininity and idealized bodies are so fraught with conflict that the preoccupation with trying to meet these ideals has rendered our bodies as sites of negativity (Bordo, 2011). Because of the feminist movement and feminist education, it is possible to critique these normative and problematic expectations imposed upon our gendered bodies and the resistances that our bodies can impose upon these normative expectations (see Cooks & Simpson, 2007; Kannen, 2013; Luke, 1997; Yuval-Davis, 2010).

How Can *You* Be Teaching This?

I have thin privilege. I have always had thin privilege. My thinness is partially related to my extraordinary height. As a woman who is 6'3", my non-normative narrow body exaggerates the presence of my thinness. The question "How can *you* be teaching this?" is a compelling one to consider. Do I have the authority to speak and teach about that which I have not experienced? I believe that I do and, in fact, I feel that I have an obligation as an educator to teach topics that affect *all* of us, as sizeism does. As my courses are overwhelmingly filled with young women, I see it as fundamental to my pedagogy to expose students to the insidious nature of body hate that proliferates in our culture, media, and social interactions. As Linda Bacon (2009) says,

> Thin privilege only exists, of course, because fat oppression exists—because we have this sick cultural idea that there is something wrong with fat and that a fat body is a marker of a defective person. This idea is so strong, so deeply entrenched in the culture, that we absorb it, it gets lodged in our psyches, and most people, fat and thin, come to believe and act as if this oppressive idea is reality. Most people want to be thin—and view thin as better. The internalization of this belief drives the body anxiety most people—fat and thin—experience. It fuels our preoccupation with trying to obtain or maintain that thin weight—and the feelings of shame if our bodies don't measure up. (p. 2)

Is it appropriate for me to speak on *behalf* of those who have experienced fat oppression? No, it is not. There is a fundamental difference between teaching and the presumption to speak *for* a group to which you do not belong. Finding this balance is crucial to anti-oppressive work (Bishop, 2002). As one way of ensuring I privilege fat voices, I incorporate readings, films, and classroom discussions that aim to give room to those who have most directly experienced sizeism and fat acceptance.

As an educator who is also focused on the feminist imperative for reflexivity in my research and teaching, I am open to discussing my own body and identities with my students. This is a risky pedagogical aim as personalizing one's pedagogy can create an avenue for personal attacks, intimate connections, and emotional exposures in the space of a classroom. I recognize that personalizing my pedagogy can have the potential to render me vulnerable, but I see how my privilege is always at work in these situations. I recognize my position of power in the classroom, my whiteness, my thinness, my assured tone of voice, and my preparedness for the exposure of my body "coming out" as privileged. I adapt Eve Kosofsky Sedgwick's (1990) language of "coming out" as a relation of privilege here to emphasize how important it is for an instructor to announce, acknowledge, and (attempt to) resist the primacy of his or her privilege. Privilege is still unacknowledged in many spaces of higher education (see Howard & Gaztambide-Fernández, 2010; Solomon, Portelli, Daniel, & Campbell, 2005; Webber, 2005), so I see it as a pedagogical imperative to "come out" as privileged, to make my privileged body a talking point as often as I feel safe in doing so, and to make tangible the lived experiences of our bodies.

Teaching fat acceptance from a thin body is understandably, and importantly, worrisome for some educators. As Patricia Boling (2011) states, "I worry that others will find me uninformed and perhaps inauthentic" (p. 112). This sentiment is often expressed by educators who teach subjects that are outside of their embodiments, particularly when the subject of discussion is an oppression that they have not experienced. As Bacon states, it makes sense for students who identify as fat not to trust instructors who appear thin. In these situations, Bacon (2009) tells her students: "We've been set up to hate each other. There's a system out there teaching us that I've got the right body, you don't, that there's something defective about you that resulted in your body, and something virtuous about how I live that resulted in my body" (p. 10). Conversely, the fat pedagogy that comes out of my thin body may be met with less resistance than if I were a fat professor. Discussions of fat acceptance that I am exposing students to could be more palatable as it may not be received as my personal agenda. As Elena

Escalera (2009) notes, fat professors may cause students "to feel discomfort with their own emotional reactions to a fat person, their beliefs about fat people, and their uncertainty of how to respond to the professor without making offensive comments" (p. 207). The privilege of my thinness negates these pedagogical dilemmas and being conscious of that privilege contributes to my reflexivity as a professor.

As educators of any body size, we cannot presume to know what others have experienced, but, as I have argued elsewhere, "[b]odies are never separate from what they do, how they are received by others, and what their relationship is to those around them" (Kannen, 2012, p. 640). We are all implicated in conversations about body acceptance, sizeism, and the cultural preoccupation with "thin" and "fat." Our constantly shifting relationships to these socially constructed ideas matter and I see it as my obligation to position this *matter*-ing as a priority in the classroom.

How Can You Be Teaching *This?*

This phrasing of the question is the most troubling one for me to analyze. Referring to women who love their bodies as "this" can dehumanize and objectify the people whose voices filled our lecture hall. While I choose not to believe that this was the student's intention, as she and I continued to talk after she had posed "the question," it became clear why she was so upset. She identified herself as an aspiring public health educator who, as she claimed, was intent on teaching against the ideas I had been lecturing on. I remember her saying, "They are killing themselves" as her tears flowed. As Noortje van Amsterdam (2013) argues,

> Eating and exercise behaviour are presented in this discourse as lifestyle choices, thus making body size a matter of individual responsibility. Those who are marked as fat are subsequently constructed as people who have failed to take the responsibility to shape their bodies to the norm of slenderness. Fat people are not only considered to be a risk for themselves (in terms of higher chances of diabetes and heart conditions), they are also constructed as a risk for society by increasing costs of medical care. (p. 158)

The discourse of fat as an individualized problem and social ill is pervasive. It is so pervasive, in fact, that this student plans to make it her life's work to educate people on how not to have the "wrong" body.

According to Samantha Murray (2009), the visibility and presence of our bodies are not considered a health issue until certain bodies are marked as wrong: "All bodies are always already visible: with regard to the 'obese' body, its pathology is inscribed onto its 'fat' flesh through the 'expert' medical interpretation of its simultaneous characterisation as 'diseased', and as a body unwilling to recognize its disease" (p. 83). As I attempted to work through ideas with the student regarding the socially constructed notions of thinness equating with health—using my own lack of physical fitness as a marker for how thinness can be misleading—I could see the student was unable to hear me. As our conversation was coming to a close, I asked her to remain in the course even though it was clearly a struggle for her so that she could be exposed to ideas that ran counter to what she believed to be true and to allow herself to learn about an alternative perspective. My plea didn't work and she dropped the course the following day.

While I initially felt as though I had failed as an instructor, it became evident throughout the rest of the term that this particular lecture had a great impact upon other students. Many students chose to base their coursework on the subject of body acceptance and weight-based oppression, while others came to my office in the following weeks to personally, and often emotionally, discuss questions that were emerging for them *through* their inquiries; disclosures of disordered eating and bodily insecurities brought relief, frustration, and, of course, tears. These tears reflected a difficult learning and reflective process for these students. Answering their questions, letting them process aloud, and directing them to resources became an integral part of our journey through the course.

Conclusion

I hope that this chapter clearly demonstrates that educators must listen to the voices of their students, especially when their students speak the unexpected. I may never know the full intention of "the question" that the student asked me, but it was important for me, and all of us doing this work, to hear. It spoke to what she, and perhaps many, students felt in our class that evening. Silence does not speak for itself. Being open to the questions that students have about new concepts—whether they come from a place that is supportive, uncomfortable, or resistant—particularly around privilege, power, and the body, is fundamental to the process of critical education.

This particular class was an introductory survey course on gender. While a contract instructor may not have much academic power, I do have the authority to choose what to include and what to exclude as subjects within the courses that I teach. Since this encounter, I feel even more of a responsibility to push the expected boundaries of familiar pedagogy. As instructors, it is important to teach that which unsettles the familiar so that we are able to introduce new ideas, present difficult challenges, and broaden the discourses that circulate on body politics in and outside of the classroom.

As an educator, I wish that the student who posed "the question" had been able to stay in the course, so that we could have tried to work through these ideas together. My reflections on "the question" have served as a reminder that while I cannot know what precisely the student meant when she asked me this question, I think that it is nonetheless crucial to our pedagogy to consider the possibilities. Since this experience, I feel that collaboration, while always a key component of my teaching, has now become a mainstay in my classroom. I want students to be aware that while I am a teacher, I am also a constant learner. They teach me. They have power. While they are experts on their own experiences, part of the challenge of education is in recognizing that one's experience does not necessarily reflect the experiences of those around us. As teachers and learners, we all need to recognize that the classroom environment is one that should be hard, but that should not make it undesirable. We can collaborate on challenging subjects, create spaces where we want to share our concerns, and enjoy working on new ideas.

References

Bacon, L. (2009, August 1). *Reflections on fat acceptance: Lessons learned from privilege.* Paper presented at the conference of the National Association to Advance Fat Acceptance. Retrieved from http://www.lindabacon.org/Bacon_ThinPrivilege080109.pdf

Bishop, A. (2002). *Becoming an ally: Breaking the cycle of oppression in people.* Halifax, NS, Canada: Zed.

Boling, P. (2011). On learning to teach fat feminism. *Feminist Teacher, 21*(2), 110–123.

Bordo, S. (2011). The body and the reproduction of femininity. In M. S. Kimmel, A. Aronson, & A. Kaler (Eds.), *The gendered society reader* (pp. 84–96). Don Mills, ON, Canada: Oxford University Press.

Cooks, L. M., & Simpson, J. S. (2007). *Whiteness, pedagogy, performance: Dis/placing race*. Lanham, MD: Lexington.

Crenshaw, K. (1994). Mapping the margins: Intersectionality, identity politics, and violence against women of color. In M. A. Fineman & R. Mykitiuk (Eds.), *The public nature of private violence* (pp. 93–118). New York, NY: Routledge.

Dyer, R. (1997). *White*. New York, NY: Routledge.

Escalera, E. A. (2009). Stigma threat and the fat professor: Reducing student prejudice in the classroom. In E. Rothblum & S. Solovay (Eds.), *The fat studies reader* (pp. 205–212). New York, NY: New York University.

Foucault, M. (1980). *Power/knowledge: Selected interviews and other writings 1972–1977*. London, England: Harvester Press.

Foucault, M. (1986). Of other spaces. *Diacritics, 16*(1), 22–27.

Foucault, M. (1990). *The history of sexuality: Vol. 1. An introduction*. New York, NY: Random House.

Frater, L. (2005). *Fat chicks rule! How to survive in a thin-centric world*. New York, NY: IG Publishing.

Garland-Thomson, R. (1997). *Extraordinary bodies: Figuring physical disability in American culture and literature*. New York, NY: Columbia University Press.

Garland-Thomson, R. (2009). *Staring: How we look*. Oxford, England: Oxford University Press.

Greenfield, L. (2006). *Thin*. New York, NY: HBO.

Hall, S. (1996). Introduction: Who needs "identity"? In S. Hall & P. DuGay (Eds.), *Questions of cultural identity* (pp. 1–17). Thousand Oaks, CA: Sage.

Hall, S. (2011). The whites of their eyes: Racist ideologies and the media. In G. Dines & J. M. Humez (Eds.), *Gender, race, and class in media: A critical reader* (pp. 81–84). London, England: Sage.

Hesse-Biber, S. N. (2007). *The cult of thinness*. New York, NY: Oxford University Press.

hooks, b. (2000). *Where we stand: Class matters*. New York, NY: Routledge.

hooks, b. (2010). *Teaching critical thinking: Practical wisdom*. New York, NY: Routledge.

Howard, A., & Gaztambide-Fernández, R. A. (2010). *Educating elites: Class privilege and educational advantage*. Lanham, MD: Rowman & Littlefield.

Kannen, V. (2012). "My body speaks to them": Instructor reflections on the complexities of power and social embodiments. *Teaching in Higher Education, 17*(6), 637–648.

Kannen, V. (2013). Pregnant, privileged and PhDing: Exploring embodiments in qualitative research. *Journal of Gender Studies, 22*(2), 178–191.

Kristjansson, M. (2011). *The fat body (in)visible*. New York, NY: Women Make Movies.

Longhurst, R. (2005). Fat bodies: Developing geographical research agendas. *Progress in Human Geography, 29*(3), 247–259.

Longhurst, R. (2012). Becoming smaller: Autobiographical spaces of weight loss. *Antipode, 44*(3), 871–888.

Luke, C. (1997). Feminist pedagogy theory in higher education: Reflections on power and authority. In C. Marshall (Ed.), *Feminist critical policy analysis II: A perspective from post-secondary education*. Bristol, England: Falmer.

McIntosh, P. (1990, Winter). White privilege: Unpacking the invisible knapsack. *Independent School*, 31–36.

Murray, S. (2009). Marked as "pathological": "Fat" bodies as virtual confessors. In J. Wright & V. Harwood (Eds.), *Biopolitics and the "obesity epidemic": Governing bodies* (pp. 78–90). New York, NY: Routledge.

Queers United. (2008). *The cisgender privilege checklist*. Retrieved from http://queersunited.blogspot.com/2008/08/cisgender-privilege-checklist.html

Rothenberg, P. S. (2005). *White privilege: Essential readings on the other side of racism*. New York, NY: Worth.

Sedgwick, E. K. (1990). *Epistemology of the closet*. Berkeley, CA: University of California Press.

Solomon, R. P., Portelli, J. P., Daniel, B.-J., & Campbell, A. (2005). The discourse of denial: How white teacher candidates construct race, racism and "white privilege." *Race, Ethnicity and Education, 8*(2), 147–169.

Valentine, G. (2007). Theorizing and researching intersectionality: A challenge for feminist geography. *Professional Geographer, 59*(1), 10–21.

van Amsterdam, N. (2013). Big fat inequalities, thin privilege: An intersectional perspective on "body size." *European Journal of Women's Studies, 20*(2), 155–169.

Varallo, S. M. (2008). Motherwork in academe: Intensive caring for the millennial student. *Women's Studies in Communication, 31*(2), 151–157.

Watkins, P. L., Farrell, A. E., & Hugmeyer, A. D. (2012). Teaching fat studies: From conception to reception. *Fat Studies, 1*(2), 180–194.

Webber, M. (2005). "Don't be so feminist": Exploring student resistance to feminist approaches in a Canadian university. *Women's Studies International Forum, 28*, 181–194.

Yuval-Davis, N. (2010). Theorizing identity: Beyond the "us" and "them" dichotomy. *Patterns of Prejudice, 44*(3), 261–280.

Notes

1   As this course focuses heavily on subject matter that may be challenging or unsettling, I inform students at the beginning of the course what topics will be covered throughout the term, including oppression, violence, and so on. In this instance, I was showing images that could also have been triggering, such as videos of women experiencing eating disorders, and so I made it known to the students that these images would be shown.

2   For further reading on identity privilege, see Frater (2005), Garland-Thomson (2009), Hesse-Biber (2007), McIntosh (1990), Queers United (2008), and Rothenberg (2005).

| FOUR

Reflections on Thin Privilege and Responsibility

Linda Bacon, Caitlin O'Reilly, and Lucy Aphramor

The three of us profit enormously from fat hatred. We start this chapter with this personal disclosure so that readers have a better frame of reference for the ideas we discuss. Put in other terms, rampant discrimination and stigmatization directed towards fat people have made our lives, as women whose bodies conform to our cultural weight standards, much easier. We're not proud of this, we didn't ask for it, and we believe that acknowledging it is prerequisite for changing the unfair system that rewards us and punishes others. In this chapter, we illustrate ways an ideology of oppression and advantage (McMichael, 2013) harms fat people while unfairly benefiting thin people. We discuss how "thin privilege" is maintained and identify strategies through which those of us who fall within the culturally normative weight range can make responsible use of our privilege and work to destabilize hegemonic, fat-phobic beliefs. In doing so, we highlight the roots of fat phobia and suggest ways to engage with the politics of identity and professionalism in the classroom.

The Ideology and Prevalence of Fat Oppression and Thin Advantage

In recent decades there has been mounting social pressure for individuals to achieve or maintain thin bodies, accompanied by exponential growth in public health initiatives attempting to reverse or cure "obesity" (Campos, Saguy, Ernsberger, Oliver, & Gaesser, 2006; O'Hara & Gregg, 2010). This has resulted in an environment where criticality and rights are sacrificed to the unchallenged authority of pseudoscience. This culture of fat hatred has fostered an alarming growth in weight bias and discrimination, such that the incidence of weight discrimination is now on par with race- and gender-based discrimination (Puhl, Andreyeva, & Brownell, 2008). Weight bias and discrimination are insidious, distorting almost all aspects of our lives, limiting opportunities and creating challenges for healthy growth and expression.

In education, for example, research indicates that teachers believe that fat students are less likely to succeed at work, more untidy, more emotional (as if that were a negative attribute), and more likely to suffer from family problems. Illustrating this, the U.S. National Education Association (2010) reports that "[f]or fat students, the school experience is one of ongoing prejudice, unnoticed discrimination, and almost constant harassment. From nursery school through college, fat students experience ostracism, discouragement, and sometimes violence. … They are deprived of places on honor rolls, sports teams, and cheerleading squads and are denied letters of recommendation" (para. 7).

Weight bias has also been well-documented in health care. Physicians ascribe the following qualities to fat patients: non-compliant, dishonest, lazy, lacking in self-control, weak-willed, unintelligent, and unsuccessful (Puhl & Heuer, 2009). Thirty-one percent of nurses said they would prefer not to care for fat patients, while 24 percent agreed that they were repulsed by fatter patients (Maroney & Golub, 1992).

Bias has also been documented in many facets of the employment sector. Fat people face discrimination in hiring preferences, promotions, employment termination, and wage inequities. As an example, fat women earn 12 percent less than non-fat females (Maroney & Golub, 1992).

More pernicious are the daily humiliations many fat people endure: the looks of disgust, the cow-calls, the bullying, the blame, and the news sources reporting that their bodies constitute a horrifying public health crisis and drain on the economy. It is often hard for fat people to escape the assumptions others make about their lifestyle choices or character and the revulsion often projected. This can contribute to self-hatred and internalized fat prejudice and detract from quality of life, health, and well-being (Puhl & Heuer, 2009).

While fatter people in contemporary society are often subjected to weight-based oppression (McMichael, 2013), thin people are conversely advantaged by this system of oppression. "Thin privilege" refers to the unearned advantages conferred to thinner people. It is a key pathway through which fat oppression is maintained. Often invisible, thin privilege fundamentally shapes our lives:

- Because of thin privilege, we can eat whatever we want in public and not be subject to concerned or snide comments about our health or "willpower."
- Because of thin privilege, regardless of our activity habits, it's unlikely that people will accuse us of being lazy.
- Because of thin privilege, we are more likely to be labeled as "healthy," and it's unlikely we will be accused of lying about our eating habits because of our body size.
- Because of thin privilege, we can open a magazine or turn on the television and see people whose bodies resemble ours more widely represented.
- Because of thin privilege, we are viewed as more attractive and have access to a larger dating pool.
- Because of thin privilege, we can go into a clothing store and be treated with respect, and have a larger choice of fashions and at cheaper prices than fatter people.
- Because of thin privilege, we can be assured that wherever we choose to go—be it a classroom, a car, an airplane, the theater, the dentist's office, a waiting room, or a restaurant—we will be able to find seats designed to accommodate our bodies.

- Because of thin privilege, we are automatically bestowed with a sense of legitimacy and objectivity when critiquing body politics, and it's unlikely that a reader will think we are making excuses for our fatness. (This list builds on the work of Peggy McIntosh, 1988.)

We could, of course, create a much lengthier list, but these few bullet points illustrate that as thin people, we reap multiple benefits from our smaller size.

It is also important to recognize that these privileges are situated within a very complex system of overlapping "intersectional" power privileges, causing a man, for instance, to experience his power and thin privilege differently from the way in which a woman might, or a wealthy woman to experience her thin privilege differently from a woman of lesser economic means. As an example, this list of thin privileges may have looked very different had it been constructed by women of color, as Jessica Wilson (2013) points out in her blog post. Many people of color are not treated respectfully in clothing stores, for example. They may have had the experience, like Wilson, of walking into a clothing store and being asked to leave their bag at the door only to find white shoppers still carrying their bags, or of being followed around a store. It is important to expand the conversation to include intersectionality, and to recognize that thin privilege is expressed differently across the weight spectrum and in different contexts.

The existence of this privilege in most contemporary Western cultures has enormous ramifications in facilitating opportunities for thin people and limiting opportunities for fat people. Consider the two examples that follow.

One of the authors (Linda) is a nutrition professor and was on a hiring committee interviewing candidates for a nutrition professorship. When it came time to discuss the lone fat candidate, one of the committee members dismissed her by saying, "Well, she really isn't the role model for someone who eats nutritiously, is she?" This assumption was based entirely on the candidate's weight. The discussion that followed made clear that had this candidate been up against a similarly credentialed thinner woman, the thinner person would have gotten the job—just by virtue of what she weighed. That's thin privilege: it limits opportunities for fat people while making career advancement for thinner people easier. Think about the many challenges this fat job candidate had probably overcome to earn her PhD in nutrition and even secure the interview in the first place. The mere act of attending an introductory nutrition course can be threatening and disempowering given the common assumptions that most nutrition instructors—and her fellow classmates—may have had about her weight and her relationship to food. It's safe to guess that she took classes taught by conventional nutrition instructors who routinely start the weight regulation section by having people calculate their Body Mass Index (BMI), which is then used as a lead-in to naming health risks for people who are in the "overweight" or "obese" categories. This is often followed by a discussion of the root causes of "overweight" and "obesity," which are, in most nutritionists' views, overeating and inactivity, and the solutions: diet and exercise.

Another very poignant example was relayed by Kate Harding, co-author of *Lessons From the Fatosphere* (2009), about the weekend her mother was dying. Kate received a call that her mother had had a massive heart attack, and she and two siblings got to their mother's bedside within hours of the call. Their other sister took two days to get there. She could have flown coach, but she couldn't afford two seats and knew that because she was fat she might be forced either to purchase two tickets or be bumped from the flight. She also knew that even if she were allowed to fly, there was a good chance she'd have to sit next to a resentful stranger giving her dirty looks. Rather than deal with the humiliation and unknown financial expense of flying, she chose to drive, hoping she could get there on time (Harding, 2010).

Thin Privilege: Invisibility and Construction

Despite the long list of privileges we as thinner women have, the concept is not often named and discussed. This invisibility has consequence: you can't fight what you don't see. For example, until that discussion with the hiring committee, Linda had not considered the degree to which her body size had aided her career advancement. When we consider airplane seats, we don't think about a dying mother waiting for her daughter to say a final goodbye and how thin privilege makes that opportunity more possible for some.

This limited awareness of thin privilege relates to theories of dominant group status (Doane, 2003) whereby the dominant group—thin people, who also often carry other sources of privilege—exert their ideological and cultural power by assigning meanings to fat and thin bodies. Thinness, in many contemporary cultures, is constructed as "normal"—which is ironic given population weight averages—while fatness is "othered" and constructed as "abnormal." Thinness is viewed as morally superior, indicative of enhanced self-control, strength of character, intelligence, and other highly valued (and male-identified) attributes; fatness is viewed as inferior and reflective of (female-identified) personal moral failings.

The system of thought that helps make thin and fat morally laden categories is known as binary thinking (also called Cartesian dualism). This sort of thinking constructs a pair of opposites with one as better or worse than its counterpart. It also describes the thinking that ranks white as superior to black, male as better than female, academic knowledge as more worthy than non-academic knowledge, and so on. This moral judgment is socially constructed, not inevitable. We only need to look back in history to understand that the fat body was not always constructed negatively. Prior to the Industrial Revolution, for example, the fat body was seen as the affluent and healthy body (Farrell, 2011). Many factors have doubtless contributed to this shift: the influence of the pharmaceutical industry over weight science research is but one example.

Helping students become aware of binary thinking and sensitized to the inherent moral judgments that are attached is one of the ways we will become aware of fat (and other) bias. As the late activist and poet Audre Lorde (1984) reminds us, there are no single issue struggles: dismantling our fat bias means becoming aware of and dismantling the system of thought that sustains this and other forms of oppression. To challenge fat phobia we must engage in critical thinking, including addressing the role of binary thinking in educating students into disconnect (Gingras & Brady, 2010).

We also must look to other ways of thinking and being that sustain this system of oppression. The construction of fatness as abnormal is in part the result of the internalized dominance of thin people, or "the assumption made by those with power that everyone shares their reality; they then operate as if their perspective were universal" (Peel School District Board, 2002, p. 4). Internalized dominance results in hegemony—the dominance of those with power or thinness over those constructed as different, or fat—such that those with thin privilege dictate the social, cultural, and medical norms related to body size. Because of the essentialist, binary construction of the thin body as the "natural" and "healthy" body, people often assume heavier individuals must be doing something wrong to fail to achieve normative status. Attention is then devoted to "curing" people of their fatness, with the argument that fat people could avoid stigma if only they lost weight. This leads us down a dangerous route of assimilation, one that contravenes standard policies on equity and diversity. The ethos of a commitment to equality is not to say that a group can have rights if they act like another group (i.e., if they assimilate). This would be tantamount to saying bisexual people should be denied equality because they could choose to live a "straight" life. Rather, fundamental human rights, such as the right to health and the right to live without stigma, should be in place for all people, not only those who are willing or able to conform to the norms of the time.

Barriers to Acknowledging Thin Privilege

Considering that thinness is constructed as the norm and thin people don't rail against daily stigmatization in a culture predicated on binary thinking, it is common for privilege to remain below our radar. Consequently, it is easy for everyone, fat and thin, to buy into the belief that our achievements are based solely on our merit, and for thin people to develop a sense of "entitlement" for what we achieve. This so-called "just world ideology" is an entrenched cognitive bias maintained by all forms of invisible privilege, one that disappears the social structures that create disadvantage and thus makes inequality appear inevitable. It is not a predestined truth that Western heads of state should be white men, it is what privilege makes most likely; it is not a course requirement that U.S. and U.K. dietitians should be thin, white, heteronormative women, it is a heady combination of classism, thin privilege, homophobia, and fat phobia that fashions this dietetic demographic. Helping our students see how the status quo is built and maintained by silence and drawing attention to the politics of representation and knowledge creation will give them a framework with which to think through the origins of disparity and the absence of fat voices speaking with agency.

If our sense of self is strongly invested in our professional identity, and that in turn is strongly invested in us being an expert, then we will likely resist ideas that contradict those we learned as we built our career. This is especially true when our sense of self-worth is tied into our accomplishments more globally. And if our personal and/or professional sense of self derives from our thin embodiment, the stakes for considering privilege and mistaken beliefs are set even higher again, more so if we have worked hard at our own body management and highly regard the values of control and restraint attributed to thin people. It would understandably be threatening to consider our success being derived in part from unearned advantages associated with thinness (and the synergistic way this impacts our experience of the world and sense of self) rather than being solely due to our merit. And we will only be able to allow for our own complicity in perpetuating oppression and peddling bad science if we can tolerate the painful feelings this engenders.

The realization that body size isn't as personally malleable as we previously believed—that the body has strong regulatory mechanisms that resist sustained weight loss (Sumithran & Proietto, 2013)—has ramifications. Not least among these are the far reaching implications for our trust in science as value free and our belief in our own objectivity.

This journey will likely only commence if we can embrace our flawed self without being overwhelmed by shame. The challenge is that when we're habituated to binary thinking our reflex response will be one of harsh self-judgment, followed by shame and disconnect. When this occurs, we have lost the opportunity to integrate our new knowledge and sense of self in a way that enables growth. However, the shame response is not inevitable: when we are habituated to mindful thinking our response will more likely be one of self-compassion. Here, we are able to stay with the acknowledgment of our complicity, the harm caused, and the painful emotions evoked because we are practiced at being warm and understanding with ourselves even in the face of the harsh reality of our shortcomings. We remain connected and we integrate our new knowledge into an abiding sense of self that does not have to be perfect to earn respect.

A classroom space that encourages enabling "good" conflict, that requires students to recognize their situatedness through ongoing reflexivity, and that supports shame management through mirroring/teaching mindfulness and self-compassion will foster criticality. So too, helping students develop a secure sense of their professional identity rather than one precariously reliant on a very bounded claim for unique expertise means they can welcome new and critical perspectives.

Dismantling Thin Privilege

While we can't make our unearned privileges disappear, by becoming conscious of our privilege we can renounce our sense of "entitlement" and use our privilege responsibly. Three strategies, educating ourselves, undoing our own internalized size oppression, and owning our identities, can assist us in being responsible with our privilege.

Educating Ourselves
Educating yourself begins with self-reflection. Consider how your life would be different if you were fatter. Think about your daily activities, whether it's meeting a new person, ordering fast food, shopping for clothes, or speaking out on weight bias. Would others view or treat you differently? Would *you* feel more or less self-conscious about others' judgments? More or less entitled in whatever you're doing?

It is also important to educate yourself about the lived experience of being fat, and to listen to what fat people say about their lives, remembering all the while that fat people are no more a homogenous group than any other, and that while someone may be willing to talk to you, it is not the role of the oppressed to educate the oppressor (Lorde, 1984) or to be an ambassador. You can do this through respectfully broaching the subject with your fat friends, or seeking out writings from within the Fat Activist or Size Acceptance community, such as through the large body of fiction that involves fat characters (Stinson, 2009). You may be surprised to learn just how differently the world treats fat and thin people, and the implications for quality of life. There is also work available on how to become an ally (Bishop, 2002).

Next, enhance your own criticality by reading up on weight myths. When we are subjected repeatedly to images of fat people as lazy and greedy, notions that weight is completely controllable by diet and/or exercise, and that fat causes people to get sick and die early, these oppressive values become deeply embedded in our psyches. However, these beliefs are just that, social constructs, and can be challenged through educating yourself with the large arsenal of critical thought that calls the weight myths into question. For instance, were you aware that people in the category "overweight" live longer than those classed as "normal" weight? If questioning that science seems far-fetched, consider that being gay was once classified as an illness, and the belief that acid causes stomach ulcers has been disproved (they're frequently caused by bacteria). Did you know that our diet and activity patterns account for less than 25 percent of our health outcomes? And that someone's postal/zip code is a more reliable indicator of likely longevity than his or her BMI? Bringing in social determinants moves us away from the "just world" thinking that shores up the status quo and fuels victim blaming. For a more holistic view of the science on social factors, weight, health behaviors, and health outcomes, see the book *Body Respect* (Bacon & Aphramor, 2014).

Readers may also want to educate themselves about the emerging field of fat studies that makes it clear that regardless of why people are fat, their weight does not detract from their inherent human right to respect. Through deconstructing societal norms around fat, scholars and activists reveal the oppressive consequences of harnessing fatness as a health issue and the harm thus inflicted (Wann, 2009).

Of course, because of the complexity of the factors maintaining fat oppression, education can't single-handedly eliminate oppressive internalized values. Even as we challenge ourselves intellectually and lessen the hold of these ideas, they leave their legacy, and we all, to varying degrees, continue to harbor prejudice. Holding this awareness can allow us to compensate.

Undoing Internalized Oppression

One of the more common ways this legacy may be felt is in our feelings towards our own bodies, and changing this relationship is an important aspect of dismantling the ideology of oppression surrounding fat bodies (McMichael, 2013). Fat phobia is itself a symptom of so-matophobia (*soma* refers to "body"). It's an ingrained legacy from Descartes' work mentioned earlier that instigated the body–mind split at the core of binary thinking. Where reason and rationality are ranked above flesh and the non-rational, body shame thrives (Aphramor, 2005). The cultural ideas that there is something wrong with fat and that a fat body is a marker of a defective person are so deeply entrenched that we absorb them, they lodge in our psyches, and most people, fat and thin, come to believe and act as if these oppressive ideas consititue reality. Thin people often also struggle with bodily discomfort and a fear of becoming fat; we can be simultaneously oppressor and oppressed. Whatever our internal struggle, we gain from thin privilege denied fatter people.

Let's put this in real-life terms. What of the thin feminist who unexpectedly gains weight in middle age and considers dieting, despite teaching her students about the social and personal harm arising from the weight-loss agenda? Or someone of any size who, despite an intellectual allegiance to the concept, struggles with body acceptance for any number of reasons, such as chronic pain or gender identity? Despite an active political commitment to fat rights and the body acceptance this entails, feelings of body ambivalence, guilt over feeling ambivalence, and fear may still surface. Injunctions such as "Love your body" fail to account for the messiness of our lived realities and can be experienced as a brutal external code against which we measure ourselves and others. Although well-intentioned, this prescription positions our body-self as an instrument, detached from the complexities of emotion, history, and situatedness, and adds one more divisive directive to the daily artillery fire of judgment, usurping our relational authenticity. If we want to create transformative learning spaces, we will have to recognize the vital role of emotion in the classroom so that we can help our students learn in a way where real life, including embodiment, is not an afterthought or optional extra, but an integral piece in their conceptual framework. For those of us in science disciplines, it is incumbent on us to communicate the fact that traditional science is one among many ways of reaching knowledge;

otherwise, we indirectly shore up the reification of the rational and an associated devaluing of the non-rational, a hierarchy generative of fat phobia (Aphramor, 2005, 2013).

In tandem with any body shame, the thin person who gains weight has a new identity to contend with, one in which the invisible privileges awarded through thinness are thrown into relief by the material fact of fat stigma. The resilience that comes from self-care and support is called for in order for this stage of personal awakening to politicized awareness to be negotiated.

So, we arrive at the need to consider our embodied self, not least to prevent burnout. There is a huge literature on mindfulness that attests to the power of body–mind connection. Our relationship with our embodied self has a profound impact on our thought processes, and vice versa. Paying attention to our physicality will influence the way our politics are articulated by and through our embodiment. There is a circularity to how transforming our relationship with our body happens when we alter our beliefs and this alters the beliefs we hold about the bodies of others, fostering relationships of mutuality and respect. Bringing back the body also destabilizes the hegemonic valorization of the intellect and creates room for us to value other ways of knowing (Aphramor, in press).

Within thin-centric constructs, embodiment is constituted as restraint, regime, and discipline with hedonism frowned upon and desire seen as suspect (Foucault, 1991). When you begin to pay attention to body–mind, take pleasure in and through your body, and accept ambivalent feelings around physicality, you will find yourself more completely reflecting your authenticity through your embodiment. Eventually, you will begin to own your right to respect and relish its embodied manifestation, rather than viewing your appearance/body-self in terms of the degree to which you conform to a socially constructed ideal of beauty and the hidden, gendered assumption that everyone wants to be "beautiful." This internal grounding will help you confront your attitudes towards fat in both yourself and others, and have compassion for the challenges of living in a fat, or otherwise marginalized, body. Mindfulness and body appreciation challenge the social constructs that dictate what an acceptable body is and what an acceptable body should do and support criticality through an enhanced awareness of new perspectives and ways of knowing (Aphramor, in press).

Identity Politics

Another important political tool to upset the hierarchical ordering of bodies is the act of re-assigning meaning to weight identity. We need to reject seeing thinness as normal and more desirable, and move towards seeing weight itself as morally neutral. Through identity politics we come to understand the importance of claiming one's identity to disrupt the traditional, often oppressive, meanings assigned to different identities.

Consider the parallel to developing a positive queer identity as a way to understand this point, as illustrated in this story: when one of the authors (Linda) was in her first year of college, she had not yet accepted her sexual identity; she was ashamed that she might be a lesbian and lived in fear that others might discover her "queerness." One day, she attended a seminar conducted by Audre Lorde; Linda didn't know that Lorde was an activist and thought she was attending an innocuous poetry reading. Lorde began by identifying herself as a black, working-class, feminist, lesbian mother and poet. The mere mention of the word "lesbian" initiated painful inner turmoil for Linda. Much to Linda's dismay, Lorde then called on a random audience member—Linda—to identify herself. On the hot seat publicly, Linda felt humiliated and scared—she was acutely conscious of what she couldn't say without profound shame. She eventually muttered something about not wanting to limit herself to particular categories, offering that she was a Caucasian woman. Lorde's (paraphrased) response provides valuable insight for understanding identity politics: "If you don't own your identity you give up your power and you allow others to control it."

Linda more recently had an opportunity to reflect on Lorde's point and the stigma of fat identity when she was reading her 9-year-old son's class work. In Isaac's school, most tests end with a question intended to help the kids clarify their values and express themselves. Recently the question was: "How would you respond if someone says: 'Your mother is fat'?" Isaac's answer began with the simple words: "So what!" Contrast that with the more common response from his classmates: "She is not!" Isaac's response illustrates that the word "fat" only has the power to shame if one believes that it is a negative identity. When we allow the dominant culture to define that identity as negative, the result is self-loathing, separation, and oppression. However, it doesn't have to be this way. When fat is viewed as a descriptive, non-pejorative term, it loses its shaming power. Through claiming our identities—whether fat or thin, or otherwise privileged and marginalized—we are able to destabilize (thin-centric) norms.

Being a Respectful Ally

As we resist a system that bestows privilege upon us, we discover that even in our resistance we have privilege. For example, many audiences attach a greater sense of legitimacy to words spoken by a thinner person—they can't write it off as a way of rationalizing fatness as they might with a fat person. This privilege of speaking out also needs to be used responsibly, and we need to take care not to inadvertently cause damage when fighting for social change. Considering that the war against fat people has been led by well-intentioned professionals (i.e., those fighting the "war on obesity"), we need to ensure that the role we play as thin people in the fat acceptance movement is negotiated through an ongoing iterative process led by fat people. We need to make sure that we don't speak *for* fat people and that our voices don't drown out the voices of fat people. We need to actively work to make their perspectives more readily heard and, when appropriate, use our voices to advance the perspectives offered by fat people. Through reaching out to the fat activism, fat studies, critical dietetics, or Health At Every Size communities, you will find guidance to help you navigate the complexities of fat oppression and avoid unintentionally causing harm. We'd also urge you to consider the personal benefits inherent in aligning yourself with any one of these communities. You don't have to feel alone in your efforts, and there's a great deal of opportunity for dialogue and support readily available.

Final Words

We can't step out of relationship so we can't ever escape or renounce the various privileges we have, whether they are based on our size, skin color, socioeconomic status, education, sexual orientation, or other attributes. But we can give a damn. By enhancing our ability to stay in connection when confronted by painful awareness, and increasing our openness to new perspectives, we are better able to acknowledge and address all forms of oppression and better placed to support others through similar growth.

References

Aphramor, L. (2005). Is a weight-centred health framework salutogenic? Some thoughts on unhinging certain dietary ideologies. *Social Theory and Health, 3*(4), 315–340.

Aphramor, L. (2013). *Well Now facilitators background reading.* Retrieved from http://www.well-founded.org.uk

Aphramor, L. (in press). *Doing nutrition justice: Teaching for transformation.* London, England: Independent Publishers Network.

Bacon, L., & Aphramor, L. (2014). *Body respect: What conventional text books leave out, get wrong or just plain fail to understand about weight.* Dallas, TX: BenBella.

Bishop, A. (2002). *Becoming an ally: Breaking the cycle of oppression.* New York, NY: Zed.

Campos, P., Saguy, A., Ernsberger, P., Oliver, E., & Gaesser, G. (2006). The epidemiology of overweight and obesity: Public health crisis or moral panic? *International Journal of Epidemiology, 35,* 55–60.

Doane, W. (2003). Rethinking whiteness studies. In A. Doane & E. Bonilla-Silva (Eds.), *White out: The continuing significance of racism* (pp. 3–18). New York, NY: Routledge.

Farrell, A. E. (2011). *Fat shame: Stigma and the fat body in American culture.* New York, NY: New York University Press.

Foucault, M. (1991). *Discipline and punish: The birth of the prison.* London, England: Penguin.

Gingras, J., & Brady, J. (2010). Relational consequences of dietitians' feeding bodily difference. *Radical Psychology, 8*(1). Retrieved from http://www.radicalpsychology.org/vol8-1/gingras.html

Harding, K. (2010). Kevin Smith: The face of flying while fat. *Salon.* Retrieved from http://www.salon.com/life/broadsheet/feature/2010/02/16/flying_while_fat-

Harding, K., & Kirby, M. (2009). *Lessons from the fatosphere: Quit dieting and declare a truce with your body.* New York, NY: Perigee Books.

Lorde, A. (1984). *Sister outsider: Essays and speeches.* Freedom, CA: Crossing Press.

Maroney, D., & Golub, S. (1992). Nurses' attitudes towards obese persons and certain ethnic groups. *Perceptual and Motor Skills, 75,* 387–391.

McIntosh, P. (1988). *White privilege and male privilege: A personal account of coming to see correspondences through work in women's studies* (Working Paper No. 189). Boston, MA: Wellesley College Center for Research on Women.

McMichael, L. (2013). *Acceptable prejudice? Fat, rhetoric and social justice.* Nashville, TN: Pearlsong Press.

O'Hara, L., & Gregg, J. (2010). Don't diet: Adverse effects of the weight centered health paradigm. In F. De-Meester, S. Zibadi, & R. R. Watson (Eds.), *Modern dietary fat intakes in disease promotion, nutrition and health* (pp. 431–441). New York, NY: Springer.

Peel School District Board. (2002). *Issue paper on the isms: Support documents for the implementation of the future we want.* Mississauga, ON, Canada: Author.

Puhl, R., Andreyeva, T., & Brownell, K. (2008). Perceptions of weight based discrimination: Prevalence and comparison to race and gender discrimination in America. *International Journal of Obesity, 32,* 992–1000.

Puhl, R. M., & Heuer, C. A. (2009). The stigma of obesity: A review and update. *Obesity, 17,* 941–964.

Stinson, S. (2009). Fat girls need fiction. In E. Rothblum, & S. Solovay (Eds.), *The fat studies reader* (pp. 231–234). New York, NY: New York University Press.

Sumithran, P., & Proietto, J. (2013) The defence of body weight: A physiological basis for weight regain after weight loss. *Clinical Science, 124,* 231–241.

U.S. National Education Association. (2010). *Report on discrimination due to physical size.* Retrieved from http://www.lectlaw.com/files/con28.htm

Wann, M. (2009). Foreword: Fat studies: An invitation to revolution. In E. Rothblum & S. Solovay (Eds.), *The fat studies reader* (pp. ix–xxv). New York, NY: New York University Press.

Wilson, J. (2013). Let's broaden the talk about thin privilege [Web log post]. Retrieved from http://mykitchendietitian.com/blog/2014/10/13/lets-broaden-the-talk-about-thin-privilege/

PART TWO

Practicing Fat Pedagogies

FIVE

Promise to Try: Combating Fat Oppression Through Pedagogy in Tertiary Education

Cat Pausé

There is no such thing as a neutral educational process. Education either functions as an instrument that is used to facilitate the integration of the younger generation into the logic of the present system and bring conformity to it, *or* it becomes the practice of freedom, the means by which men and women deal critically and creatively with reality and discover how to participate in the transformation of their world. (Freire, 2003, p. 34, emphasis in original)

Education can liberate *and* oppress, emancipate *and* domesticate (Freire, 2003). This chapter explores ways that those who teach tertiary education reinforce *and* resist fat oppression. We live in a world where slimness is privileged (LeBesco, 2003; Wann, 1998) and slim bodies are read as good bodies: disciplined, active, attractive, and successful (Jutel, 2005). In contrast, fat bodies are read as bad bodies: undisciplined, lazy, disgusting, and undesirable (Murray, 2008). The anti-fat attitudes that result from these beliefs influence the lives of individuals of all sizes in employment settings, health care settings, and educational settings. They can be found in the interactions between classroom participants (teacher—student, student—teacher, student—student) and in the treatment of bodies within the subject material, given normative messages about bodies and the subsequent reinforcement of anti-fat attitudes are common (Smith, 2012). Educators committed to social justice must make room for body size to have a place in their praxis alongside their commitment to working on issues of gender, race, class, ability, sexual orientation, and beyond (hooks, 1994).

Whether to integrate social justice within the tertiary classroom is a choice for each faculty member who shapes a syllabus. Some make this commitment eagerly and work to disrupt oppression. Many dispute that this opportunity exists or see it as too much of a burden, or disregard it altogether. Others may look upon pedagogies of social justice as desirable, but lack the knowledge and skills to implement them in their classrooms (Guthman, 2009). Social justice pedagogies can be approached in multiple ways and include disrupting oppression or, at the very least, not (re) producing oppression. Those who teach fat studies courses are able to engage in fat pedagogies that both disrupt fat oppression and promote social justice for all individuals regardless of size (Watkins, Farrell, & Hugmeyer, 2012). But how do those of us not teaching courses in fat studies incorporate body size justice into our classroom? How may we recognize that the bodies of our students, and the bodies involved in our subject area, are political?

In this chapter, I consider various ways that those in a range of disciplines might include fat politics in our classrooms (e.g., Koppelman, 2009). Issues I consider include providing fat friendly classrooms, introducing issues of fat politics, and ensuring that course material and assessment do not reinforce fat oppression and shame. Special attention is given to exploring how social media may be used as tools for engaging in fat pedagogy (Harding & Kirby, 2009).

While I identify as a fat studies researcher, I am not currently teaching fat studies courses. In many tertiary education institutions, the financial climate does not foster the space to introduce new courses and calls into question the validity of courses seen as suspect because of their connections to identity politics and activism. And unfortunately, this is making subjects that are seen by the status quo as unnecessary, such as gender studies, vulnerable (Fisher, 2010). I do receive student requests, however, to teach courses in fat studies, and I hope that one day that will become part of my workload. In the meantime, I am often asked to give guest lectures and workshops around my university. I have been invited into business classes to discuss weight discrimination in employment, counseling classes to discuss provider bias impact on fat patients, education classes to discuss how anti-fat attitudes in teachers impact students of all sizes, and nutrition classes to discuss what fat activism means for students' future professional practice.

The level of interest, from colleagues and students alike, in fat studies is not surprising to me. Many students are drawn to courses about bodies. As noted by Patricia Boling (2011), "Students find deeply resonant arguments that bodies are cultural artefacts socially constructed by the particular expectations and practices of the time and place in which one lives" (p. 110). Of course, conversely, some students may resist taking such courses because of the risk it may pose to their own identity management (Pausé, 2012; Watkins et al., 2012).

The discipline of fat studies has arisen to challenge normative assumptions and discourse in the scholarship of fat bodies (namely, "obesity" studies). Fat studies works to disrupt stereotypes that surround people living in fat bodies by denaturalizing fatness and rejecting essentialist epistemologies. The scholarship within fat studies situates fatness within "the context of rights and exclusions" (Garland-Thomson, 2005, p. 1557).

Courses in fat studies have been offered at a range of institutions, including Oregon State University, George Washington University, Macquarie University, and Rutgers University. Patti Lou Watkins, Amy Farrell, and Andrea Doyle Hugmeyer (2012) examined the offerings of four fat studies courses in tertiary education settings (along with two courses centered on "Health At Every Size," and six other courses that adopted a critical perspective on mainstream obesity discourses). They found that fat studies courses were described as interdisciplinary and intersectional, exploring how body size interacts with other identities (such as gender, race, class, and ability) to position some people into places of power and others into places of oppression. The courses privileged the role of social construction in understandings of fatness, and critiqued mainstream discourses of "globesity." Critical examinations of mainstream notions of fat may be also found in health classrooms that center a "Health At Every Size" perspective, such as the nutrition classes taught by Linda Bacon (Watkins et al., 2012). Other courses in the areas of feminist theory, women's studies, and literature have been found to be complementary to the pedagogies and theories of fatness (Boling, 2011).

Fat studies (like queer studies, women's studies, and Māori studies) is a marginalized discipline within academia. Scholars in these fields are often stigmatized by the academy, and their work is often dismissed as not being valid scholarship (Waitere, Tremaine, Wright, Brown, & Pausé, 2011). Outside of academia, concerns are raised that identity scholarships, like fat studies, focus more on politics than on academic rigor (Binder, 2010). Some have countered this concern by arguing that any subject can be taught in way that compromises rigor, and suggest that identity scholarships may in fact do a better job of presenting a challenging and critical pedagogy than more traditional disciplines (North, 2010).

Universities, as producers and distributors of knowledge, are conservative institutions, functioning largely to reproduce existing ways of knowing and structures of power (Angell & Price, 2012). Within the classroom, professors set the agenda of a course and are responsible for the topics that are addressed and the materials that are consumed as well as the areas that are excluded. This is an incredible position of power, as students take seriously the issues presented and implicitly acknowledge the lesser importance of the ones that are not (Boling, 2011). Educators committed to social justice work to synthesize research, teaching, and activism through pedagogies that place social justice at their core (Wilcox, 2009).

Building on the work of Elisabeth Grosz (1994), many have developed arguments to support the acknowledgment of the body's role in lived experience and knowledge production (Wilcox, 2009). Rejecting the Cartesian split of the active mind and the passive body, these scholars focus on embodiment and its interactions with epistemology, ontology, and methodology. Within any classroom, the bodies of the teacher and of the students play important roles, even if ignored (Tirosh, 2006). But we cannot disregard the role that bodies play in the classroom, as both students and professors read the bodies of those around them (Fisanick, 2007). As Christina Fisanick suggests, "The body has everything to do with the way in which we see ourselves as professors and the ways in which our students and our colleagues perceive us and expect us to perform" (p. 245). While those in the academy might like to suggest that legitimacy, advancement, and position are based on the merits of the mind alone, the role that the body plays in these arenas has been demonstrated as important (American Association of University Women, 2004; Basow, 1998; Benton, 2004; Escalera, 2009; Fisanick, 2007; Patton 2014).

In some classrooms, bodies are acknowledged as sites of knowledge and analysis. In fields related to health and sport, for example, body pedagogies are common (Cliff & Wright, 2010). Body pedagogies, according to John Evans, Emma Rich, Brian Davies, and Rachel Allwood (2008), are "conscious activity taken by [a curriculum], designed to enhance an individual's understanding of their own and/or others' corporeality. [These pedagogies] define the significance, value and potential of the body" (p. 17). The body pedagogies found in many health and sport classrooms unfortunately sit in direct contrast to fat pedagogies as they reinforce fat oppression. Teaching students that there are only a handful of acceptable bodies serves to reproduce anti-fat attitudes as well as attitudes that inspire fear and disgust around dis/abled bodies and queer bodies.

Fat Oppressive Classrooms

Based on my own experiences with colleagues in health, social sciences, and the sciences, I share three examples of fat oppression that was embedded in their teaching. I do so not only to demonstrate how readily fat oppression is reproduced in university classrooms but also, in two of the examples, to demonstrate how interventions by those of us committed to fat pedagogy can make a difference in helping colleagues notice and then address the fat oppression in their teaching materials, assignments, or practices.

College of Health

A colleague teaching courses in nutrition invited me to review the PowerPoint slides she used when she lectured on "obesity." As a scholar who engages with critical theory, she had already integrated critical literature into her material (e.g., Bacon & Aphramor, 2011; Flegal, Kit, Orpana, & Graubard, 2013), which ensured that her curriculum acknowledged that there are dissenting views. Unfortunately, the images she was using in the slides reinforced fat oppression. To accompany the material on "obesity," for example, she had illustrated her slides with "headless fatties" (i.e., images of fat people without heads). As Charlotte Cooper (2007) explains, depicting fat people in this way results in the objectification of fat bodies. It makes them less than human, not worthy of dignity or respect. After a discussion of this, she updated the slides to remove the torsos, and she began inviting me into her classroom to give a regular lecture. So, that is a good news story. But far more common is the reinforcement of fat oppression in classrooms that explicitly deal with bodies and health. And for many, if not most, faculty and students in those classrooms, this kind of oppression usually goes unnoticed.

College of Social Sciences

An assignment from a sociology class asked students to consider the impact of environmental racism on personal health outcomes. In the assignment, students are asked to consider the impacts of socioeconomic status on health by considering the same scenario for two different women. Woman A is a well-paid professional with a flexible schedule who owns her home; Woman B is an hourly worker who rents in a high-crime area. In the instructions, the students learn that both women have recently decided they wanted to "lose weight and get healthy." The assignment instructs the students to consider the resources available to both women to achieve their goal along with the possible challenges they will face. The students are asked to conclude by making an argument for "who is more likely to get healthy."

In this assignment, we have an intersection of gender, class, and size (and possibly race), but only two of these are outwardly acknowledged in the prompt. We also have conflation of body size and health. The assignment reinforces the myth that weight loss results in better health and, as such, is an important goal, which encourages fat shaming. In this particular example, I suggested that the assignment prompt be revised to remove the conflation of body size and health and the fat shaming. The assignment now instructs the students that the woman's goal is to "begin exercising regularly and eating more nutritious meals." In the revised assignment, the same learning objectives are being addressed and students are still able to demonstrate acquisition of course concepts; while the healthism of the assignment remains, I am pleased that their work at least no longer reinforces fat oppression.

College of Sciences

Lastly, consider this assignment from a statistics course. The assignment in question was part of the section on comparing group means. The students are given information about 20 people and how long it takes them to consume a Big Mac meal; 10 of the people are identi-fied as "overweight." The students are instructed to use SPSS (a statistical software package) to determine whether there is a significant difference between length of eating time for the two groups, and then draw conclusions from the analysis. The data are set up to lead to results that demonstrate that the "overweight" group eats at a much faster rate than the "non-overweight" group. The students then draw on their own "everybody knows" logic about fat people and their behaviours to speculate on the relationship between this (fabricated) finding and indi-vidual body size and future health. I encouraged revision of the assignment in order to remove the negative reinforcement of a fat stereotype, and pointed out that all of the individuals in the simulated study are eating the same fast food meal, highlighting a common fallacy made when assessing body size and health: fat people who eat fast food are derided for making poor choices whereas non-fat people who eat the same food are left alone. Unfortunately, the as-signment was not amended, as I failed to convince my colleague of the oppression inherent in the design.

Fat Friendly Classrooms

Once faculty members have worked to rid their course materials and classroom of materials that reinforce fat oppression, they may decide that they want to take their commitment to size justice to the next level. They may wish to achieve this by developing curricula and practices that are body size neutral. There are a number of ways to do this.

Faculty members can work to create spaces that are safe for people of all sizes. This can be done by avoiding the use of language or attitudes that reinforce body shame and fat hatred, and challenging them when they do arise in the classroom. Also, attention to ensuring that appropriate physical spaces are being used is critical. We do a great disservice to our students when we ignore the role that physical comfort plays in their learning. Are the spaces we provide accessible to all students? Are they fat friendly, able to accommodate a range of body sizes? I spent much of my own tertiary education squeezing my body through narrow rows and into desks that were too small for me, and the message received is, "You don't belong here. You aren't wanted." As Ashley Hetrick and Derek Attig (2009) share, "Desks hurt us. … [Desks] are highly active material and discursive constructions that seek to both indoctrinate students' bodies and minds into the middle-class values of restraint and discipline, and inscribe these messages onto the bodies that sit in them" (p. 197). Size appropriate accommodation for stu-dents and teachers alike should be provided within educational settings.

Fat Positive Classrooms

Another option for faculty is to embrace a fat pedagogy wholeheartedly and actively work to construct a classroom that promotes fat liberation. In the same way that professors can avoid reinforcing fat oppression in their course materials, they can also ensure that when bodies are included in the curriculum, a wide range of body types and sizes are present. These curricula should be intersectional in their approaches to material (Gillborn, 2015; Pausé, 2014b) and present diverse fat bodies and experiences as normative and desirable. Faculty members should consider using images of fat people (but not "headless fatties") when preparing and presenting visual materials; head to the "Stocky Body Image Library" for a range of choices if needed (Gurrieri, 2013). Include stories and narratives produced by fat people when assigning readings. Watch films about fat people's lives or that place fat bodies in the center rather than at the margins.

If one makes a commitment to engaging with fat pedagogies in the classroom, I recommend making this explicit to students. Susan Koppelman (2009) asserts, "What is printed on a syllabus is at best an approximation of what actually happens in a classroom" and "reading the syllabus can tell us much about the intentions and attitudes of its author" (p. 213). Listing classroom assumptions in the syllabus or administration guide is a clear message of the expectations and tone of the course (Lord, 1982). Assumptions for a fat positive classroom could include statements such as "the fat body is a normal model of a human body" and "the subjective experience of fat individuals is valid and important" (see Mohr, Matthews, & Emmanuelle, 2011, or Nowell, 2013, for other great suggestions).

You may be wondering whether fat pedagogies are appropriate for your classroom. I would suggest that many courses and other educational activities have opportunities to engage in fat pedagogies. They may not engage with fatness directly, but these curricula could engage in broader discussions of what shapes our cultural understandings of fatness and the fat body. Topics could include the social construction of bodies and/or health, connections between morality and health, historical perspectives of beauty and/or body size, and physical representations of bodies in everyday culture.

Social media provide great tools for promoting fat pedagogies in a classroom. These tools, especially Web 2.0 tools, are becoming more common in their use in tertiary education (Stein, Shephard, & Harris, 2011; Stiler & Philleo, 2003). The openness of the Internet allows for individuals to engage in oppositional politics free of boundaries and limitations (Kahn & Kellner, 2005). Many in the fat activist community have embraced social media as tools in their movement (Harding & Kirby, 2009; Pausé, 2014a). Requiring students to engage in social media as part of their course and directing them to fat friendly sites are ways to make it more likely that students will consider the intersections of experiences and be exposed to diverse perspectives and points of view.

It is extremely important that disciplines across academia bring fat pedagogies into the classroom. Very few students will have the opportunity, even if they desire it, to complete a course dedicated solely to fat studies. Just as fat studies courses must acknowledge the intersections of body size with race, class, gender, ability, sexual orientation, and beyond (Pausé, 2014b), courses in other disciplines that consider such social justice issues must also acknowledge the myriad ways these intersect with body size. But incorporating fat pedagogies should not, and is not, limited to courses with social justice foci. Any course may engage fat pedagogies by providing safe spaces for individuals of all sizes, ensuring that pursuit of higher education is for every body.

References

American Association of University Women. (2004). *Tenure denied: Cases of sex discrimination in academia.* Washington, DC: AAUW Educational Foundation.

Angell, K., & Price, C. (2012). Fat bodies in thin books: Information bias and body image in academic libraries. *Fat Studies, 1*(2), 153–165.

Bacon, L., & Aphramor, L. (2011). Weight science: Evaluating the evidence for a paradigm shift. *Nutrition, 10*(9), 2–13.

Basow, S. (1998). Student evaluations: The role of gender bias and teaching styles. In L. H. Collins, J. C. Chrisler, & K. Quina (Eds.), *Career strategies for women in academe: Aiming Athena* (pp. 269–271). Thousand Oaks, CA: Sage.

Benton, T. H. (2004, August 30). On being a fat professor. *Chronicle of Higher Education.* Retrieved from http://chronicle.com/article/On-Being-a-Fat-Professor/44595/

Binder, E. (2010, November 3). "Fat Studies" go to college. *The Daily Beast.* Retrieved from http://www.thedailybeast.com/articles/2010/11/03/fat-studies-colleges-hot-new-course.html

Boling, P. (2011). On learning to teach fat feminism. *Feminist Teacher, 21*(2), 110–123.

Cliff, K., & Wright, J. (2010). Confusing and contradictory: Considering obesity discourse and eating disorders as they shape body pedagogies in HPE. *Sport, Education and Society, 15*(2), 221–233.

Cooper, C. (2007). Headless fatties. Retrieved from http://charlottecooper.net/publishing/digital/headless-fatties-01-07

Escalera, E. (2009). Stigma threat and the fat professor: Reducing student prejudice in the classroom. In E. Rothblum & S. Solovay (Eds.), *The fat studies reader* (pp. 205–221). New York, NY: New York University Press.

Evans, J., Rich, E., Davies, B., & Allwood, R. (2008). *Education, disordered eating and obesity discourse: Fat fabrications.* Oxford, England: Routledge.

Fisanick, C. (2007). "They are weighted with authority": Fat female professors in academic and popular cultures. *Feminist Teacher, 17*(3), 237–255.

Fisher, A. (2010, December 1). Axing gender studies "setback to rights." *Stuff.* Retrieved from http://www.stuff.co.nz/national/education/4407891/Axing-gender-studies-setback-to-rights

Flegal, K. M., Kit, B. K., Orpana, H., & Graubard, B. I. (2013). Association of all-cause mortality with overweight and obesity using standard Body Mass Index categories: Systematic review and meta-analysis. *Journal of the American Medical Association, 309*(1), 71–82.

Freire, P. (2003). *Pedagogy of the oppressed.* New York, NY: Continuum.

Garland-Thomson, R. (2005). Feminist disability studies. *Signs, 30*(2), 1557–1587.

Gillborn, D. (2015). Intersectionality, critical race theory, and the primacy of racism: Race, class, gender, and disability in education. *Qualitative Inquiry, 21*(3), 277–287.

Grosz, E. (1994). *Volatile bodies: Toward a corporeal feminism.* Bloomington, IN: Indiana University Press.

Gurrieri, L. (2013). Stocky bodies: Fat visual activism. *Fat Studies, 2*(2), 197–209.

Guthman, J. (2009). Teaching the politics of obesity: Insights into neoliberal embodiment and contemporary biopolitics. *Antipode, 41*(5), 1110–1133.

Harding, K., & Kirby, M. (2009). *Lessons from the Fat-O-Sphere: Quit dieting and declare a truce with your body.* New York, NY: Penguin.

Hetrick, A., & Attig, D. (2009). Sitting pretty: Fat bodies, classroom desks, and academic excess. In E. Rothblum & S. Solovay (Eds.), *The fat studies reader* (pp. 197–204). New York, NY: New York University Press.

hooks, b. (1994). *Teaching to transgress: Education as the practice of freedom.* New York, NY: Routledge.

Jutel, A. (2005). Weighing health: The moral burden of obesity. *Social Semiotics, 15*(2), 114–125.

Kahn, R., & Kellner, D. (2005). Oppositional politics and the Internet: A critical/reconstructive approach. *Cultural Politics, 1*(1), 75–100.

Koppelman, S. (2009). Fat stories in the classroom. What and how are they teaching about us? In E. Rothblum & S. Solovay (Eds.), *The fat studies reader* (pp. 213–220). New York, NY: New York University Press.

LeBesco, K. (2003). *Revolting bodies? The struggle to redefine fat identity.* Boston, MA: University of Massachusetts Press.

Lord, S. (1982). Teaching the psychology of women: Examination of a teaching–learning model. *Psychology of Women Quarterly, 7*(1), 70–80.

Mohr, P., Matthews, B. R., & Emmanuelle, C. (2011). Teaching resource: Fat studies. *Feminist Teacher, 21*(2), 168–170.

Murray, S. (2008). *The fat female body.* New York, NY: Palgrave Macmillan.

North, A. (2010, November 4). Should "fat studies" be taught in school? *Jezebel.* Retrieved from http://jezebel.com/5681887/should-fat-studies-be-taught-in-school

Nowell, M. (2013, September 27). Sociology of fatness: Critical perspectives for teaching sociology (and anthropology). *Conditionally Accepted*. Retrieved from http://conditionallyaccepted.com/2013/09/27/sociology-of-fatness/

Patton, S. (2014, April 3). I'm the biggest man on campus. *The Chronicle of Higher Education*. Retrieved from https://chroniclevitae.com/news/426-i-m-the-biggest-man-on-campus

Pausé, C. J. (2012). Live to tell: Coming out as fat. *Somatechnics, 2*(1), 42–56.

Pausé, C. J. (2014a). Causing a commotion: Queering fatness in cyberspace. In C. J. Pausé, J. Wykes, & S. Murray (Eds.), *Queering fat embodiment* (pp. 75–88). London, England: Ashgate.

Pausé, C. J. (2014b). X-static process: Intersectionality within the field of fat studies. *Fat Studies, 3*(2), 80–85.

Smith, E. S. (2012). Making room for fat studies in writing center theory and practice. *Praxis: A Writing Center Journal, 10*(1), 1–7.

Stein, S. J., Shephard, K., & Harris, I. (2011). Conceptions of e-learning and professional development for e-learning held by tertiary educators in New Zealand. *British Journal of Educational Technology, 42*(1), 145–165.

Stiler, G. M., & Philleo, T. (2003). Blogging and blogspots: An alternative format for encouraging reflective practice among pre-service teachers. *Education, 123*(4), 789–797.

Tirosh, Y. (2006). Weighty speech: Addressing body size in the classroom. *Review of Education, Pedagogy, and Cultural Studies, 28*, 267–279.

Waitere, H., Tremaine, M., Wright, J., Brown, S., & Pausé, C. J. (2011). Choosing to resist or reinforce the new managerialism: The impact of performance based research funding on academic identity. *Higher Education Research & Development, 30*(2), 205–217.

Wann, M. (1998). *FAT!SO?* Berkeley, CA: Ten Speed Press.

Watkins, P. L., Farrell, A. E., & Hugmeyer, A. D. (2012). Teaching fat studies: From conception to reception. *Fat Studies, 1*(2), 180–194.

Wilcox, H. N. (2009). Embodied ways of knowing, pedagogies, and social justice: Inclusive science and beyond. *National Women's Studies Association Journal, 21*(2), 104–120.

SIX

Teaching Fat Studies in a Liberal Arts College: The Centrality of Mindfulness, Deep Listening, and Empathic Interpretation as Pedagogic Methods

Amy E. Farrell

For the past five years I have taught Fat Studies as an intermediate-level, cross-listed American studies and women's and gender studies course at Dickinson College in the United States. Dickinson is a small (about 2,400 students), highly selective undergraduate college that prides itself on its international programs, its commitment to sustainability, and its strong interdisciplinary offerings. In the past decade, it has also been listed as one of the "fittest" schools by *Men's Fitness* based on its physical education requirement, its exercise and recreational facilities, and its food options. This latter ranking got national attention (including articles in *USA Today* and segments on NBC News and the *Today Show*) as well as significant "press time" on our own website and admissions materials. Despite its emphasis on "fitness" (which for most people not in the Health At Every Size movement translates into thinness), Dickinson is also one of the first colleges in the United States to offer a fat studies course, in contrast to "obesity studies" or "health and obesity" courses. While colleagues at other institutions have detailed the problems they faced in having a fat studies course approved, at my own institution both the provost and my departments were quick to support the course, just as they had provided both financial and collegial backing for my own research in the field (Watkins, Farrell, & Hugmeyer, 2012).

From the beginning, Fat Studies has been a tremendously popular course, with more than 100 students signing up each year for a course that is capped at 25. With no prerequisites, students range from first-years to seniors. Priority goes to American studies and women's and gender studies majors; the rest of the students come from across the disciplines: psychology, health studies, biology, art history, political science, environmental studies, business and management, sociology, history, theater, and English. Students arrive to class passionate about the topic; many of them seem to live, eat, and breathe concern about fat, voicing experiences with disordered eating and extraordinary attention to their own and others' body size and fitness. Few students of size sign up for the course; I voiced my concern about this to writer and activist Marilyn Wann who suggested that it may not feel particularly safe for students to "out" themselves as fat within a college setting that prides itself on fitness, especially if they don't know that fat studies offers a critical perspective on dominant understandings about weight and health.

During the first semester I taught the course, I noticed two strong, problematic student reactions. The first reaction was anger. Students were quick to raise their hands, voices trembling, dismissing the scholarship that challenged our dominant paradigm of fat and illness and that connected fat discrimination to other forms of oppression. The other reaction was confusion. A few students continually gave quizzical looks and struggled to respond to my questions and assignments. At the end of the semester, some students noted in their evaluations that they "didn't understand" or "didn't get" what we were discussing until very far into the semester. I do not think that these two reactions of anger and confusion were because the students were too high strung or impolite (in the first case) or because the course was too difficult or that they were ill prepared or unintelligent (in the second case.) Rather, I think it was infuriating and/or incomprehensible because it simply challenged too many deeply held beliefs and ideologies. They simply could not "get" the premise of a class that ran in such opposition to "common sense" knowledge—that "obesity" is an "epidemic" that needs to be controlled, either through prevention or through weight loss. I would suggest, in fact, that the course itself generated "stigma threat." In teaching for social justice, one of the first challenges faced is overcoming students' reluctance or unwillingness to engage in the subject matter because of strongly held prejudices or the "stigma threat" generated by the instructor or the subject matter (Escalera, 2009; Goffman, 1963). That is, confronted with an idea— or a person—that carries a stigmatized identity, students will often react with nervousness and hostility, thereby preventing themselves from considering new ideas and points of view. The use of the word "fat," the discussions about the experiences of fat people, the activisms that fat people enacted—all were so overwhelming to many students that they simply could not comprehend our readings or could not discuss them without becoming irritated, even furious.

This chapter focuses on the methods I used—both in terms of syllabus design and pedagogic style—to navigate the stigma threat and obstacles that emerged in teaching Fat Studies. Drawing from student evaluations and open-ended student responses, all of which were anonymous, I discuss in particular the importance of deep listening and mindfulness, empathic interpretation, and an intersectional, historically focused approach in teaching about fat stigma and fat activisms. These methods might also be used, I conclude, to address the hostile atmosphere that fat professors face in academia, inasmuch as they encourage the open discussion of fat oppression and fat discrimination.

Stigma Threat and the Professor

In discussing my methods in teaching Fat Studies, it's essential, if uncomfortable, to reflect on my own body size privilege. As a 51-year-old white woman who is not thin but whom others do not necessarily identify as "so fat that I have to ask for an airplane seatbelt extender" as the writer Judith Moore (2005, p. 1) puts it in her very painful memoir *Fat Girl*, I have not had to deal with the kind of embarrassed looks, nervous stammering, and outright hostility and distrust that Elena Andrea Esclarera (2009) describes in her essay in *The Fat Studies Reader* on fat professors and stigma threat. A recent article in the *Chronicle of Higher Education* describes the hostile atmosphere that fat professors face in academia:

> Overweight professors across academe describe similar battles to achieve self-acceptance, full inclusion in academic life, and genuine respect from students and colleagues. Some struggle daily to navigate campus spaces that don't comfortably accommodate their size. Some stand in front of classrooms and wonder whether their bodies influence how students perceive their minds. … Yet larger professors often grapple with these concerns in isolation and silence. On a national level, discussions of obesity have become increasingly common—and, at times, increasingly contentious. But many fat professors, along with allies in the emerging field of fat studies, feel that colleges and universities have yet to hold productive conversations on the topic, especially when it comes to "fat shaming" and how size influences hiring, tenure, and promotion decisions. (Patton, 2014, para. 8)

And, as Escalera discussed in her article, it's not just hiring, tenure, and promotion that are affected by fat shaming; pedagogy and learning in the classroom are also involved. (Of course, all of these connect, particularly as student evaluations are usually key to tenure and promotion decisions, particularly in small, liberal arts colleges.)

My own experience teaching fat studies, however, is one of body size privilege and what Peggy McIntosh (1989) articulated years ago as white skin privilege. Students seem to perceive my 51-year-old white woman's body as acceptable, not young, not old, not thin, not fat, with no particular axe to grind when it comes to fatness. This apparent "neutrality" is one that Escalera points out is impossible for fat professors, which creates a vulnerability that makes teaching about fat particularly difficult.

Deflecting Stigma Threat Through Deep Listening

Despite the significant advantages that I carry into the classroom in terms of my size, age, and skin color, the subject matter itself generates intense stigma threat. To displace this anger and confusion, I begin class by asking students to note and observe their own affective and intellectual reactions to the material without engaging in them. I explain to students that we will be reading a range of perspectives, studies, and opinions that will not mesh with what they have generally heard. On the first day of class we list everything they know and associate with fatness. This typically generates a long list of health problems (arthritis, diabetes, heart attacks), psychological attributes (laziness, lack of willpower, depression), aesthetic issues (ugly, deformed), and solutions (diets, surgeries, pharmaceuticals, support groups). In the latest iterations of the course, a few students have also listed discrimination and stigma on the board, but these ideas are always in the minority.

After generating these lists, I explain that in this class students will be exploring contrarian points of view to this common sense information about fatness. Everything on the board, I explain, will be interrogated, from the connection between fatness and illness to the association of fatness with laziness, psychological problems, and lack of beauty. We will even question the questions, I explain, asking why our culture focuses so much on body size, how the framing of questions shapes the problem itself, and who benefits and who loses from a fixation on fatness. Instead of challenging these ideas, or arguing with them (or me), I ask that students allow the new ideas to roll around in their heads, to figure out how to explicate them, to feel unrushed to come to some definitive opinion. I want them to luxuriate in listening. At the end of the semester they should feel free to agree or disagree with the materials, but for now, they should just be alert to their thoughts and reactions, perhaps even voice them, but mainly they should practice listening.

This technique allows space for the students to consider new ideas that can often be more difficult if students are using all their thoughtfulness to challenge the material before they even can consider it. Arguing, I've found, is counterproductive, particularly before they have had an opportunity to read and understand other perspectives. My tactic, then, is to deflect this tendency to rush to argument in order to allow students to think without agitation, to *ponder*. In recent years, many scholars have focused their research on the importance of mindfulness and contemplation within academic settings. Tobin Hart (2004) writes that contemplation is a

> third way of knowing that complements the rational and the sensory. The contemplative mind is opened and activated through a wide range of approaches—from pondering to poetry to meditation—that are designed to quiet and shift the habitual chatter of the mind to cultivate a capacity for deepened awareness, concentration, and insight. (p. 29)

Today, students experience constant chatter from physicians, professors, parents, friends, and advertisers, and on every form of media, about the dangers of "obesity," about the importance of weight loss, about diets, products, and medical procedures to change one's body. It is crucial to get past that chatter in order for students to be able to comprehend some different points of view about fat and body size. Hart (2004) describes a number of techniques that faculty use in their classes to encourage contemplation—meditation, free writing, poetry writing. For me, what has worked is a shift in tone, one that emphasizes deep listening. When students begin to argue with the material, I thank them for the important issue they raise and then I ask them to imagine they are asking the question (or raising the challenge) to the author who wrote the article or book we are reading. How would that author respond to this question? Students then need to turn to the readings themselves, search through them, think about them, to articulate a response.

The class readings work first to *denaturalize* contemporary understandings of fatness. The idea that fat is bad, ugly, and dangerous is so powerful and deeply rooted in history (Farrell, 2011) that it's essential to allow students to see some other possibilities. After I introduce the field of fat studies with the first chapters in the 2009 *Fat Studies Reader* (by Marilyn Wann, Esther Rothblum, and Sondra Solovay), we discuss Don Kulick and Anne Meneley's 2005 collection of essays, *Fat: The Anthropology of an Obsession*. We compare the experiences of fat valorization in Niger in the 1980s with the culture of fat talk among Swedish high school girls in the 1990s; we contrast the valorization of olive oil compared with the love for Spam in Hawaii; we discuss whether pornography that focuses on fat women eating should be seen as liberatory for those women. The point of these discussions is not to get to a "right" answer, but rather to allow students to realize that there are indeed *a lot* of ways to think about fat.

At this point we turn to a multiweek focus on fatness and stigma. We read Erving Goffman (1963) to identify some of the key points about how stigma surrounding a "discredited attribute" works to decrease "life chances." We discuss how people will go to "extraordinary lengths" to decrease stigma—and then we link this to fatness, in particular reading about the ways that stigma might help to explain some of the horrible headlines we regularly read about the dangers of fatness. We explore the development of fat stigma in the United States to illuminate the ways that ideas about fat are neither natural nor inevitable, but rather the result of cultural beliefs, struggles, and hierarchies. We discuss the ways that stigma connects with race (Sapphire, 1996), with class (Ernsberger, 2009), and sexualities (Bergman, 2009; Vade & Solovay, 2009). By the middle of the semester, I ask students to choose their own example of fat stigma to analyze; most recently, students have written on such topics as the Strong4Life campaign in Atlanta, the film *Precious*, the TV show *Here Comes Honey Boo Boo*, and a series of People for the Ethical Treatment of Animals (PETA) ads.

Encouraging Empathic Vision

The first unit in the course, then, focuses on bypassing students' initial resistance to the ideas articulated within the field of fat studies. The second unit pushes students to understand the history of fat stigma and the way that it works in contemporary culture. The third unit on fat activism changes direction, moving students from that abstract understanding of fat denigration and discrimination to a process of empathic interpretation based on the ideas of "empathic vision" that visual culture scholar Jill Bennett (2005) describes. Bennett and other scholars such as Roewan Crowe and Michelle Meagher (2012) explain that traditional art criticism positions the visual scholar or critic as the expert who locates the correct meaning in the work. In contrast, Crowe and Meagher articulate a new way of responding to the work, one that wonders "how it feels to *be* with the work of art, to think about the *effects* of a work of art, and to consider what a work of art might *do*" (p. 9). They urge a "critical and self reflexive empathy as a mode of engagement" (p. 6) with art. This is my goal in the final unit: to move students to a place of empathic vision, of critical and self-reflexive empathy. After we read articles that analyze the overall goals, the discursive tactics, and material strategies of various activists—Do they embrace the abject, the idea that fatness is "gross," for instance, or do they articulate a position of respectability? Is the group led by a "normal," to draw from Goffman again, or by fat people themselves?—students are required to research, write, and present on the goals, strategies, and tactics of a fat activist individual or group that they have researched. That is, students move to a place where they must think through the work of fat activists in order to be successful, which means that they must consider the ideas of fat activists rather than engaging in mockery, derision, or hostility.

By far the most powerful part of the class that encourages empathic interpretation is the short residency by a fat activist that I have been able to organize, drawing on resources of my own departments as well as co-sponsorships with other departments and organizations on campus. During the past five years I have organized visits by Marilyn Wann, Paul Campos, S. Bear Bergman, Hanne Blank, Jeanette dePatie, Ragen Chastain, and, most recently, Susan Stinson, the poet and novelist whose works include *Belly Songs* (1993), *Fat Girl Dances With Rocks* (1994), *Martha Moody* (1995), *Venus of Chalk* (2004), and *Spider in a Tree* (2013).

Stinson's visit provides a very illuminating window through which to see this process of empathic interpretation. During her visit to Dickinson, she took part in three events: a reading of *Belly Songs* in my Fat Studies class; a reading and discussion at the Women's and Gender Resource Center of selections from *Belly Songs*, *Venus of Chalk*, and *Spider in a Tree*; and, finally, a reading at our local independent bookstore from her newest novel, *Spider in a Tree*. Besides being a beautiful writer, Stinson is a very memorable reader of her own work. As she describes herself, she is "visually interesting," a fat white woman in her 50s, with long gray hair and pointed glasses. On the day she visited Dickinson she wore a tight-fitting patterned dress over black leggings. While she read, she gestured sensuously, moving her hands in the air and down her body; she swayed to the rhythm of the words. She was mesmerizing.

All my Fat Studies students saw her in our class in the morning; many also attended the other events. I required students in my intermediate-level American Studies Workshop in Cultural Analysis course to attend at least one of the events. In that class, as preparation, we read an excerpt from *Spider in a Tree*, a novel that focuses on the life and work of the eighteenth-century American theologian Jonathan Edwards. We discussed the ways that Stinson represented his slaves and challenged deeply rooted stereotypes of black people, but we did not discuss her fat-oriented poetry or novels.

The day after Stinson's visit I asked students in both classes to write for 5 minutes to this prompt: "What was your reaction to Stinson? What was your experience like, listening to her read?" I explained that they should be completely honest, that they didn't need to put their names on their sheet, and that I wouldn't be grading it. After they finished writing, I explained that I would like to use their writings for a paper I was planning to present and then publish. If they were willing to share what they wrote they should pass their papers forward; if not, they didn't need to pass it on. (I counted the responses, and only one student in each class didn't pass in the sheets.)

The results were fascinating. Students in the Fat Studies class described being "taken aback," "shocked," "surprised," "challenged," and "overwhelmed" when Stinson first started reading. Her "extraordinary movements … caught me off guard," one student wrote. Students were acutely aware of their own and others' reactions and could describe them with precision. As one wrote, "I saw a few people hiding back smiles and chuckles and I can't help but think that it was because they felt uncomfortable."

They thought about their own limits to their understanding, how different it was to understand something abstractly versus in person, and how their feelings towards their own bodies influenced how they experienced Stinson. As one student wrote:

> I have been sympathizing with a movement against fat phobia, but this is different than actually empathizing with a person. I have found it much easier to connect with an issue or a movement than with another human being. It made me realize that overcoming stigma requires changing not just how we see others, but how we see ourselves. That sympathizing with a social movement, and not human beings can perpetuate the "othering" of those stigmatized.

Students wrote about understanding Stinson's poetry in a much deeper way listening to her read it. One poem, for instance, "Pretty Fat," begins with the stanza

> so and so fat so fat fat so fat
> so so so so fat so fat so so fat
> fat fat so fat so fat so so so fat
> so fat fat fat fat fat. (1993, p. 35)

In personal correspondence with me, Stinson explains that she wrote this poem precisely to elicit this reaction:

The poem 'Pretty Fat' has been, for me, for years, for decades, a key part of my own strategy to make the conversation possible. The word fat, there in the room with us, so many times. The repetition and what all it can release. The lingering on the body, and the movement through the poem to a place of opening, of graciousness in flab—unheard of thing. (personal communication, August 29, 2014)

Students explained that it was hearing the poem directly from Stinson, her presence, her voice, her recitation, that allowed them to reach a deeper level of understanding. As one student wrote, "I didn't understand the 'fat so' poem until she read it and it was an obvious reclamation of offensive terms used against her." Listening, deeply listening, then, had allowed this student to understand, to comprehend in a way that hadn't been possible earlier. Another student described it this way:

Her first poem ["Pretty Fat"] made me want to cry. I felt like I could hear the hurt behind those words she grew up listening to and I sat there envisioning a young Stinson being labeled those intentionally hurtful words. The way she spoke them in such an accusatory and passionate manner also made me feel like she was saying these words to us. This kind of performance forced me to … think about the ways in which I ridicule my own body.

Another student was quite self-reflexive about her own conflicted response. In particular, she speaks about her own budding awareness of the unfairness of thin privilege:

I sat in the front row center when she came to visit. I was wearing a dress with black tights right in front of this fat woman also wearing a dress with tights. Immediately I felt guilty. Here I was in my nice dress and my thin body in front of this fat woman who would never look the way I looked in her dress. I felt guilt for even having that thought. For the first time, I felt like a complete outsider for my weight. Normally when people are bigger than me it makes me feel more confident in my own weight, but this time I felt privileged in a different way—in a guilty way. It was hard for me to cope with my reaction, because Susan Stinson was so open and comfortable in her body, so I should have respected her, but I was very conflicted and self-conscious of my own visible reaction to her performance.

Students wrote about identifying with Stinson, no matter their body size. In particular, her poem "The Line" resonated with many students. This piece portrays a young fat teenager waiting in line at a church youth group game. She sneaks out the back before she can be humiliated. As one student articulated:

As someone who has had issues with body image, it was comforting to see her act so confidently and speak with almost an authority on body image and self-confidence through her work. Her poem on the church bag-drag game spoke to me, as I was one who would make every attempt to get out of any activities that I thought would put a spotlight on my weight and lack of athleticism.

Even those who were thin felt a connection: "Despite our different experiences with our body shapes I had a large sense of empathy towards her. With my health issues and lack of athleticism I have had to 'sneak out the back' plenty of times." Other students discussed how discouraged they felt at their reactions:

> I am still uncomfortable with the word fat. I still feel like this is an offensive term. While I know Stinson identifies herself as fat I did not feel like I could address her in that way. In this class we've talked about how fat studies aims to reclaim the word fat, and I do not think I have been able to do this yet.

Another wrote, "I felt myself take a step backward and feel more uncomfortable in her presence during her performance which was discouraging. ... I know I have to work on my mindset for the future."

In contrast to these deeply reflective remarks about their own reactions, about how the entire class interacted with her, about the building of and limits to their own empathy from the Fat Studies students, one thing stood out among the responses from the students in the American Studies Critical Analysis class: *no one* mentioned she was fat, that she was "visually interesting," or that they had powerful responses to her presence. Their responses were short, terse even, polite. They discussed how "passionate" she was, how impressive and admirable it was that she had written so much. Only a few gave hints of something else: "She did not necessarily have a professional tone" one student wrote. Another wrote, "At times I felt uncomfortable during her presentation." Neither of these students, however, elaborated on what sparked their impressions or analyzed their own reactions.

To me, this is a powerful difference. The Fat Studies class, learning about fat denigration, fat stigma, and fat discrimination in the "abstract" were primed to identify and reflect on powerful "affective" responses to fatness in action. Perhaps part of their reaction was based on what Stinson (personal communication, August 29, 2014) described in an email to me as "one of the gifts of fiction." Reading fiction, she wrote, "can cultivate empathy, the willingness to enter inner lives that are not one's own." In addition, they had also been primed to engage in deep listening, with focused attention, rather than what Hart (2004) calls "passive listening," involving "casual attention" (p. 36). Their comments were honest, substantive, passionate—one could see the building of understanding, the formation of empathic vision. The other students were polite, and "knew" not to mention her body size or her style as it might be considered "irrelevant" or "insulting."

To return to Patton's (2014) *Chronicle* article discussed at the beginning of the chapter, it is no wonder that there have been very few "productive conversations" about body size in the academy. It is a taboo, embarrassing subject. It took a class primed to think about body size to talk about it, to *ponder its cultural meanings,* to even be able to mention that Susan Stinson was fat. It didn't mean that her body size didn't influence the second group's responses; it just meant that their reactions were so powerful and "normalized" that they knew not to mention it or to code it as "unprofessional." For us to have "productive conversations" in our institutions, we will need to work to bring out affective responses, not just bury them, to challenge the stigma threat, not just ignore it. Encouraging a contemplative state of mind, I would argue, does just that.

Acknowledgments

Many thanks to my students for sharing their responses, and, especially, to Susan Stinson for her extraordinary generosity in allowing this open, frank, and difficult discussion to take place. Thanks also to my intern Johanna Fleming for help with the final formatting.

References

Bennett, J. (2005). *Empathic vision: Affect, trauma, and contemporary art.* Stanford, CA: Stanford University Press.

Bergman, S. B. (2009). Part-time fatso. In E. Rothblum & S. Solovay (Eds.), *The fat studies reader* (pp. 139–142). New York, NY: New York University Press.

Crowe, R., & Meagher, M. (2012). Feelingful encounters: Feminist engagements with artist Rosalie Favell. Unpublished manuscript.

Ernsberger, P. (2009). Does social class explain the connection between weight and health? In E. Rothblum & S. Solovay (Eds.), *The fat studies reader* (pp. 25–36). New York, NY: New York University Press.

Escalera, E. A. (2009). Stigma threat and the fat professor: Reducing student prejudice in the classroom. In E. Rothblum & S. Solovay (Eds.), *The fat studies reader* (pp. 205–212). New York, NY: New York University Press.

Farrell, A. E. (2011). *Fat shame: Stigma and the fat body in American culture.* New York, NY: New York University Press.

Goffman, E. (1963). *Stigma: Notes on the management of a spoiled identity.* New York, NY: Simon & Schuster.

Hart, T. (2004). Opening the contemplative mind in the classroom. *Journal of Transformative Education, 2*(1), 28–46.

Kulick, D., & Meneley, A. (2005). *Fat: The anthropology of an obsession.* New York, NY: Penguin.

McIntosh, P. (1989). White privilege: Unpacking the invisible knapsack. *Race, Class, and Gender in the United States: An Integrated Study, 4,* 165–169.

Moore, J. (2005). *Fat girl: A true story.* New York, NY: Hudson Street Press.

Patton, S. (2014, April 3). I'm the biggest man on campus. *Chronicle of Higher Education.* Retrieved from https://chroniclevitae.com/news/426-i-m-the-biggest-man-on-campus#sthash.BdNUNjmr.bTFFS8SC.dpuf

Rothblum, E., & Solovay, S. (2009). *The fat studies reader.* New York, NY: New York University Press.

Sapphire. (1996). *Push.* Toronto, ON, Canada: Random House.

Stinson, S. (1993). *Belly songs: In celebration of fat women.* Northampton, MA: Orogeny Press.

Stinson, S. (1994). *Fat girl dances with rocks.* San Francisco, CA: Spinster Ink Books.

Stinson, S. (1995). *Martha Moody.* San Francisco, CA: Spinster Ink Books.

Stinson, S. (2004). *Venus of chalk.* Ann Arbor, MI: Firebrand Books.

Stinson, S. (2013). *Spider in a tree.* Easthampton, MA: Small Beer Press.

Vade, D., & Solovay, S. (2009). No apology: Shared struggles in fat and transgender law. In E. Rothblum & S. Solovay (Eds.), *The fat studies reader* (pp. 205–212). New York, NY: New York University Press.

Watkins, P. L., Farrell, A. E., & Hugmeyer, A. D. (2012). Teaching fat studies: From conception to reception. *Fat Studies, 1,* 180–194.

SEVEN

Weapons of Mass Distraction in Teaching Fat Studies: "But Aren't They Unhealthy? And Why Can't They Just Lose Weight?"

Esther D. Rothblum

As co-editor of *The Fat Studies Reader* and editor of *Fat Studies: An Interdisciplinary Journal of Body Weight and Society*, I include fat studies as a topic in all my university courses in women's studies, psychology, and LGBT studies. In addition, my colleagues often invite me to speak about fat studies in their classes. The good news is that a few universities now offer specific fat studies or Health At Every Size courses (see Watkins, Farrell, & Hugmeyer, 2012). In my own lectures, I focus on control of women's appearance in general; the history of fat; media focus on weight; the "war on obesity"; weight and capitalism; the intersection of weight with gender, race, and sexual orientation; weight stigma in employment; weight anti-discrimination laws; and the creation of fat studies. Yet I have found that it is impossible to talk about fat oppression without being asked about the health risks of fat and why fat people can't just lose weight. These two questions are so often the focus of students that I have termed them "weapons of mass distraction." This chapter focuses on how to deal with these issues in a manner that doesn't distract from the substantive content of fat pedagogy.

Placing Weight Obsession Into Historical and Cultural Focus

In my teaching, I begin by examining appearance norms across time and culture, and emphasize that women in particular have always been told how to look. Susan Brownmiller (1984) offers an excellent review of the ways in which women's appearance is controlled and manipulated in her book *Femininity*; I list some of her points on slides in my teaching as follows:

- Women are expected to look and dress in ways that immobilize them;
- These constricting norms are thought to be the invention of women themselves;
- Without conformity to these norms, women are considered ugly or immoral by men;
- Without conformity to these norms, women cannot marry or function in society;
- These norms exaggerate the smallness of a feature that is already smaller in women than in men;
- These norms are considered trivial when in fact non-conformity to this fashion has vital consequences for women;
- The constricted body part or article of clothing is considered highly erotic by men;
- The medical establishment endorses the practice as health promoting while at the same time treating large numbers of women for medical complications resulting from this practice.

To illustrate these factors, I use the examples of women wearing tight corsets made of whalebone in Western cultures and the practice of binding girls' feet in China; both practices symbolized women's beauty and wealth in recent centuries. Even though women's waists are already smaller than those of men, and so are women's feet, these practices further exaggerate the smallness of women's features. I point out that women with bound feet couldn't walk or run, and that corseted women would faint when moving quickly because the pressure of the corset impeded their lung capacity. Yet women who didn't engage in these practices couldn't marry, and physicians at the time viewed corsets as a healthy method for strengthening women's spines.

In my experience, describing outdated appearance norms provides students some distance from these topics and thus allows students to understand the role of cultural and social control. Students often express shock when I describe some of the details of these practices. I then ask how the current obsession with weight fits into Brownmiller's criteria, and students are able to describe some of the parallels. They point out that women generally weigh less than men, yet women experience greater pressure to be thin than men. They state that thinness is a major criterion for women's beauty and marriageability. Sometimes students add that weight loss programs make women feel weak and tired—a form of immobilization. They may also mention that the medical profession focuses on "ideal" weights yet treat numbers of young women for eating disorders or fatalities from extreme weight loss programs.

Next I define the term *fat* and delve into the history of fat, including presenting slides of "Venus figures" from as far back as 40,000 years ago. I discuss Laura Fraser's (2009) chapter "The Inner Corset: A Brief History of Fat in the United States" from *The Fat Studies Reader*, in which she states,

> Once upon a time, a man with a thick gold watch swaying from a big, round paunch was the very picture of American prosperity and vigor. A hundred years ago, a beautiful woman had plump cheeks and arms, and she wore a corset and even a bustle to emphasize her full, substantial hips. Women were *sexy* if they were heavy. In those days, Americans knew that a layer of fat was a sign that you could afford to eat well and that you stood a better chance of fighting off infectious diseases than most people. If you were a woman, having that extra adipose blanket also meant you were probably fertile, and warm to cuddle up next to on chilly nights. (p. 11; emphasis in original)

Fraser focuses on how the image of "fat as good" prior to the 1880s in the United States changed to "fat as bad" by the 1920s. I ask students what could account for this change, and focus on three of Fraser's points: food production increased so that fatness was no longer a sign of wealth, weight became associated with morality, and there was a wave of immigrants into the United States during that period so that people of northern European descent "wanted to distinguish themselves, physically and racially, from stockier immigrants" (2009, p. 12).

As part of the history of fat, I end this section by describing the formation of the National Association to Advance Fat Acceptance (NAAFA), the Fat Underground, and the *Fat Liberation Manifesto* (Freespirit & Aldebaran, 1973). I describe that Surgeon General C. Everett Koop declared "war on obesity" in 1995 as part of the *Shape Up America Campaign* with over $1 million in funding from Weight Watchers, Jenny Craig, and Slimfast (Lyons, 2009). In this way, I also draw an association between weight and profit in capitalist societies.

Linking Weight to Income

It is imperative for an understanding of weight and health to discuss economic factors. I tell students that research in "developed" nations finds that poor people are fat and rich people are thin, and that this association is particularly pronounced for women. I ask students why they think that weight is inversely correlated with income. Nearly always (well, always, really), students believe that poor people are fat because of their inability to afford nutritious food or memberships in fitness clubs. They point out that poorer people have lower levels of education and therefore may not know which foods are high in carbohydrates, calories, or sugar. And poor people might work several jobs, they add, and so have no time to exercise. In other words, they assume that poverty causes fatness. First you are poor, and due to poverty (poor nutrition, less exercise), one becomes fat.

In fact, my research on employment discrimination and that of others has shown that there is stronger evidence for the opposite direction of causality—fatness leads to poverty due to discrimination and downward social mobility. A large body of research has shown that fat people, especially girls and women, are negatively evaluated by children, adolescents, and adults, as well as by physicians, medical students, and nutritionists, and even landlords discriminate against heavier renters (see Wann, 2009). Heavier applicants are less likely to be accepted into elite universities (Canning & Mayer, 1966), and less likely to receive financial support for college from their parents (Crandall, 1991, 1995). In the work setting, fat people are less likely to be hired, perceived as having undesirable traits, more harshly disciplined on the job, given inferior assignments, paid less, viewed as liabilities for employee health benefits, and fired for not losing weight (see Fikkan & Rothblum, 2005). Additionally, fat women are more adversely impacted by employment discrimination than fat men, including in hiring, promotion, performance evaluation, and salary (see Fikkan & Rothblum, 2012). In sum, as Paul Ernsberger (2009) has written: "While there is evidence that poverty is fattening, a stronger case can be made for the converse: fatness is impoverishing" (p. 26).

Furthermore, in the case of heterosexual women, thinner women tend to marry wealthier men (see Fikkan & Rothblum, 2012). In contrast, men are considered "marriageable" based on economic success rather than appearance. I tell students that if I had two sisters, one thinner and the other fatter than I am, my thinner sister would be more likely to get accepted to an elite university, get her tuition paid by our parents, marry a more successful man, and have greater success in her career.

It is also important to mention the intersection of race, ethnicity, and income in the United States. Given the strong relationship between weight and income, Paul Campos (2004) has argued that fat prejudice is a subtle way to discriminate against poor people (and thus also people of color) without being viewed as overtly racist and classist. Media depictions of fat children and adults often use words that are "code" for race or ethnicity. Natalie Boero (2009, p. 116) describes how media chastise mothers who give their children "pan dulce" (Mexican sweet bread) or "collard greens smothered in fatback" (part of traditional African American southern cooking).

Finally, it is vital to mention that a multibillion-dollar weight loss industry has a lot to lose (no pun intended!) if people become satisfied with their weight. The diet food, diet soda, diet book, diet cookbook, cosmetic surgery, bariatric surgery, diet spa and retreat, and fitness club mega-industries are quick to voice their objections in the media whenever a study shows that weight is unrelated to health or that diets don't work. A major contradiction common in the media, possibly driven by media's ties to industry, is to report on a research study that indicates diets don't work or "obesity" is genetic and then to imply (usually in the last paragraph) that all that is needed is a stricter diet, better self-control, or other variables that blame the individual for the weight. In other words, the body of the article is indicating that weight is not under personal control, whereas the ending advocates for personal weight loss. For example, the *Washington Post* (Squires, 1994) reported on the "obesity gene," confirming that "obesity" is genetic. Yet a textbox in this cover story is entitled "setting a goal for weight loss gets harder with age" and focuses on the weight loss progress of one man who wanted to lose weight in time for his fiftieth birthday.

Exposing Methodological Flaws in the "But Aren't They Unhealthy" Myth

I begin this section by pointing out that there are plenty of media stories about "the obesity epidemic" but also plenty about our increasing life expectancy, yet these two topics are never presented together. For example, an article entitled "Epidemic of Obesity" in the *San Francisco Chronicle* stated, "Some 40 to 50 percent of food eaten by kids is consumed at school, and school cafeterias often offer prepackaged, unhealthy food" (2012, p. E10). Yet 6 months earlier, an article in the same newspaper entitled "Americans Are Living Longer, Need More Services" had a very different slant: "The number of Americans at least 90 years old has tripled in recent decades. … People are living longer for a variety of reasons—with better and more available medical care and improved nutrition topping the list" (2011, p. A9). It is interesting that the same newspaper describes nutrition as poor in the first example and good in the second one.

Research on Weight and Health Does Not Control for Income
Given the strong association between weight and income, it is perplexing how rarely studies control for income. Research comparing fat and thin people is simultaneously comparing poor and rich people. Especially in the United States, where there is no national health plan,

poor people are less likely to have adequate health insurance and access to quality health care. Consequently, they may wait longer to see a health care provider and may put off preventive health care because of its high cost.

Dieting Is Associated With Health Problems, and Heavier People Are More Likely to Diet

Fat people in the United States have dieted more than thin people, and dieting (even when it's a so-called healthy diet, whatever that might be) is associated with health risks. Research on laboratory animals demonstrates that putting animals on a diet (i.e., limiting available food until they have lost a certain amount of weight and then letting them eat freely until they have regained the weight) is associated with a host of health problems, including high blood pressure, craving fat, high cholesterol, heart disease, and death (see Rothblum, 1990). Furthermore, with each subsequent "diet," it takes animals longer to lose the weight and a shorter time to regain it. The same is true of people.

Fat People Are Reluctant to Seek Medical Treatment Because of How They Are Treated in Health Care Settings

An additional factor that increases health risks is that fat people report negative experiences in medical settings and thus are more likely to avoid or delay medical care. Research has shown that medical students and physicians hold negative attitudes towards fat people (see Fikkan & Rothblum, 2012). Fat people report disrespectful treatment, embarrassment at being weighed, negative attitudes of providers, unsolicited advice to lose weight, and medical equipment that does not fit their size as reasons for avoiding visits to the doctor.

Examining Myths About Weight and Mortality

A discussion of weight and health is not complete without some focus on mortality since fat people are often told that they will die. I remind students that, unfortunately, all of us will die—the mortality rate is one per person. I show a cartoon from *The Onion* (1997) that states: "World Death Rate Holding Steady at 100%." Ernsberger (2009) has reviewed studies on weight and mortality. He reports that research that finds fat people at *lower* risk for mortality than thin people includes studies of German construction workers, San Francisco longshoremen, residents of rural Scotland, residents of Fiji, and elderly populations. Studies that find no connection between weight and mortality include research on Black people in Charleston, South Carolina, Black women insured by Kaiser Permanente; residents of rural Italy; residents of American Samoa; and Maoris in New Zealand. Finally, studies that do find fat people at high or moderate risk for mortality are those of life insurance policyholders; Harvard alumni; residents of Framingham, Massachusetts; American Cancer Society volunteers; residents of Finland; and White women in Charleston, South Carolina. Ernsberger points out that it is this last group of studies—focusing on privileged populations—that are most often cited in textbooks and in the media.

Exposing Methodological Flaws in the "But Why Can't They Just Lose Weight" Myth

For college students who are young and who have generally not experienced serious health problems, critiques of the connections made between weight and health may be less threatening than critiques about dieting. College students are typically dieting for reasons of attractiveness, not to improve health. In every classroom there will be many students who are currently dieting, and informing them that diets don't work in the long run is discouraging. In my experience, they will push back with stories of how well their own "healthy" diets are working; for that reason, in general, I don't leave much room for student discussion when I review this topic.

Weight Loss Programs Have High Attrition

It is logical to assume that the effectiveness of dieting is assessed by weighing all participants before and after a weight loss program. But in fact most weight loss studies have considerable attrition, as participants drop out of treatment, particularly if they are in the waiting list control group, don't like the treatment condition to which they are randomly assigned, or are not losing weight (see Rothblum, 1999). This means that the post-treatment and follow-up data are based on those participants who stuck with it, who were willing to attend the treatment sessions regularly and engage in the activities associated with the treatment, and who were able to lose weight.

How Is "Success" Measured?

In many areas of medical and health intervention, success is defined as change from "clinical" to "normal" levels. Take the case of smoking cessation programs. No matter how many packs of cigarettes participants are using on a daily level, the success rate of the program is defined as the percentage of smokers who quit, who don't smoke at all. Similarly, depression treatment programs admit people who have scores at the clinical level on depression scales and then measure success by the percentage who score below that level after treatment.

If weight loss programs used these criteria, none of the results could be published. People don't lose enough weight to move from Body Mass Index (BMI) scores at the "overweight" and "obese" levels into "normal weight" BMIs (for a critique of the BMI in general, see Ernsberger, 2012). Instead, "success" is defined in number of pounds lost. Imagine if smoking cessation programs counted the number of cigarettes smoked pre- and post-treatment.

People Do Not Keep Off the Weight They Lose

Commercial weight loss programs typically do not publish long-term, follow-up data, but among research studies, the long-term (5 years or more) failure rate of diets is 90 to 95 percent (Gaesser, 2009). In the early 1990s, my graduate student Jeanine Cogan examined the results of 50 published weight loss programs (Cogan & Rothblum, 1993). The typical participant across all of these studies was a White, middle-class woman who was 48 percent over "average" weight before treatment, who lost 12.8 pounds during a 13-week treatment program, and then regained 4.3 pounds over the next 6.5 months. To put this into context, I tell students that if the participant's "ideal" weight should be 120 pounds according to BMI charts, then at nearly 50 percent over that average she would weigh about 180 pounds. That meant that her weight would decrease to about 167 pounds after treatment, and then rise back to 171 pounds 6 months later. I ask students whether a change from 180 to 171 pounds would make a difference in this woman's health or even affect her clothing size. Certainly she would be nowhere near the "normal weight" category according to the BMI. There has been little research about how people feel about their repeated failures in losing weight. As early as 1958, Albert Stunkard stated, "Most obese persons will not stay in treatment of obesity. Of those who stay in treatment most will not lose weight and of those who do lose weight, most will regain it" (p. 79). More than 60 years later this statement is still true.

The Health at Every Size Movement and Strategies for Overcoming Student Resistance

A logical ending to the discussion of the myths about health and dieting is introducing students to the Health At Every Size (HAES) movement, a public health initiative that focuses on health for all people, regardless of body weight (see Bacon, 2008; Burgard, 2009). HAES emphasizes improving nutrition and enjoying food, and also the joy of movement instead of adherence to a structured exercise program. HAES clinicians strive to end bias against fat people, and underscore the fact that we cannot tell people's health or fitness level just by looking at them. Health is defined as physical, emotional, and spiritual well-being, and HAES clinicians focus on everyone appreciating their body and its appearance.

Deb Burgard (2009) describes how regimens that are prescribed for fat people would be defined as eating disorders if thin people engaged in them. She also states:

> If people have to do things in their day-to-day life in order to achieve a particular weight that a study says would be healthier, and the things they have to do (like stomach surgery, starving, or exercising 4 hours a day) are not compatible with loving self-care, then by definition, that is not a "healthy" weight for that individual. It would be like starving a St. Bernard because a study of dogs shows that greyhounds live longer. We are genetically like different breeds of dogs, but we can't tell what breed we are by looking. (p. 44)

HAES practitioners de-emphasize weight and dieting, and argue that if diets don't work in the long run, we are doing people a disservice by promoting such failure experiences. It is not easy to take on the multibillion-dollar weight loss industry in one lecture, or even one semester. Over the years I have used a few strategies for overcoming student resistance. First, I begin by stating that I have two areas of research, one mainstream and the other radical. I tell students that my "mainstream" research is on lesbian studies! I was hired by my current university for a position in lesbian studies; not that long ago professors would have been fired for coming out as sexual minorities. I explain that my "radical" research area is fat studies. This statement not only implies that what is considered radical today may become mainstream in the future, but also introduces the term "fat" early on.

Conclusion

As a fat woman myself, I realize that students would be more convinced by a thin professor. So I explain that in any area of oppression, the earliest scholars were usually white, middle- or upper-middle-class men, simply because members of oppressed groups (women, people of color, working-class people) experienced barriers to entering the academy. Thus, there are some prominent thin scholars who have conducted research in fat studies, yet it is a mark of success when members of an oppressed group begin to write and teach about themselves. I also remind students that there is great room for fat allies to do good work to help address fat oppression. For example, thin people are sometimes more likely to hear fat-oppressive comments directed at fat people behind their backs and can, and need to, become fat-affirmative activists.

In sum, discussions of weight, health, and dieting cannot be ignored in fat pedagogy as long as our society is obsessed with these factors. As a social scientist and researcher on weight stigma, I have had to become well-versed in medical studies on the association among weight, health, and dieting. I thus encourage all educators interested in pursuing fat pedagogy to check out the Yahoo! Groups site ShowMeTheData.com wherein researchers analyze the results and potential confounds of current health and medical studies. With such information at hand, educators engaged in fat pedagogy can feel more confident in addressing typical forms of resistance and provide an environment that can foster a paradigm shift in attitudes about weight and stigma.

References

Americans are living longer, need more services. (2011, November 18). *San Francisco Chronicle*, p. A9.

Bacon, L. (2008). *Health at Every Size: The surprising truth about your weight.* Dallas, TX: Benbella.

Brownmiller, S. (1984). *Femininity.* New York, NY: Fawcett Columbine.

Boero, N. (2009). Fat kids, working moms, and the "epidemic of obesity": Race, class, and mother blame. In E. D. Rothblum & S. Solovay (Eds.) *The fat studies reader* (pp. 113–119). New York, NY: New York University Press.

Burgard, D. (2009). What is "Health At Every Size"? In E. D. Rothblum & S. Solovay (Eds.) *The fat studies reader* (pp. 42–53). New York, NY: New York University Press.

Campos, P. (2004). *The obesity myth: Why America's obsession with weight is hazardous to your health.* New York, NY: Gotham.

Canning, H., & Mayer, J. (1966). Obesity: Its possible effect on college acceptance. *New England Journal of Medicine, 275,* 1172–1174.

Cogan, J. C., & Rothblum, E. D. (1993). Outcomes of weight-loss programs. *Genetic, Social, and General Psychology Monographs, 118,* 385–415.

Crandall, C. S. (1991). Do heavy-weight students have more difficulty paying for college? *Personality and Social Psychology Bulletin, 17,* 606–611.

Crandall, C. S. (1995). Do parents discriminate against their heavyweight daughters? *Personality and Social Psychology Bulletin, 21,* 724–735.

Epidemic of obesity. (2012, May 10). *San Francisco Chronicle*, p. E1.

Ernsberger, P. (2009). Does social class explain the connection between weight and health? In E. Rothblum & S. Solovay (Eds.), *The fat studies reader* (pp. 25–36). New York, NY: New York University Press.

Ernsberger, P. (2012). BMI, body build, body fatness, and health risks. *Fat Studies, 1,* 6–12.

Fikkan, J., & Rothblum, E. D. (2005). Weight bias in employment. In K. D. Brownell, R. M. Puhl, M. B. Schwartz, & L. Rudd (Eds.), *Weight bias: Nature, consequences, and remedies* (pp. 13–28). New York, NY: Guilford Press.

Fikkan, J., & Rothblum, E. D. (2012). Is fat a feminist issue? Exploring the gendered nature of weight bias. *Sex Roles, 66*(9), 575–592.

Fraser, L. (2009). The inner corset: A brief history of fat in the United States. In E. Rothblum & S. Solovay (Eds.), *The fat studies reader* (pp. 11–14). New York, NY: New York University Press.

Freespirit, J., & Aldebaran. (1973). *Fat liberation manifesto.* Los Angeles, CA: The Fat Underground.

Gaesser, G. (2009). Is "permanent weight loss" an oxymoron? The statistics on weight loss and the National Weight Loss Registry. In E. Rothblum & S. Solovay (Eds.), *The fat studies reader* (pp. 37–40). New York, NY: New York University Press.

Lyons, P. (2009). Prescription for harm: Diet industry influence, public health policy, and the "obesity epidemic." In E. Rothblum & S. Solovay (Eds.), *The fat studies reader* (pp. 75–87). New York, NY: New York University Press.

Rothblum, E. D. (1990). Women and weight: Fad and fiction. *Journal of Psychology, 124*, 5–24.

Rothblum, E. D. (1999). Contradictions and confounds in coverage of obesity: Psychology journals, textbooks, and media. *Journal of Social Issues, 55*, 355–369.

Squires, S. (1994, December 6). Setting a goal for weight loss gets harder with age. *The Washington Post*, p. 10.

Stunkard, A. J. (1958). The results of treatment for obesity. *New York State Journal of Medicine, 58*, 79–87.

Wann, M. (2009). Foreword: Fat studies: An invitation to revolution. In E. Rothblum & S. Solovay (Eds.), *The fat studies reader* (pp. ix–xxv). New York, NY: New York University Press.

Watkins, P. L., Farrell, A. E., & Hugmeyer, A. D. (2012). Teaching fat studies: From conception to reception. *Fat Studies, 1*, 180–194.

EIGHT

Creating Space for a Critical Examination of Weight-Centered Approaches in Health Pedagogy and Health Professions

Pamela Ward, Natalie Beausoleil, and Olga Heath

It has been argued by critical obesity scholars that as a society we are suffering from "obesity panic." As a population, we are taught that "overweight" and "obesity" are disease producing, hence weight beyond the ideal is something to be feared. This fear, according to the literature, is derived from a healthist perspective in which people are held responsible for their health outcomes and commitment to health-promoting behaviors (Crawford, 1980). In keeping with this approach, "obesity" is viewed to be the product of a lack of discipline and disregard for one's health, resulting in disdain for fat that ultimately produces intolerance and weight stigma (Guthman, 2009; Jutel, 2009; Rich & Evans, 2005). The role of pedagogy in the production and perpetuation of "obesity" discourse is gaining increasing attention within the literature. It is well-documented that health professionals who are educated within a dominant medical paradigm that defines "obesity" as an "epidemic" often demonstrate negative perceptions of "overweight" and "obesity" that translate into negative attitudes towards larger patients (Mold & Forbes, 2013).

Critical pedagogy provides us with tools to challenge broadly held assumptions regarding fat and provides students with the means to engage in a more balanced examination of the issues (Amsler, 2011; Connolly, 2014). In this chapter, we provide reflections on our approaches as educators to addressing "obesity" from a critical perspective in undergraduate nursing and medical curricula, a graduate program in community health, as well as in interprofessional education for health professionals, students in the health professions, and practicing educators. We discuss how we integrate our pedagogical approach and utilize our positions as educators to work within the very structures that produce and reinforce dominant discourses of health.

Why Do We Need Critical Pedagogy? "Obesity" as a Contestable Construct

According to Jan McArthur (2010), the underlying premise of critical pedagogy is "the belief that education and society are intrinsically interrelated and that the fundamental purpose of education is the improvement of social justice for all" (p. 493). A goal of critical pedagogy is to open up ways of examining issues that disrupt traditional modes of thought and "transform inequitable, undemocratic, and oppressive institutions and social relations" (Cameron, 2014, p. 100). While we contend that a critical approach may be effective in challenging dominant notions of health, such an approach is often not deliberately employed within health education experiences and clinical placement settings. As noted by Richie Neil Hao (2011), "schooled knowledges and disciplines still continue to influence students based on dominant ideals" (p. 271). In terms of "obesity," students within professional programs and practicing health professionals are expected to possess knowledge of health risks, potential outcomes, and strategies to prevent and treat this "condition." Drawing upon the work of Michel Foucault (1972), we consider these professionals to be educated in a "regime of truth" in which dominant discourses or "languages" of health construct the healthy body as thin and toned. These discourses are also embedded in pedagogical practices, shaping the knowledge base and views of our students and their mentors.

Medical knowledge of "obesity" is derived predominantly from positivist research that defines "obesity" as disease (Park, Falconer, Viner, & Kinra, 2012). Students are often educated within this perspective in the classroom and clinical settings with little attention given to other ways of examining the issue. Moreover, very little consideration is given to body size as a complex issue that is impacted by numerous intervening factors. Students are taught that "obesity" is a problem of individual behavior that can be resolved through an intense and "responsible" focus on healthy lifestyles that achieve a balance between caloric intake and energy expenditure (Rich & Evans, 2005; Shea & Beausoleil, 2012). Within this paradigm, those who do not achieve this balance are viewed as lazy and irresponsible (Gard & Wright, 2005; Hopkins, 2012; Jutel, 2009). This perspective results in pervasive fat stigma within the general population, including the health professional community (Puhl & Heuer, 2009). We contend that this uncomplicated pedagogical approach may restrict students' ability to grapple with the complexities of "obesity" and inhibit them from engaging in practices that disrupt the status quo.

Therefore, as educators we incorporate new ways of thinking into our teaching. While a critical obesity approach has not been dictated in the curricula from which we teach, we have integrated critical elements in ways that are strategic and opportunistic. First, we utilize Megan Boler and Michalinos Zembylas' (2003) notion of "pedagogy of discomfort" to challenge dominant beliefs about "obesity," working to elicit feelings of discomfort that might compel students, teachers, and health professionals to consider their own biases and discursive truths. Second, we utilize teaching strategies that encourage critical reflection, dialogue, and sharing of experiences and opinions. In the next section we elaborate on these strategies through reflections on our approaches.

Pamela's Perspective

I am a nurse educator at the Centre for Nursing Studies where I teach in the Bachelor of Nursing (Collaborative) Program of Memorial University of Newfoundland (MUN). While educated within the biomedical paradigm, I was introduced to feminist poststructural work in my doctoral program. I used this approach in my doctoral research that considered the embodied experiences of children in "obesity" treatment. This provided me with tools to engage critically with the subject and explore how "obesity" discourses were utilized and resisted by the children and health professionals involved. This perspective also shaped my teaching in that it shed light on how health professionals are schooled in dominant discourses of health that may negatively impact patients. It also enhanced my ability to reflect not only upon the issues at hand but also upon my own pedagogical journey. Thus, while providing me with tools to critically explore issues that impacted the population, it also facilitated a change in my teaching and an active engagement with students and the subject matter. Furthermore, it motivated me to infuse a critical "obesity" perspective into my various teaching roles.

I utilize a number of strategies to integrate a critical approach into teaching about "obesity." First, I search for occasions within the formal nursing curriculum where issues related to "obesity" are presented. For example, there are various places where issues of food, lifestyle, and the pathology of "obesity" are discussed in depth. Also, I find ways to introduce students to critical perspectives early in their program because students' preconceived ideas about "obesity" affect their attitudes towards larger patients (Waller, Lampman, & Lupfer-Johnson, 2012). Teaching within an introductory health promotion course, for example, allows me to insert this perspective into discussions of the social determinants of health, the promotion of positive body image, and the impact of the environment on health and the body with particular attention to issues such as food security. Within this course I also utilize a video exercise in which students explore how bodies are constructed as beautiful and the role advertising and large corporations play in the promotion of the thin ideal. Students are asked to reflect upon the messaging, the contradictions, the potential impact on health, and the motives behind the advertising. Finally, within this course, students are provided with an opportunity to explore "obesity" messaging in an assignment that requires them to utilize social media to provide three key health promotion messages. They must consider what they are promoting, how they are constructing health, and the implications of their messages on the population that engages with them.

While introducing a critical obesity approach in the first year of the nursing program is important, I also recognize that students are otherwise immersed throughout their program in a biomedical paradigm where fat stigma is pervasive (Mold & Forbes, 2013). I therefore attempt to interrupt the status quo by inserting a critical perspective into guest lectures in other courses and sharing with colleagues who teach about "obesity." I purposefully request to conduct presentations within faculty forums where I discuss my philosophical framework, findings from my research, and presentations on the evolving "obesity" literature. Within these sessions I provide examples of critical and mainstream literature and promote open discussion and critical debate. As a result, a number of faculty members have voiced interest in this issue and regularly seek guidance in teaching about "obesity."

While the classroom is vital in engaging students in critical discussions of health, students are also in a position to grapple with new perspectives in their clinical placements. I thus take advantage of opportunities to infuse critical perspectives in clinical placements as well. For example, I coordinate a fourth-year community assessment course in which I assign students to agencies that deal with issues related to "obesity," eating disorders, and body image. Students are challenged to consider the needs of particular aggregates in relation to the promotion of positive body image, the Health At Every Size (HAES) paradigm, and the prevention of eating disorders. Many students also engage in curriculum development exercises for schools where they must challenge the practice of promoting what Erin Cameron et al. (2014) refer to as the "schooled healthy body." This exercise is particularly challenging for the students because they must question their own preconceived ideas of health as well as those of the institutions in which they are working. In doing so, I encourage them to begin with the critical literature. I meet with students regularly to discuss the meanings they derive from the literature and encourage them to interview people who can provide further insight. The students then critically analyze the literature in relation to their own data. This process, while eliciting moments of discomfort for the students, most often results in an evolving sense of confidence. Students, when given the tools and permission to move outside of the dominant paradigm, begin to recognize their abilities to engage with other ways of knowing and to challenge some of the dominant notions of health they took for granted throughout their education. While these exercises do not completely negate the powerful messages embedded in "obesity" discourse, it is my hope that they help students recognize that these messages can be resisted and changed.

Natalie's Perspective

I teach in the Division of Community Health and Humanities in the Faculty of Medicine at MUN. Trained as a sociologist, my research has always been feminist and critical, incorporating insights from ethnography, ethnomethodology, cultural studies, postmodernism, and poststructuralism. My approach to teaching undergraduate and graduate students is also inherently critical. My sociological focus on the body precedes my joining the Faculty of Medicine and it influences my approach to teaching about health. Jan Wright (2014) asks: What is health education about? How can a critical scholar navigate teaching a medical curriculum that takes the body as focus of study without much discussion about the social production of the body itself? Wright suggests that as critical scholars in the field of the body, our teaching needs to be about health knowledge and its production.

It has been easy to teach from a critical perspective at the graduate level. There are structural reasons for this. When teaching graduate seminars we have more time, whole semesters in fact, to examine the biomedical model of health and its hegemonic discourses from a critical sociology of knowledge perspective. Graduate students know of my critical approach and overall expect me to provide such a perspective and do not manifest much resistance. More often than not they embrace this critical approach. Graduate students taking my courses are a self-selected group as they usually choose these courses, rather than being required to take them. I have been able to use critical obesity scholarship in special topic courses and reading courses. For instance, in 2008 I created the graduate course Critical Studies of the Body, Weight, and Health in Contemporary Western Society. I have taught this course to graduate students in community health and humanities as well as in gender studies, psychology, and humanities in the Faculty of Arts. The creation of such a course that is "on the books" as opposed to a reading course with a generic title contributes, I think, to the establishment of critical obesity scholarship as a legitimate field of teaching in our university.

Only one of my graduate courses is mandatory and it focuses on advanced qualitative research methods and methodologies. In this course, I review the various paradigms and approaches in interpretive qualitative research. I do not hide my preference for critical, postmodern, and poststructural approaches and I also cover arts-based research. I encourage students to engage in experimental writing and to review their usual ways of writing, as suggested by Laurel Richardson (2004). Interestingly, Richardson's paper has turned out to be a favorite for students over the years and some students went as far as saying that it was a revelation for them, crucial and life-changing. This course requires students to reflect on their own theoretical assumptions, their personal and disciplinary backgrounds, and their ways of learning and doing research. In other words, I emphasize that they work to become reflexive students and researchers. Reflexivity is, for me and many other researchers, an inherent part of doing critical research. In this course, I also invite students to question their own assumptions about the social production of health, embodiment, and healthy or unhealthy bodies. These students come from a range of disciplinary backgrounds and they are choosing qualitative or mixed methods approaches for their own graduate research projects. They may or may not have any formal critical (including feminist) background. While some students have been puzzled with my approach and expressed some resistance, the vast majority have embraced the approach. Based on my numerous years of experience, I now firmly believe that when given the tools and opportunity, students welcome the possibility to think critically about their own fields of study and their own lives.

Teaching a critical perspective to our undergraduate medical students has proved to be more challenging for several reasons. First, the undergraduate medical curriculum is organized very differently from graduate courses. Although medical students are required to take courses in community health and humanities, we have only a few hours per semester to deliver our teaching. Moreover, and most important, the undergraduate medical curriculum is based on objectives dictated by the Medical Council of Canada (MCC), which has traditionally championed a biomedical approach to health and the body. This approach is at the forefront of defining large bodies as diseased and deviant and the MCC directives and objectives do not include an alternative discourse on large bodies. Second, students enter our medical school clearly expecting to be taught in a biomedical paradigm. While there is some diversity among medical students, the majority come from a natural science background. (Students must have completed an undergraduate degree before entering medical school.) For many students entering medical school, the healthy body is the thin body and challenging this assumption is problematic. I surmise that in medicine as well as in physical health education, students have a moral investment in viewing thinness as a sign of health (Cameron, 2014). Furthermore, many medical students have never been exposed to critical thinking about the body specifically and the production of knowledge more generally.

While critical obesity scholarship and fat studies do not figure officially in the undergraduate medical curriculum at MUN, some of us nonetheless have been able to bring critical insights into our teaching. For instance, some colleagues and I have conducted "lunch and learn" sessions on "obesity" from a critical perspective. These sessions were optional, but students who attended manifested a great interest in learning about a different perspective on "obesity." In the formal curriculum, colleagues and I have been able to talk about fat people as a marginalized population because of the weight stigma and discrimination they encounter in health care, other institutions, and social relations. At times, we have also exposed students to the writings of critical public health scholars who have analyzed and denounced Canada's narrow-minded health promotion focus on lifestyles and "obesity" instead of tackling the most important determinants of health (Raphael, 2008).

Interestingly, the recent CanMEDS competency framework positions physicians not only as medical experts but also as communicators, collaborators, managers, health advocates, scholars, and professionals. Learning these roles requires that students be exposed to knowledge beyond the biomedical perspective. In fact, these roles that take them beyond their medical expertise require social, cultural, and political understanding only available from other disciplines and other paradigms (Kuper & D'Eon, 2011). I propose that this opening to knowledge outside of the biomedical perspective is a place to begin bringing critical thinking about body, health, and weight to the undergraduate medical curriculum.

Olga's Perspective

I teach in interprofessional education (IPE) where health professional students learn from, with, and about each other (Barr, Koppel, Reeves, Hammick, & Freeth, 2005). Trained as a clinical psychologist, my approach to research has been positivist. My thinking has been increasingly impacted by recognition of the value and importance of adopting a critical and qualitative lens as a complementary perspective in understanding research participant, client, and student experiences. For me, teaching students from multiple professions in the same room is an opportunity to offer an alternative perspective in a situation in which students are already out of their comfort zone and therefore perhaps more open to thinking in a divergent and critical manner.

Health professionals are generally trained in silos despite having to work together in teams in clinical settings. Until recently, health professional education did not teach about the knowledge and skills needed to function effectively as team members (Kuper & D'Eon, 2011). IPE can highlight client and professional stereotypes that negatively impact care and encourage students to examine the impact they have on their provision of care (Blair, Steiner, & Havranek, 2011). Here I will highlight the activities we have designed and inserted into the IPE curriculum that prompt students and faculty to consider paradigms other than the positivist for understanding "obesity."

The undergraduate IPE curriculum at MUN has been in place for 8 years and has been grounded in a positivist paradigm in which the assumptions in the clinical content of learning activities are not questioned. In 2011, there was an opportunity to revamp our IPE. This allowed us to focus on the stereotyping of clients and how this plays out in team dynamics and ultimately impacts client care. The new format for IPE is a series of 8 half-day themed sessions over 2 years in which students spend the majority of their time with the same small interprofessional group of students and a facilitator. This promotes the development of trust and safety, an ideal environment in which to challenge dominant discourses. The four themes are team functioning, team communication and stereotyping, team conflict, and highly functioning teams. The sessions are designed to be highly interactive, experiential, and reflective. This format provides the opportunity to insert a critical perspective on "obesity" within the second theme focused on team communication and client stereotyping. Specifically, we wanted to provoke students into acknowledging stereotypes about particular client groups in the context of clinical practice. While none of us likes to admit to holding stereotypes, the literature suggests that health professionals engage in stereotyping and that it affects client care (Blair et al., 2011; Lam, 2008; Smedley, Stith, & Nelson, 2003). We feel that it is important to use these sessions to sensitize students to the fact that even if they feel that they do not stereotype, they nonetheless could find themselves in a situation in which this could happen.

The team communication and stereotyping theme session began with a plenary session in which we introduced students to the complexities associated with communicating with other professionals given multiple barriers (e.g., power hierarchies, physical separation, schedules, conflict), the impact of stereotyping, and strategies to help avoid stereotyping and associated communication pitfalls. Students then met in their small, facilitated groups wherein they were assigned a scenario related to various stereotypes. They were asked to develop a team project in which they role-play a team discussion about their assigned stereotype, its impact on care, and a plan to address this issue. We deliberately chose to include "obesity" as one of the stereotypes because we felt that students needed to be aware of how "obesity panic" discourses impact their thinking and, more important, their care of clients with larger bodies. The scenario given to the students read as follows:

> Denise Roche has an appointment with the fertility team. She has been unable to conceive for 2 years despite reproductive counselling from her family doctor. Ms. Roche is 30 years old, 5'5", weighs 204 pounds, with a BMI of 34. The team meets to review Ms. Roche's file before her appointment. Several team members note her weight and suggest that they tell her she must lose weight before they assess her.

In the facilitated session, my students began by questioning whether this was even a stereotyping issue. They saw the scenario as representing a medical reality—this client was "obese" and therefore at greater risk of health and pregnancy complications. They suggested that requiring weight loss was in both her and her potential child's best interests. The students were clearly, and understandably, processing the case from a mainstream perspective.

In the ensuing discussion I introduced students to literature that questions mainstream assumptions about the impact of weight on health and highlights the importance of focusing on health behaviors instead of weight. This represented a new way of thinking for these students and there was some skepticism expressed. In response to the skepticism, there was also discussion (which I initiated and that was expanded upon by a couple of students) about the patriarchal and patronizing approach the team had displayed in stipulating that it was better for the patient and her potential unborn child to deny treatment until she had achieved what they felt was an appropriate weight. The comment that seemed to provoke attitude change for most was my stating that this scenario could be seen as analogous to suggesting that because African Americans are more prone to hypertension, and hypertension is a risk factor in pregnancy, that an African American woman who requests fertility treatment should first get her hypertension under control without ever assessing whether she was in fact hypertensive. Interestingly, it was in the context of a racial analogy that students began to recognize that weight, like race, should not be conflated with health.

The key factor that helped students unpack the "obesity" stereotype seemed to come from them coming to recognize that "obesity" is not a disease and that weight is not synonymous with health. This allowed them to appreciate how denying a client access to treatment based on weight would be discriminatory. These students then developed a role-play to present to their peers and to faculty members. The role-play took the form of a team discussion in which some members took the mainstream approach and others argued from a critical perspective. Their conclusion was that this client must be assessed on the basis of her health and not her weight, a powerful message for an entire medical school class and other professional students in the room.

Working Collaboratively

While working individually to develop our fat pedagogies has strengthened our teaching, we also have availed ourselves of opportunities to teach together. This demonstrates how different professionals can collaboratively engage in critical discussions of health and learn from one another. For example, in our medical undergraduate course Health and Illness, Beliefs, Cognitions and Behaviours, we teach sessions together, offering a critical perspective on "obesity" while fulfilling the course objectives related to the discussion of the role of cultural/social contexts and exploring dominant discursive representations of health and illness. We ask students to consider how people experience health and illness, to listen to patients' stories, and to be attentive to how health professionals and their clients utilize dominant discourses in understanding health. In this course, we are able to deconstruct ideas of the "healthy body" and raise issues of stigma and discrimination. We also demonstrate how ideas of the healthy body are gendered, using an existing curriculum case study about an adolescent male who wants to "bulk up," and linking this case to relevant critical literature on the production of the masculine body.

Conclusion

In this chapter, we utilized our own reflections to illustrate how we, as professionals from different backgrounds, have integrated critical approaches in our teaching. Our stories demonstrate that the work of health educators and health professionals does not have to occur in separate philosophical silos. As we have demonstrated in this chapter, health educators can change the present health professional training milieu by recognizing the need for critical fat pedagogy. We must do this by drawing on research that not only provides attention to, and room for, the exploration of embodied experiences of those in non-normative bodies but also by challenging long-held assumptions about the relationship between weight and health. We must work together and accept a broader approach that incorporates different ways of knowing sensitive to issues of stigmatization and the "do no harm" philosophy. We contend that learners at all stages need to be provided opportunities to learn how to critically analyze various perspectives, including practicing professionals who mentor students who can be reached by integrating a critical perspective into postlicensure interprofessional education.

References

Amsler, S. S. (2011). From "therapeutic" to political education: The centrality of affective sensibility in critical pedagogy. *Critical Studies in Education, 52*(1), 47–63.

Barr, H., Koppel, I., Reeves, S., Hammick, M., & Freeth, D. (2005). *Effective interprofessional education: Argument, assumption and evidence.* Oxford, England: Blackwell.

Blair I. V., Steiner, J. F., & Havranek, E. P. (2011). Unconscious (implicit) bias and health disparities: Where do we go from here? *The Permanente Journal, 15*(2), 71–78.

Boler, M., & Zembylas, M. (2003). Discomforting truths: The emotional terrain of understanding differences. In P. P. Trifonas (Ed.), *Pedagogies of difference: Rethinking education for social justice* (pp. 110–136). New York, NY: Routledge.

Cameron, E. (2014). A journey of critical scholarship in physical education teacher education. In A. Owens & T. Fletcher (Eds.), *Self-study in physical education teacher education* (pp. 99–115). New York, NY: Springer.

Cameron, E., Oakley, J., Walton, G., Russell, C., Chambers, L., & Socha, T. (2014). Moving beyond the injustices of the schooled healthy body. In I. Bogotch & C. M. Shields (Eds.), *International handbook of educational leadership and social (in)justice* (pp. 687–704). New York, NY: Springer.

Connolly, B. (2014). Critical pedagogy and higher education: "Really useful civic engagement." *The All Ireland Journal of Teaching & Learning in Higher Education, 6*(1), 1–14.

Crawford, R. (1980). Healthism and the medicalization of everyday life. *International Journal of Health Services, 10*(3), 365–388.

Foucault, M. (1972). *The archaeology of knowledge and the discourse on language.* New York, NY: Pantheon.

Gard, M., & Wright, J. (2005). *The obesity epidemic: Science, morality, and ideology.* New York, NY: Routledge.

Guthman, J. (2009). Teaching the politics of obesity: Insights into neoliberal embodiment and contemporary bio-politics. *Antipode, 41*(5), 1110–1133.

Hao, R. N. (2011). Rethinking critical pedagogy: Implications on silence and silent bodies. *Text and Performance Quarterly, 31*(3), 267–284.

Hopkins, P. (2012). Everyday politics of fat. *Antipode, 44*(4), 1227–1246.

Jutel, A. (2009). Doctor's orders: Diagnosis, medical authority and exploitation of the fat body. In J. Wright & V. Harwood (Eds.), *Biopolitics and the obesity epidemic: Governing bodies* (pp. 60–77). New York, NY: Routledge.

Kuper, A., & D'Eon, M. (2011). Rethinking the basis of medical knowledge. *Medical Education, 45*, 36–43.

Lam, R. (2008). *Made in Sinai health equity competencies: Delivering healthcare to diverse communities, community consultation summary findings. A project of the Mount Sinai Hospital Diversity and Human Rights Committee.* Toronto, ON, Canada: Mount Sinai Hospital.

McArthur, J. (2010). Achieving social justice within and through higher education: The challenge for critical pedagogy. *Teaching in Higher Education, 15*(5), 493–504.

Mold, F., & Forbes, A. (2013). Patients' and professionals' experiences and perspectives of obesity in health-care settings: A synthesis of current research. *Health Expectations, 16*(2), 119–142.

Park, M. H., Falconer, C., Viner, R. M., & Kinra, S. (2012). The impact of childhood obesity on morbidity and mortality in adulthood: A systematic review. *Obesity Reviews, 13*(11), 985–1000.

Puhl, R. M., & Heuer, C. A. (2009). The stigma of obesity: A review and update. *Obesity, 17*(5), 941–964.

Raphael, D. (2008). Grasping at straws: A recent history of health promotion in Canada. *Critical Public Health, 18*(4), 483–495.

Rich, E., & Evans, J. (2005). "Fat ethics": The obesity discourse and body politics. *Social Theory & Health, 3*(4), 341–358.

Richardson, L. (2004). Writing: A method of inquiry. In A. N. Hesse-Biber & P. Leavy (Eds.), *Approaches to qualitative research: A reader on theory and practice* (pp. 473–495). New York, NY: Oxford University Press.

Shea, J. M., & Beausoleil, N. (2012). Breaking down "healthism": Barriers to health and fitness as identified by immigrant youth in St. John's, NL, Canada. *Sport, Education and Society, 17*(1), 97–112.

Smedley, B. D., Stith, A. Y., & Nelson, A. R. (Eds.). (2003). *Unequal treatment: Confronting racial and ethnic disparities in healthcare.* Washington, DC: National Academies Press.

Waller, T., Lampman, C., & Lupfer-Johnson, G. (2012). Assessing bias against overweight individuals among nursing and psychology students: An implicit association test. *Journal of Clinical Nursing, 21*(23/24), 3504–3512.

Wright, J. (2014). Beyond body fascism: The place for health education. In K. Fitzpatrick & R. Tinning (Eds.), *Health education: Critical perspectives* (pp. 233–248). New York, NY: Routledge.

NINE

The Enemy Within: Teaching "Hard Knowledges" About "Soft Bodies" in a Kinesiology Faculty

Moss Norman and LeAnne Petherick

In her contribution to the *The Fat Studies Reader*, Susan Koppelman (2009, p. 213) asks, "Are there already stories about fat people in the [university] curriculum? Which stories? Which courses?" In answering her questions, Koppelman surveys syllabi from postsecondary social sciences and humanities courses in the United States. We argue, however, that her question could also be meaningfully posed to the interdisciplinary field of kinesiological sciences. And so, in this chapter we ask, what stories are being told about fat people in kinesiology? Although it may not be apparent at first glance, kinesiology is full of stories about fat bodies. The problem, however, is that these stories are not told using fictional prose, but rather rely upon the seemingly objective language of positivist science, a language that gives these stories the appearance of an unassailable "truth."

By now, all of us living in the Western world will be quite familiar with the story about fat people that kinesiology tells. It's a story about how the number of fat people is increasing worldwide at an alarming rate, that fat people are addicted to food and technology, and that fat people don't engage in enough physical activity. Heard that one? Of course you have, it's one that's told everywhere—in the newspapers, on television, on the Internet, in doctors' offices, and indeed, in our kinesiology courses. Let us not forget that this story is deadly serious because it ends in an all-out "war on obesity" that translates into an all-out war on fat people. So if you were thinking the stakes weren't high, you're wrong, they're deadly, because there are no wars without causalities. You may be saying to yourself, "Of course the stakes are deadly, obesity kills!" And if you are, then you may well be a student or faculty member in kinesiology. In fact, we hope you are, because this chapter is directed at you.

Following other critical fat scholars (e.g., Gard & Wright, 2005), we want to tell a different story. We don't want to retell the story about how "obese" people are killing themselves through gluttony and sloth, nor do we want to rehash the slightly more sophisticated version of this story that talks about how "obesegenic environments" are killing fat people, a story that has its own set of flaws (Kirkland, 2011). This is a war that deploys blame, shame, and fear (Rich, 2011) as its weapon of choice, while using a battle strategy that focuses attention on fat bodies and, in so doing, shifts the focus away from other complex and systemic determinants of health, such as racial, gender, and class oppressions, and the broader structural relations (i.e., deregulation of markets, retrenchment of welfare models of governance, processes of neoliberal capitalist globalization) that perpetuate such oppressions (McGibbon, 2012). Rather, individuals bear the burden of blame and are made to feel shame for the size and shape of their bodies, and it is individuals who must change their ways of eating and exercising. This is where kinesiologists enter the fray, as frontline combatants in this war, diligently modifying the exercise behaviors of all those "lazy" fat people.

In this chapter, we[1] start with an overview of how the relationship between science and technology in kinesiology has intensified in response to broader social and political contexts, particularly the "obesity epidemic." We then set out to disrupt some of the prevailing "obesity truths," which requires that we interrogate our assumptions about positivist science and its approach to human movement. Next, we discuss how approaches to movement and the body within kinesiology curriculums are both dominant and seductive but also, we argue, destructive for the fat bodies that they aim to "save" and "transform." We conclude with some solutions on how to teach and do human movement and health in different, potentially fat-positive, ways.

A Spoonful of Exercise Helps the Medicine Go Down

"It is difficult to get a man [*sic*] to understand something when his job depends on his not understanding it" (Upton Sinclair cited in Wann, 2009, p. xviii).

If, as Karl Newell (2007) suggests, physical activity is kinesiology's "raison d'être for having a distinct ... degree granting unit ... in higher education" (p. 8) then we argue that the "obesity epidemic" is the "cause" that gives kinesiology its professional integrity, if not moral authority. Indeed, the language of doom and gloom that has fueled "obesity crisis" rhetoric (Gard & Wright, 2005) has given kinesiology, with its promise of delivering more active, healthier lifestyles, an intensified focus and purpose within the contemporary medical-industrial-academic complex (Pringle & Pringle, 2012). Within the context of this complex, physical activity becomes exercise, and exercise becomes medicine, and the embodied pleasures of human movement are swapped for techno-scientific and measurable deliverables (Pronger, 2002) of, for example, exercise Frequency, Intensity, Time, and Type (i.e., the FITT principle). Nowhere is this techno-scientific approach to activity more evident than in the biomedical language that accompanies its transition into medical clinics, where it is now common to talk about "exercise as medicine" and "prescribing exercise," thus giving the distinct impression that activity can be dissociated from the complex social, cultural, and embodied relations in which it is always already embedded and instead taken like any other medically prescribed pill-type remedy. More often than not, the "disease" that exercise prescription seeks to remedy is "obesity" and the inactive lifestyles that supposedly produce it.

Rather than challenging biomedicalized, techno-scientific approaches to activity, kinesiology curricula more or less uncritically adopt the "exercise as medicine" mantra and, along with it, take up dominant obesity discourse (Evans et al., 2008) that socially constructs fatness as a health pathology that is, in part, correctable through the prescription of exercise by a professionally trained exercise specialist—that is, a kinesiologist. In this way, the discipline of kinesiology and its practitioners have a lot to gain by "not understanding" the complexity and contradictions of dominant obesity discourse (Pringle & Pringle, 2012). Nevertheless, we argue that it is absolutely crucial to our disciplinary integrity that kinesiological curricula take up a critical stance towards dominant obesity discourse, a theme that we explore in more detail below.

"Obesity" Science, Stories, or Myths?

We opened this chapter by suggesting that kinesiology is full of stories about fat people, even though we often don't think of them as such. In fact, it might seem strange to refer to the lessons about body weight and its relationship to health that are taught in kinesiology classes as "stories." After all, these aren't stories, they are scientific "truths," they are facts that emerge from rigorous scientific studies—or are they? Our challenge in this section will seem foreign to readers unfamiliar with postmodern critiques of positivist science generally, and evidence-based health knowledge more specifically (Murray, Holmes, Perron, & Rail, 2008). Nevertheless, we build a case that these postmodern perspectives are important for understanding the "obesity" stories—what Geneviève Rail (2012) more critically refers to as "obesity myths"—told in kinesiology, as well as the consequences these stories have for the people they name and supposedly know. Central to the postmodern critique is the notion that scientific fact is not a found reality, uncovered through objective and neutral experimentation, but rather is the effect of persuasive argumentation. One of the ways that scientific truth is produced is through systematically excluding those complicating stories that render the emergence of one truth an impossible ideal.

This is not to suggest, however, that modernist science is useless or ineffective. The fact that the techno-scientific approach to the body works, that it has the ability to powerfully shape human performance and health, for example, is undeniable. Nevertheless, we must recognize that the production of scientific facts, such as the various "obesity truths" that we aim to challenge in this section, are always embedded within social, cultural, and political processes that make the standard of objectivity an impossible ideal. In drawing attention to scientific truths as the outcome of conflict, we displace the notion of "one truth" in favor of the idea that there are multiple and competing truths, and that science is but one, albeit socially privileged, way of recounting the story among many different truth-stories.

Within the current context, "obesity" discourse has come to be "one of the most powerful and pervasive discourses influencing ways of thinking about" our own bodies as well as the bodies of others (Rich, Monaghan, & Aphramor, 2011, p. 2). One of the core assumptions of "obesity" science is that, when submitted to rigorous scientific measures, the body can be made to "tell its story." In other words, the body can be made to speak the truth about its health status through submitting it to a battery of relatively easily administered tests, such as the Body Mass Index (BMI), Waist-to-Hip Ratio, and skin fold caliper measurements. While appealing in their simplicity, these tests are not without their flaws. Measuring body weight and shape is a relatively easy endeavor but measuring body fat is far more complicated, expensive, time consuming, and ultimately less reliable (Gard & Wright, 2005). Given this, body weight and shape are often used as proxies for body fat, but these proxy measurements do not tell us with any certainty how much fat is on the body nor do they speak definitively about the health status of the bodies measured. Instead, they provide some understanding of the relative risk of certain health outcomes (e.g., heart disease, diabetes) as measured against broader population trends. These tests give us a *partial truth* and not the whole story, yet this partial truth is often taken up as the *sole truth.*

The BMI is a highly contested and controversial measure of "obesity" and its relationship to health (Gard & Wright, 2005). Critics of the BMI have undermined the credibility of this measure on three fronts: it does not measure what it is often assumed to measure (i.e., body fat); there is no simple relation between BMI and health; and the complex and contested relationship between body size, health, and the BMI is oversimplified into "obesity truth" claims that are, given the reliability of the BMI, largely unfounded (Evans & Colls, 2009). Despite this, the BMI remains the principal measure for "defining and diagnosing overweight and obesity and forms the basis for obesity policy projections and targets" (Evans & Colls, 2009, p. 1051). In other words, despite its flaws being well-known, the BMI stubbornly persists as the principal technique for producing evidence of what has been called a global "obesity pandemic" (Gard, 2011).

Our goal in talking about the contested terrain of "obesity truths" is not to enter into the struggle to find the one "truth." Rather, we ask why, given the contradictory and inconclusive state of "obesity science" (Bombak, 2014), kinesiology as a discipline continues to resort to the oversimplified message that fat equals unhealthy and exercise equals cure? Part of the answer lies in the legitimacy that obesity epidemic discourse bestows on kinesiology. But to stop here is too simple in that it suggests that kinesiologists are deliberately ignoring best evidence and maliciously deceiving the public about the threat that "obesity" represents. In reality, the circumstances are far more complex and involve social and cultural factors that go well beyond scientific truth. As others have argued (e.g., Gard & Wright, 2005), what makes obesity discourse so powerful and pervasive is that it taps into and intensifies already existing moral assumptions (i.e., fat people are lazy and irresponsible) and aesthetic ideals (i.e., thin is attractive and fat is unappealing) about fatness that congeals into "common sense" knowledge about fat people and fat bodies (Rich, 2011). Therefore, it is not just that we *know* fat bodies to be "unhealthy" based on rudimentary and flawed measurement techniques, but we also *feel* that they are "immoral" and "unappealing"—"disgusting" even—and these felt or visceral knowledges shape how we relate not only to "obesity" science claims but also to our own bodies and the bodies of others. Indeed, the complex entanglement of science, morality, and affective knowledges converges to foreground some "obesity" stories while silencing others.

The "Obesity as Usual" Curriculum

The stories told in the kinesiology curriculum are in fact *about* fat bodies and seldom—if ever—are there stories *from* fat people. In other words, the stories that are told about fat bodies are usually ones that devolve down into quantified measurements of body weight and shape, as opposed to the diverse gendered, sexed, raced, classed identities which make up experiences of fatness, as well as the lived embodied desires, fears, pleasures, and agonies of living as a fat person. In kinesiology, it is the biomedically objectified bodies of fat people that do all of the talking, not fat people themselves!

We want to be careful here because this is not a simplistic plea to open the storytelling floor as it were, although this is definitely an important part of the solution (Koppelman,

2009; Wann, 2009). Having people of different body sizes and shapes tell their story is more difficult than it at first sounds. This is partly because fat people are often perceived to be dishonest (Puhl & Heur, 2011). This means that when fat people try to tell their stories, thin people (including many kinesiologists) don't necessarily "hear" their stories, but rather think they are hearing stories that are designed to deliberately mislead. For instance, we can imagine a scenario in which a fat person describes exercise rooms and gyms as hostile spaces that they are afraid to enter, let alone exercise in. Despite the fact that exercise spaces have been consistently identified in the literature as hostile spaces for fat people (Norman, 2009; Rice, 2007; Sykes, 2011; Sykes & McPhail, 2008), some exercise experts might hear this story of fear as an "excuse." In this way, stories from fat people are discredited as are fat people themselves, and therefore the stories that fat people have to share are effectively silenced or erased from the kinesiology curriculum.

This mistrust and discrediting of the stories of fat people is partly a result of the fat body dominantly being understood as an excessive, undisciplined, and thus irrational body (Braziel & LeBesco, 2001), whereas the thin, taut body is constructed as controlled, mindful, and rational. The suspicion of the fat body is a generalized cultural and institutional suspicion that emerges from deeply held cultural beliefs about body size and shape and its relationship to the self. For fat people, this means that they operate from a deficit discourse, where their stories are, from the get-go, assumed to be less truthful than the stories of thin people. This construction of the fat subject as irrational and dishonest is especially problematic in an educational context, given that the "foundation for classroom interaction is reason," as Elizabeth Ellsworth argues (1989, p. 301).

While the ideal of classroom dialogue filled with diverse voices and perspectives is a good one, it is in fact a very difficult, if not impossible, ideal to achieve. Ellsworth (1989) suggests classroom dialogue is premised on the misguided assumption "that all members have equal opportunity to speak, all members respect other members' rights to speak and feel safe to speak, and all ideas are tolerated and subjected to rational critical assessment against fundamental judgements and principles" (p. 314). However, we have just unravelled how the fat body is approached with suspicion, is often silenced, and is ultimately constructed as irrational within our dominant kinesiology curricula. In other words, the very size and shape of the fat person's body marks them as irrational and thus discounts them from participating in dialogue. If fat people do speak, in order to be heard they are compelled to stick with the dominant kinesiological storyline about fatness (that it is unhealthy and inactive); if they offer alternative views about fatness, such as the story about the contradictory and inconclusive evidence that underlies "obesity science" that we discussed earlier, they risk being viewed with suspicion or accused of having a self-serving agenda.

It is important to recognize that it is not just fat people who are silenced in such discussions, but all alternative stories that do not adhere to the supposedly truthful story of "obesity science." Kinesiology students are not a homogenous group, and as a whole they will have varied and deeply personal experiences with body weight and shape, perhaps having friends, family, or experiences of their own that do not easily align with the relatively simple story of energy balance and personal control that is told in our courses. These experiences are often also discounted as anecdotal and non-scientific, therefore peripheral to the main story that is rooted in "obesity truth." Thus, the ideals of equal opportunity, respect, safety, and tolerance of multiple perspectives are more or less empty ideals when the ground rules for speaking assume the precondition of rational and reasonable argumentation. This being the case, how can alternative stories about fatness and health be introduced into kinesiological dialogues when a rational approach to the body, its weight, and its relationship to health are the preconditions for speaking in the first place? Storytelling spaces are never neutral spaces; rather, they are always embedded in what may be difficult-to-discern power relations that enable some stories (i.e., "obesity truths") and silence others (i.e., messy stories of lived, embodied experiences). Acknowledging these power relations is only part of the task, however. The other is considering how to disrupt and alter these relations so that multiple perspectives can emerge in the kinesiology curricula and classroom.

Solutions: Disrupting the "Obesity as Usual" Curriculum

In our teaching, we primarily use two tactics for prying apart "obesity truths." Our first tactic is to start not with the "problem of obesity," but rather with the body itself. In doing so, we work to undermine and disrupt the received naturalistic view of the body. The naturalistic perspective assumes that there is one biological body that, when submitted to rigorous methods, will reveal its truth or tell its story. This perspective is absolutely core to what we teach in our kinesiology curriculum, where the body is understood as a fleshy mass of bone and tissue that is represented as a machine that can be manipulated through various regimes of diet and exercise. Our tactic here does not involve dismissing the biological body altogether, but rather it highlights that it is but one way, among many ways, of knowing the body. In order to draw attention to those other, less apparent ways of knowing our bodies, we emphasize what the students already feel in their everyday embodied practices. Here, we point out that the naturalistic body is the one that our students *know* through their studies, but it is not necessarily the body that they *feel* when they engage in their daily, embodied practices of sport, exercise, and physical activity. We do various exercises to get them thinking *through* the body as opposed to thinking *about* the body. For example, we ask them to describe their own bodies in narrative form or to visualize a particularly enjoyable bout of exercise. These exercises can make some of our students who are well-trained in adopting an objective approach to the bodies of others quite uncomfortable when that gaze is turned back upon their own bodies. For us, this discomfort is an important component of our pedagogy.

Their stories are full of embodied sensations, emotions, feelings, pleasures, and pains as well as reflections about the environment, friendships, and family. The moving bodies they describe and visualize are not of the same order as the singular and knowable body outlined in their physiology, anatomy, and biomechanics labs. The body they recount is a messy, porous, and complex one that extends beyond the borders of the skin, is touched by and touches the environment in which it plays, emotionally opens out to those other bodies that it exercises alongside, that literally ingests the space around it as it gasps for air, and so on. We use these exercises to highlight to our students that the moving body is a "complex, multifaceted, multidimensional phenomenon that cannot be reduced to any one domain or discourse, be it biological, psychological, social or cultural" (Williams cited in Blackman, 2008, p. 32). We assert that it is particularly important to remind our students of the embodied, felt relations that are associated with human movement given kinesology is dominated by an objectivist, naturalistic approach to movement which makes it too easy to forget the multidimensional aspects of embodiment.

We also remind our students that many—if not most—of them chose kinesiology as a discipline because of past experiences of sensual, embodied pleasures derived from sport and physical activity, and not for purely instrumental purposes, such as measuring steps taken and calories expended. That does not mean students do not have instrumental understandings of their bodies, of course. It is important to recognize that in the contemporary moment, the physically fit body has been appropriated by the industrial-medical-academic complex, giving rise to what Brian Pronger (2002) refers to as fascistic desires to control and discipline the body into a socio-culturally privileged form; this "body fascism" has a pleasure of its own. Nonetheless, there are other non-reductive and non-instrumental desires that simultaneously course through the moving body, and these desires are central—albeit often unacknowledged—to the passions that bring kinesiologists to the profession in the first place. Drawing out the multiple pleasures and desires that simultaneously flow through the moving body allows us to ask our students: what is lost when we quantify movement in terms of steps taken, duration, distance traveled, calories expended, and hitch movement to clearly defined objectives, such as weight maintenance or loss? And what happens when these objectives, such as weight loss, are not achieved? Is this a complete failure or is there something else to be gained in movement itself?

If movement equals weight loss, the fat moving body cannot take pleasure in the here and now of its own embodied movements; rather, its pleasure is perpetually deferred to a future when weight will have been lost and health supposedly secured. Fat activists staunchly oppose this view, suggesting that the fat moving body has its own set of sensual and erotic pleasures that are too often discredited in our contemporary fat-phobic context (Colls, 2007; Rice, 2007). The question, therefore, is this: do we, as a profession, want to curtail, police, and discipline the sensual pleasures of the fat moving body, chaining them to objective measures and outcomes, or do we want to stimulate, foster, and incite the pleasures of fat movements that disrupt, challenge, and undermine dominant "obesity as usual" discourses? Moreover, we ask our students to consider what such a socially and culturally transgressive space would look like. However, we must admit that pointing to multidimensionality only goes so far, as we have found that our students are generally quite reluctant to fully relinquish the notion of the "truth" about fatness and its relationship to health.

Our second tactic builds upon the first, but this time positions "obesity science" and its truths as its primary target. Here, we deliberately introduce students to the multiple contradictions and inconsistencies that inform "obesity epidemic" rhetoric more generally and "obesity science" specifically. In so doing, we refuse to peddle simplified and reductive truths about body weight and shape and its relationship to health (Gard, 2011), instead unraveling the irreducible complexity of the science behind the causes and consequences of "obesity." This creates what Richard Pringle and Dixie Pringle (2012) refer to as "discursive confusion" (p. 153) among the students, whereupon realizing the complexity of "obesity truths" themselves, students are displaced from their position as passive recipients of knowledge, and forced to actively engage in evaluating the validity of "obesity truth" claims. Once these truths are subjected to closer interrogation, there is a greater chance that students will be able to better see and challenge some of the "elementary moralities" (Evans & Colls, 2009, p. 1060) that underlie them.

This is a more difficult task than it at first sounds because, as we mentioned earlier, "obesity truth" is a hybridized concoction of science, morality, and ideology (Gard & Wright, 2005), and many students and faculty alike have internalized these truths to the point where they are accepted without question. However, while this concoction of science and ideology is what makes these "obesity truths" so powerful and pervasive, it is also exactly what makes them vulnerable (Evans & Colls, 2009). If you will recall our argument earlier, the truth of "obesity science" is founded more on the erasure of uncertainty than it is on some universally applicable knowledge. If we can help students see the complexity that must be actively erased in order for the "one truth" to crystallize then we can pry open the "obesity canon" and allow for alternative stories to emerge. For instance, if we can get students to shift from thinking of the body as a purely biological entity to the body as the outcome of ongoing interactions between the biological *and* the social, cultural, and historical, then they have a far more complex and messy story about the body than the purely naturalistic representation allows for. Therefore, our primary objective with this tactic is to disrupt—even if only temporarily—the myth of one story about body size, shape, and exercise, thus allowing for alternative, multiple, and partial stories to emerge within the classroom.

In our approach to teaching in kinesiology, then, we ask students to constantly ask how the stories that we hold to be true or that we cherish in kinesiology function in the world. We want students to ask, how does my story about the body and movement shape how I approach the otherness of others? How does my story enable the movement practices of some, while constraining or even oppressing others? Does my story work towards allowing others who are different from myself to feel the bodily pleasures of movement or does it foreclose those pleasures? Our purpose in asking these questions is to produce a level of confusion that refuses to sediment into a known certainty—that is, into the notions that fatness is unhealthy, exercise can help fat people lose weight, and so on. This is what Ellsworth (1989) describes as "pedagogy of the unknowable" (p. 318). The discomfort of not knowing the truth of the other and recognizing that one's own perspective is always partial does not necessarily lead to paralysis, but we hope may potentially compel student-soon-to-be-professional practitioners to engage more critically and thoughtfully with dominant and pervasive "obesity truths" and the effects they have for fat people.

References

Blackman, L. (2008). Regulated and regulating bodies. In L. Blackman (Ed.), *The body: Key concepts* (pp. 15–35). New York, NY: Berg.

Bombak, A. (2014). The "obesity epidemic": Evolving science, unchanging etiology. *Sociology Compass, 8*(5), 509–524.

Braziel, J. E., & LeBesco, K. (2001). *Bodies out of bounds: Fatness and transgression.* Berkeley, CA: University of California Press.

Colls, R. (2007). Materializing bodily matter: Intra-action and the embodiment of "Fat." *Geoforum, 38*(2), 353–365.

Ellsworth, E. (1989). Why doesn't this feel empowering? Working through the repressive myths of critical pedagogy. *Harvard Educational Review, 59*(3), 297–324.

Evans, B., & Colls, R. (2009). Measuring fatness, governing bodies: The spatialities of the Body Mass Index in anti-obesity politics. *Antipode, 41*(5), 1051–1083.

Evans, J., Rich, E., Davies, B., & Allwood, R. (2008). *Education, disordered eating and obesity discourse: Fat fabrications.* New York, NY: Routledge.

Gard, M. (2011). *The end of the obesity epidemic.* New York, NY: Routledge.

Gard, M., & Wright, J. (2005). *The obesity epidemic: Science, morality and ideology.* New York, NY: Routledge.

Kirkland, A. (2011). The environmental account of obesity: A case for feminist skepticism. *Signs, 36*(2), 463–485.

Koppelman, S. (2009). Fat stories in the classroom: What and how are they teaching about us? In E. Rothblum & S. Solovay (Eds.), *The fat studies reader* (pp. 217–220). New York, NY: New York University Press.

McGibbon, E. (2012). *Oppression: A social determinant of health*. Winnipeg, MB, Canada: Fernwood.

Murray, S., Holmes, D., Perron, A., & Rail, G. (2008). Towards an ethics of authentic practice. *Journal of Evaluation in Clinical Practice, 14*(5), 682–689.

Newell, K. (2007). Kinesiology: Challenges of multiple agendas. *Quest, 59*(1), 5–24.

Norman, M. (2009). *Living in the shadow of an "obesity" epidemic. The discursive construction of boys and their bodies* (Doctoral dissertation). University of Toronto, ON, Canada.

Pringle, R., & Pringle, D. (2012). Competing obesity discourses and the critical challenges for health and physical educators. *Sport, Education and Society, 17*(2), 143–161.

Pronger, B. (2002). *Body fascism: The salvation in the technology of fitness*. Toronto, ON, Canada: University of Toronto Press.

Puhl, R. M., & Heur, C. A. (2011). Public opinion polls about laws to prohibit weight discrimination in the United States. *Obesity, 19*(1), 74–82.

Rail, G. (2012). The birth of the obesity clinic: Confessions of the flesh, biopedagogies, and physical culture. *Sociology of Sport Journal, 29*(2), 227–253.

Rice, C. (2007). Becoming "the fat girl": Acquisition of an unfit identity. *Women's Studies International Forum, 30*(2), 158–174.

Rich, E. (2011). Exploring the relationship between pedagogy and physical cultural studies: The case of new health imperatives in schools. *Sociology of Sport Journal, 28*(1), 64–68.

Rich, E., Monaghan, L., & Aphramour, L. (2011). *Debating obesity: Critical perspectives*. New York, NY: Palgrave Macmillan.

Sykes, H. (2011). *Queer bodies: Sexualities, genders and fatness in physical education*. New York, NY: Peter Lang.

Sykes, H., & McPhail, D. (2008). Unbearable lessons: Contesting fat phobia in physical education. *Sociology of Sport Journal, 25*(1), 66–96.

Wann, M. (2009). Foreword: Fat studies: An invitation to revolution. In E. Rothblum & S. Solovay (Eds.), *The fat studies reader* (pp. ix–xxvi). New York, NY: New York University Press.

Note

1 Importantly, both authors self-identify as having bodies that fall within the normatively slender range and thus benefit from the privilege associated with slenderness, particularly in a kinesiology faculty that increasingly defines itself through the "war on obesity."

TEN

"Obesity" Warriors in the Tertiary Classroom

Lisette Burrows

Large-scale quantitative studies purporting to measure and report rates of "obesity" among particular populations have proliferated in the past decade, fueling policy and practices focused on ameliorating what many regard as an "obesity crisis" (Gard, 2007; Gard & Wright, 2005). Children and young people are positioned in much of the latter work as both the cause of escalating "obesity" rates and as the solution to these. On the one hand, children's avowedly sedentary, digitally saturated lifestyles together with their propensity to eat energy-dense foods are posited as contributing to the "obesity" problem. On the other, children are regarded, by virtue of their youthful promise, as hopes for a fat-free future (Gard & Pluim, 2014; Vander Schee & Boyles, 2010).

Given this context, health and educational professionals are unsurprisingly regarding schools as superlative sites for teaching young people about the perils of "obesity" and fostering "healthy" approaches to eating and exercise (Burrows & Wright, 2007; Welch & Wright, 2011). Undergraduate physical education students, too, are increasingly linking their aspirations to teach with a desire to solve the "obesity problem." Anecdotally, their writing, thinking, and practices suggest that many envision themselves as "obesity warriors"—prospective teachers who have the knowledge, skills, and commitment to turn the tide on childhood "obesity."

In this chapter, I interrogate my own endeavors to challenge New Zealand undergraduate physical education students' normative perceptions about fat, to raise questions about the wisdom of focusing their teaching on "obesity" prevention, and to encourage an understanding that size is not *all* that matters in the holistic education of young children. While cognizant that some may label what follows as simply "anecdotal" reflections and that much has been written already about reflective practice in education, I nevertheless consider interrogation of one's practice to be a worthwhile exercise (Moon, 1999). I hope that rather than conveying "flights of an individual's reflective fantasy" (Atherton, 2010, para. 30), these musings may contribute to an emerging collaborative intellectual and professional conversation about how educators may rein in the excesses of weight-related oppression in schools and tertiary environments. I begin by declaring what I think I "know" of my students before they come to my classes and then map some of the pedagogical moves I have made during the past decade.

Student Baggage

When offered the choice to interrogate any health or physical education issue, half of my class members choose childhood "obesity" year after year. When asked to write an essay exploring what physical education can contribute to a child's education, almost every essay mentions "obesity" prevention as a key rationale for school-based physical education. When asked to reflect on what they believe about health and physical education and what and who have shaped those beliefs, most mention a desire to curb the "obesity" problem in New Zealand and elsewhere. The course thus begins with a dedicated cohort of "fat-busters," young people who are committed to the notion that (1) "obesity" is a problem for everyone everywhere; (2) "obesity" is the outcome of overeating and underexercising; and (3) they, armed with the correct knowledge, are able and willing to curb the presumed rising tide of "obesity." Much, but not all, of their undergraduate course work (e.g., exercise prescription, injury prevention, rehabilitation, physical activity and health, and exercise psychology) consolidates this disposition for them. So too does their inevitable immersion in a culture where fat is widely regarded as abhorrent (Campos, 2004; Evans, Rich, Davies, & Allwood, 2008; Murray, 2008), where health and fitness are inextricably linked to the Body Mass Index (Ross, 2005), and where levels of public concern about the "obesity problem" are unprecedented.

As if the aforementioned "evidence" was not compelling enough, added to the mix for the students I work with is an institutional resistance to different views on "obesity" (Cameron, 2014). Academics who challenge "obesity" orthodoxies have been vilified privately and publicly in New Zealand and abroad. On one occasion at my institution, two international experts who raised questions about the veracity of "obesity" science were accused of sullying the university's reputation. Their alternate views were cast as "mad," "crazy," "unscientific," and/or embarrassing. Conversely, experts bearing the imprint of epidemiological science are gifted generous institutional and media support. In 2014, two "leading sports scientists" wrote an open letter to the *New Zealand Medical Journal* complaining that ill-prepared and "slack" teachers were incapable of enacting physical activity imperatives in their classes. They hailed mandatory exercise for children in schools as a partial solution for the "obesity epidemic" (Broughton, 2014). These sorts of stories and the academic credibility attached to them further entrench our aspirational PE teachers' already sedimented perceptions that physical education and, by default, they as its teachers, have a key role to play in "obesity" prevention. As Michael Gard and Carolyn Pluim (2014) have convincingly argued, this presupposition is rather misguided.

The final piece of baggage that my students bring with them is potentially their response to my own embodiment (Throsby & Evans, 2013). Hardly the picture they envisage as symbolic of a healthy specimen, adorned in clothes and jewelery not "normally" befitting a physical educator, my colleagues tell me that my students will have already pegged me as "slightly off beam" before I open my authoritative teacherly mouth. I am not sure about this observation, but raise it here as a possibility. Having witnessed the different responses my students display to a range of embodied identities I have paraded in front of them during my teaching career, I concede that different "looks" do yield different reactions.

In sum, my students, then, are skilled at reading dispositions from bodies, familiar with the plethora of biomedical pieces that map the extent and escalation of the "obesity" problem. They have grown up in times when "obesity" concerns are "everyday" concerns and study in places that confirm what they "know" from both scholarly and everyday encounters with "obesity." They are committed "obesity" warriors, passionate about their cause, and fueled with what they perceive to be certain knowledge that will equip them to do something to solve the "problem." Granted, this picture painted is a prototype, a caricature of what my students bring, and obviously not representative of each and every student's basket of knowledge and experience. Nevertheless, there are times when boxes are useful and this may be one of them. In what follows I tease out the strategies I have harnessed in an attempt to disrupt rather than sediment these core understandings.

Philosophy Up Front

A premise of the courses I teach is that every issue in health and/or physical education has, of course, multiple perspectives. Another premise is that subjectivity is a movable feast and that any behavior, perspective, or attitude is necessarily shaped by the discourses one has access to. Understanding how discourses contour one's capacity and desire to do, be, and think in particular ways is a bedrock underpinning for all my course work. Engaging students in thinking "otherwise," unsettling sedimented perceptions, examining how "truths" are produced, developing their capacity to question orthodoxies, and fostering their willingness to always ask the "so what?" question are explicit goals of the courses. I am clear about what drives our collective work and what will be rewarded in terms of assessment outcomes.

Being up-front about what defines the courses one teaches is non-negotiable in my mind. Students have a right to know where one's coming from, not so they can mirror one's own disposition in their assignment work, but rather so they come to know that all of the knowledge they engage with at university and elsewhere is contoured by its communicator's worldview. Nothing is "neutral." Rather, everything is, as Michel Foucault (1983) would say, "dangerous" (p. 256). Fostering an intellectual curiosity, a desire to imagine their social worlds in ways that are cognizant of both the dangers and the delights within them is apposite here. If nothing else, a course that embraces any version of fat pedagogy should endeavor to elicit this, I believe.

I am not convinced the aforementioned up-front declaration, my endeavor to clearly map my aspirations for the course, and my efforts to clarify expectations of what and how students will learn make any difference at all. I continue to receive assignments that privilege one perspective over others. Without specified readings, students, in the main, seem to retreat to what they "know" already, drawing on academic papers they may have read in other courses. On occasions, they refer to the existence of an alternate view on "obesity," but simply in passing. That is, while bolstering their "obesity" argument with 10 empirical pieces based on work in the United States, they say things like "of course there are other views" before moving swiftly on to reiterate findings from the U.S. studies. My urging to think beyond the square, to always consider knowledge "in context," does not appear to translate into actually attempting this. I suspect there are at least two potential reasons for this reluctance to consider any positions other than those with which they are already familiar. First, I am not convinced students necessarily understand what their lecturers mean by "critical engagement." Simply acknowledging the existence of other views does not suffice. Second, I wonder whether a mistaken presumption that academic writing requires certainty, an expression of arguments as "facts," as how things "are," gets in the way of students communicating the uncertainty, contradictions, and messiness of obesity that wide reading would unearth. Phrases such as "the world is facing an obesity crisis" and "childhood obesity levels are escalating" permeate students' essays. Simply prefacing these statements with phrases such as, "it is suggested by ..." or "according to ..." would alleviate that certainty and permit (at least on paper) a sense of openness to the possibility that whoever made that statement may not be the only authority on the matter.

Reworking Obesity Science

As Erin Cameron (2014) and others have suggested (e.g., Gard & Wright, 2005), interrogating the veracity of "obesity" science, one of the most compelling pieces of evidence in students' cadre of "obesity" armory, is now a familiar strategy for critical fat pedagogues. Fortunately the resources for facilitating such an interrogation are expanding by the year. Paul Campos' (2004) *The Obesity Myth: Why America's Obsession With Weight Is Hazardous to Your Health*; Michael Gard and Jan Wright's (2005) *The "Obesity Epidemic": Science, Ideology and Morality*; Gard's *The End of the Obesity Epidemic*; John Evans, Emma Rich, Brian Davies, and Rachel Allwood's (2008) *Education, Disordered Eating and Obesity Discourse: Fat Fabrications*; Deborah Lupton's (2013) *Fat*; and latterly Gard and Pluim's (2014) *Schools and Public Health: Past, Present, Future* are among those texts that afford plenty of rich resources for students to begin the process of untangling the "truths" so widely promulgated about "obesity." A surfeit of journal articles, too, offers alternate perspectives on "obesity" science. Aware of our undergraduates' propensity *not* to read, I also endeavor to present my own argument about what critiques of "obesity" science might mean for the truth status of positions derived from biomedical science. Aware that many students have been forewarned of my propensity to advance strange sociological arguments in the face of the "hard" evidence that students have hitherto been presented with, I am careful to ensure that epidemiological scholars who themselves have challenged the veracity of biomedical accounts of "obesity" are part of the suite I introduce students to.

Perplexed, puzzled, and incredulous faces meet me when sharing critiques of "obesity" science. In 15 years, I have had few students actually engage with the counter-arguments and actively seek to convey these in oral or written presentations. Given the outlined endeavors, this may be a function of my incapacity to convey the possibility of alternate views in my speech and/or my demeanor. As one of the fat pedagogues in Cameron's (2014) research commented:

> I'm learning that there are certain ways of saying things, a certain language or certain argument that you can put your work into where people are more receptive. ... You want people to be receptive and so you have to kind of guide them through what you're trying to say. (p. 140)

I concur, but have yet to find a way (or ways) that elicits this receptiveness. Indeed, I suspect, as is the case with all pedagogy, that there will be different strokes for different folks. Recently, I listened to a teacher talk about a variety of dispositions one can embrace when teaching health education. He used religious metaphors to categorize these as fundamentalist, evangelical, devout, believer, non-practicing, agnostic, atheist, and others. I suspect I have ranged across the gamut of these. Perhaps this is all one can do—give different approaches and ways of saying things a go and then see what happens, who is hailed by the discourse, and who is repelled by it. Indeed, it is more than likely not a matter of either embrace or repel, but rather the chance to interrupt and shift perception along a continuum that may well encompass extremes at both ends of the "obesity" position scale.

Policy Pushing

In New Zealand where I teach, we have a health and physical education curriculum that explicitly embraces a holistic view of health and well-being and a requirement that teachers work to elicit critical thinking from their students (Gillespie & Culpan, 2000; Sinkinson, 2011). Senior school assessment tasks privilege the capacity to interrogate taken-for-granted understandings about health and physical activity and reward those who can understand any given phenomenon from multiple perspectives. Underpinning values of this curriculum include striving for innovation, inquiry, and curiosity by thinking critically, creatively, and reflectively; diversity; equity; and respect for human rights. Key competencies include "thinking." As the writers put it, "intellectual curiosity is at the heart of this competency" (Ministry of Education, 2007, p. 12). The document, its philosophy, its vision, and its implied pedagogy are usefully paraded in front of my students as a compelling rationale for thinking broadly and critically about what they think, what they do, and the potential effects of their pedagogies on the young people at the center of their practice. When all else fails, I wheel the curriculum document out, point to its dictates, and raise questions about how subscribing to narrowly defined prescriptions for health, judging fat children's habits, and teaching in ways that convey a certainty around health imperatives gel (or not) with mandated curriculum imperatives.

In essence, in this mode I am policy pushing—wielding a legal document as a weapon in my anti-fat bias armory. In terms of health, the key message I try to convey is that health education is education about health rather than for health (Robertson, 2005). This distinction is fundamental, in my view, to any attempt to inspire critical fat pedagogies. As long as undergraduates continue to regard their forthcoming role as one of ameliorating health problems, advocating disease prevention, or making young people healthy, the allure of public and educational health strategies premised on anti-fat science or morality will be challenging to shift.

Pretending

Drawing from an activity primary school teachers have used to encourage young children to rethink their understandings of health (Cosgriff, Burrows, & Petrie, 2013), I often ask students to adopt an identity (either fictional or non-fictional) and debate the "obesity" issue from that perspective. A favorite is the "Paul Campos versus Kelly Brownell" debate. Paul is a law professor from Boulder, Colorado, while Kelly is director of Yale University's Rudd Center for Food Policy and Obesity. These are two characters with distinctly different views on the "obesity" issue. I supply students with six days' worth of an actual debate, which ran in the *Los Angeles Times* in 2007, and ask them to "be" their designated person and argue a case from what they imagine and can see from scripts is their perspective.

The discomfort is palpable. Nervous giggles and comments like "this is too hard," " I can't do this," and "this doesn't feel right" pepper the pre-debate dialogue. Some enjoy the permission that playing a "character" gives them to think differently and verbalize thoughts hitherto unexpressed, something rendered more possible via the opportunities that "pretending" presents. Akin to dressing up or donning a mask, being someone other than oneself seems to facilitate an openness to experiment. This taking sides, this requirement to be someone one's not, to step in another's shoes and defend that person, means adopting, at least for a moment, an alternate perspective, and not one that can simply be written or privately pretended, but rather a public expression of an "other." This strategy is compelling and potentially productive of a window to comprehending difference in ways other strategies I have tried are not.

Hearts

Given that most of my research in the past decade has been squarely focusing on understanding the place and meaning of health in young people's lives, the notion of showcasing children's views on health, "obesity," fatness, and fitness with my undergraduates is an uncomplicated pedagogical decision. As academics, we are expected to undertake research-informed teaching, to bring the supposed expertise we gather through research activities to the classroom. This imperative is not the only thing that drives my desire to place young people's views front and center, however. Cognizant of the vast literature pointing to the power of "story" to shift hearts and minds, aware of the embodied nature of learning, and having witnessed firsthand the affect and effect hearing children's views yielded for teachers I was working with on a research project (see Petrie, Burrows, & Cosgriff, 2014), I thought that confronting students with stories from "real" people (children and adults) might prompt shifts in thinking, feeling, and believing hitherto impossible. Charlotte Cooper (2007) refers to the proliferation of news and documentary coverage featuring "headless fatties," that is, shots of fat people that show their bodies but not their heads. She writes of the need to humanize fatness, to bring the heads back into the picture.

Convinced that this kind of humanizing work would do the trick, I have tried showcasing fat news broadcasters, fat scholars, fat activists, and fat runners speaking about the discrimination they are subject to. I show students commentary from young children during which the children talk of their confusion, guilt, worry, and disgust associated with fat and the avowed contributors to this (exercise and food). I show pictures that children have drawn illustrating their equation of health with body size and fitness with non-fatness. And, perhaps most compellingly, from my point of view, I air numerous exemplars of children and young people's resistance to ubiquitous health messages, and their capacity to recognize the contradictions and uncertainty embedded in health messages that simply don't make sense given their local experiences, family circumstances, peer relations, and lived contexts. Undergraduate physical education students' responses to these airings are surprising.

First, children's so-called resistance to health messages is, more often than not, reinterpreted as evidence of either children failing to "get the message," families failing to support their children's new learning, and/or simply reflective of poor teaching. Second, material that points to the ways health knowledge gets folded into kids' bodies, sometimes prompting an unhealthy obsession with portion size and/or what they eat, prompts delight at the ways children are "getting it," that is, understanding health teaching. Third, material that points to the ways children are castigated by others for indulging in unhealthy eating practices (e.g., eating pies) and/or being fat is received by some as boosting the case for fat-busting. That is, the ill treatment that young people experience as a consequence of being fat is reframed as yet another reason they need to get thinner. Losing weight, in effect, is represented as a bullying prevention strategy. Fourth, research that depicts the links children draw between thinness and health, fatness and moral turpitude, and non-fatness and a "good" life (see Burrows & Wright, 2004) is more often received as unsurprising and not particularly problematic. That is, these tropes are familiar and therefore "normal" for many undergraduates. Finally, attempts to humanize fatness, to prompt reflection on the sense of entitlement others display in demonizing fat people via airing commentary from those who have been the target of vicious blogging and media tend to evoke one of two responses. That is, either a startled silence or responses that suggest students feel sorry for "the fatties" while simultaneously regarding them as deluded, misguided, and still fat.

In so saying, while not deliberately planned by me, there are occasions over the years where personal experiences of students or those to whom they are close have yielded palpable shifts in thinking about "obesity," about fat, and about health. In a task that asks students to reflect on what they believe about health and physical education and who/what has shaped these beliefs, one student in 2014 wrote about a "turning point" she experienced while while visiting the doctor:

> I was told that I was dangerously overweight. ... The doctor suggested that I lose 20 kilos in 3 months to be considered healthy in relation to the BMI statistics. I knew BMI is only one health indicator and is not accurate for people who fall outside of a normal height and muscle range. It also sent alarm bells off in my head about the dangers of losing that weight in such a short amount of time.

While clearly this experience could have prompted a shift in the other direction—that is, understanding oneself as "overweight" and taking action to ameliorate this—for this student, the injustice of the doctor's attitude together with her capacity to read what she heard alongside what she knew from her studies evoked a rupture, a questioning of medical expertise, and a resolve never to visit this kind of "professionalism" on others in her practice. Perhaps it is the degree of closeness to one's own circumstance that permits stories to "touch" and to provoke thinking and being otherwise. For most of my students a lived experience of feeling or being fat is not available to them. Perhaps stories recited from people whom students have no relationship with nor understanding of exacerbate rather than ameliorate the othering they engage in.

Concluding Brief

Deana Leahy (2009) refers to the increasing assortment of confronting health pedagogies applied in school health education classrooms as "disgusting pedagogies"—pedagogies that are designed to elicit fear, loathing, and disgust. In a sense, some of the tactics I described earlier could be regarded as these, except rather than seeking student disgust in relation to fat, fatty food, or sedentary living, my agenda is provoking disgust at the ways those who are labeled fat are constructed and treated by the lay public, professionals, and their communities. At one level, the possibility of this descriptor being applied to my work is abhorrent to me. Is deploying the tools of the tyrannizer in service of different ends an ethical practice? Troubling, too, is the degree of pompousness I detect in the pedagogical reflections I have conveyed thus far.

Is imagining that one's pedagogy and one's belief in a version of social justice might shift the hearts and minds of anyone a form of unbridled arrogance? I think that sometimes the critical project risks descending into a brand of "unless you are capable of thinking as cleverly as me, you aren't with the programme thinking. This, to my mind, is as constraining as the orthodoxies some of us rail against. Health is lived, not learned; it is experienced, not necessarily intellectualized all the time. Whatever efforts are applied at the abstract, rational domain need to be complemented by the recognition that it is an always already diverse cadre of embodied identities we work with. A place for the local, the situated, the lived stories of undergraduates *and* their relation to established knowledge is needed. The trick is engaging both hearts and minds.

Karen Throsby and Bethan Evans (2013) capture a critical fat pedagogue's conundrum beautifully with the following:

> The challenge of knowing when, and if, to speak out is an inescapable element of the complex social and familial relations of everyday life. … To speak out, however politely, can lead to discord and confrontation; to not speak out allows the presumption of agreement, producing complicity through inaction. (p. 332)

This dilemma is precisely the one I have grappled with. I consider that I have oscillated from seizing every opportunity, speaking loudly, authoritatively, and persuasively to surreptitiously sneaking the "speaking out" into course tasks and suggested readings. As signaled throughout this chapter, assorted forms of speaking out have yielded variable results. Perhaps impacting a rare few is all I can do. If so, does it make challenging fat truths a worthless exercise? I think not. "Complicity through inaction" is not an option in tertiary education in my view. One fewer teacher pushing weight-based oppression in schools is worth an effort.

References

Atherton, J. (2010). *Reflection on reflection*. Retrieved from http://www.doceo.co.uk/heterodoxy/reflection.htm#ixzz39gLXYh5g

Broughton, C. (2014). Make exercise at school mandatory: Academics. *The Press*. Retrieved from http://www.stuff.co.nz/national/health/10347451/Make-exercise-at-school-mandatory-academics

Burrows, L., & Wright, J. (2004). The good life: New Zealand children's perspectives of health and self. *Sport, Education and Society, 9*(2), 193–205.

Burrows, L., & Wright, J. (2007). Prescribing practices: Shaping healthy children in schools. *The International Journal of Children's Rights, 15*(1), 83–98.

Cameron, E. (2014). *Throwing their weight around: A critical examination of faculty experiences with challenging dominant obesity discourse in post-secondary education* (Doctoral dissertation). Lakehead University, Thunder Bay, ON, Canada.

Campos, P. (2004). *The obesity myth: Why America's obsession with weight is hazardous to your health*. New York, NY: Gotham Books.

Cooper, C. (2007). Headless fatties. Retrieved from http://charlottecooper.net/publishing/digital/headless-fatties-01-07

Cosgriff, M., Burrows, L., & Petrie, K. (2013). "You'll feel fat and no one will want to marry you": Responding to children's ideas about health. *Set: Research Information for Teachers, 1,* 21–28.

Evans, J., Rich, E., Davies, B., & Allwood, R. (2008). *Education, disordered eating and obesity discourse: Fat fabrications*. London, England: Routledge.

Foucault, M. (1983). On the genealogy of ethics: An overview of work in progress: Afterword. In H. L. Dreyfus & P. Rabinow, *Michel Foucault: Beyond structuralism and hermeneutics* (2nd ed., pp. 253–280). Chicago, IL: University of Chicago Press.

Gard, M. (2007). Is the war on obesity a war on children? *Childrenz Issues: Journal of the Children's Issues Centre, 11*(2), 20–24.

Gard, M., & Pluim, C. (2014). *Schools and public health: Past, present, future*. Lanham, MD: Rowman & Littlefield.

Gard, M., & Wright, J. (2005). *The "obesity epidemic": Science, ideology and morality.* London, England: Routledge.

Gillespie, L., & Culpan, I. (2000). Critical thinking: Ensuring the "education" aspect is evident in physical education. *Journal of Physical Education New Zealand, 44*(3), 84–96.

Leahy, D. (2009). Disgusting pedagogies. In J. Wright & V. Harwood (Eds.), *Biopolitics and the obesity epidemic: Governing bodies* (pp. 172–182). London, England: Routledge.

Lupton, D. (2013). *Fat.* New York, NY: Routledge.

Ministry of Education. (2007). *The New Zealand curriculum.* Wellington, New Zealand: Learning Media.

Moon, J. (1999). *Reflection in learning and professional development: Theory and practice,* London, England: Routledge.

Murray, S. (2008). *The "fat" female body.* London, England: Routledge.

Petrie, K., Burrows, L., & Cosgriff, M. (2014). Building a community of collaborative inquiry: A pathway to re-imagining practice in health and physical education. *Australian Journal of Teacher Education, 39*(2), 45–57.

Robertson, J. (2005). *Making sense of health promotion in context of health and physical education curriculum learning.* Paper prepared for the Ministry of Education's New Zealand Curriculum Marautanga Project. Retrieved from http://nzcurriculum.tki.org.nz/Archives/Curriculum-project-archives/References

Ross, B. (2005). Fat or fiction: Weighing the obesity epidemic. In M. Gard & J. Wright (Eds.), *The obesity epidemic: Science, morality and ideology* (pp. 86–106). New York, NY: Routledge.

Sinkinson, M. (2011). Back to the future: Reoccurring issues and discourses in health education in New Zealand schools. *Policy Futures in Education, 9*(3), 315–327.

Throsby, K., & Evans, B. (2013). "Must I seize every opportunity?" Complicity, confrontation and the problem of researching (anti-)fatness. *Critical Public Health, 23*(3), 331–344.

Vander Schee, C. F., & Boyles, D. (2010). "Exergaming," corporate interests and the crisis discourse of childhood obesity. *Sport, Education and Society, 15*(2), 169–186.

Welch, R., & Wright, J. (2011). Tracing discourses of health and the body: Exploring pre-service primary teachers' constructions of "healthy" bodies. *Asia Pacific Journal of Teacher Education, 39*(3), 199–210.

PART THREE

Researching Fat Pedagogies

Fat Bullying of Girls in Elementary and Secondary Schools: Implications for Teacher Education

Hannah McNinch

Bullying in schools is linked to various forms of oppression: racism, homophobia, sexism, and classism, to name a few (Walton, 2005). However, one form of bullying that remains barely addressed, and indeed is blatantly tolerated if not perpetuated by adults in power, is related to body size. In an attempt to understand this phenomenon better and to raise awareness, I focused my Master of Education thesis research on fat bullying in elementary and secondary school contexts. I used a qualitative approach and interviewed six female pre-service teachers (i.e., students in the final year of their Bachelor of Education [BEd] program who spend significant time in schools on practicum and who will soon be certified teachers). Using pseudonyms to protect their identities, I analyzed their retrospective accounts of being bullied on the basis of being labeled fat and their future plans for addressing fat bullying as teachers. Using critical discourse analysis, the results revealed systemic oppression of fat youth through bullying and exclusion that was often tolerated, and occasionally even encouraged, by staff in health and physical education (HPE) settings such as gymnasiums, outdoor fields, and the girls' change room, as well as other environments including classrooms, the cafeteria, and recess space. Further, I found that these participants, although once victims of fat bullying, reproduced fat-phobic discourse when discussing their experiences and future plans, thereby creating the possibility that they themselves might unwittingly reinforce fat phobia when they become teachers.

In the end, my research shed insight into how school environments foster the oppression of fat youth. For the purposes of this chapter, I briefly discuss four themes that emerged from my research: physical education and activity in school environments; other school environments; assigning responsibility; and participants' future students. I conclude with recommendations for pre-service teacher education that are grounded in the analysis of the experiences of the participants.

Physical Education and Activity

Being fat can lead to both social exclusion and bullying in elementary and secondary school (Gesser-Edelsburg & Endevelt, 2011; Taylor, 2011; Weinstock & Krehbiel, 2009; Wykes & Gunter, 2004). All my participants reported feeling such exclusion and all participants admitted to engaging in weight loss endeavors not only to escape bullying but also to feel as though they belonged in school. Jamie Lee Peterson, Rebecca Puhl, and Joerg Luedicke's (2012) research provides evidence that "weight-related bullying appears to be heavily concentrated in school settings including the classroom, cafeteria, playground, locker-room, and hallways" (p. 177). The participants in my study described bullying experiences in every one of these school environments as well.

The Gymnasium and Outdoor Field

The study was not primarily focused on participants' experiences in their physical education classes, but nevertheless their multiple negative memories of that environment emerged strongly. One participant recalls being told by a peer, "Maybe if you lost a few, then you could do better on your fitness test." Many of the participants shared that they initially enjoyed being active in school, but as the bullying continued they felt that their bodies were on display solely for the purpose of public ridicule. Participants reported not just verbal bullying, but also social exclusion and assumptions about what they were or were not capable of based on their size. As Erin Cameron et al. (2014) indicate, "many students remember their physical education experiences as negative and derived from frameworks predicated upon competition and the shaming of 'unfit' bodies" (p. 697). Participants learned to compare their bodies and their abilities with those of other students and could certainly see how privilege was afforded to "fit" and thin bodies in these environments.

Sports Teams

The privileging of "fit" students, particularly athletic students, was not reserved just for the gymnasium. Patrick Brady's (2004) research echoes what most participants already knew very well: "athletes, or jocks as they are more commonly known, stood at the apex of the hierarchy" (p. 359). Participants described feeling discriminated against as they witnessed teachers and administrators favor athletes in school generally and on teams in particular. One participant noted how she rarely got to play and when she did, other players never passed the ball to her. She quickly saw an athletic hierarchy in her school: "The emphasis [the school] put on if you were on a sports team, you were the kind of end all and be all" and noted that "it was really great" when she herself actually made it onto a team. Participants' recollections of being cut from teams and spending more time on the bench versus the court or the field echo the finding of Peterson et al. (2012) who found that teachers often discourage fat youth participation. Activities that presumably are meant to motivate students instead harmed them.

The Girls' Change Room

Another highly charged school environment for participants was the change room. Theoretically, environments like the gymnasium and field enable teachers and coaches to witness bullying and intervene (not that any did, according to the participants). The change room, however, is a mostly unsupervised social environment. For the participants, change rooms became a place where students contrasted bodies, with participants comparing themselves with thinner peers very unfavorably and feeling frustrated with their own bodies. They thus felt compelled to change elsewhere, to hide in corners of the room, or to change their clothes while remaining as covered as they could. Two participants resorted to changing in the bathroom stalls within the change room or in other bathrooms altogether. One participant recalled other girls locking the stalls on purpose so that she could not change in privacy.

Pavica Sheldon (2010) notes that "comparison with thin attractive models ... [leads] to lowering of body esteem as long as participants considered models to be similar with them" (p. 279). In the change rooms, participants compared themselves with peers of the same age whom they perceived as not only thin and popular but also as model students in their schools; these comparisons were a source of great frustration and shame and led one participant to take HPE in the summer term so she could change at home and other participants from not engaging in any public physical activity at all.

Other School Environments

While the HPE curriculum places emphasis on the body so that it perhaps more understandably could be a prime site for fat bullying, participants fell victim to fat bullying in other school environments as well. The earliest memory of fat bullying described by a participant in my study was in Grade 3. Fat phobia, alas, seems to blossom early in girls' lives; as Hayley Dohnt and Marika Tiggemann (2005) described, there is a correlation between the time when girls enter school and the point at which they start to become more body conscious.

Classrooms
Despite teacher presence, classrooms provided little safety for participants, as there were few interventions from adult staff to stop the bullying. Participants shared stories of being bullied physically (pinching, poking) as well as verbally through fat-phobic and dehumanizing taunts. One participant's experience of being compared to an earthquake immediately reminded me of Paulo Freire's (1970) explanation of oppression as coming from a failure to recognize another as human. Even when participants were called the more common "fatso" or "fatty," they were being dehumanized by being reduced to a solute.

Recess and the Cafeteria
Recess and food breaks are meant to give students a break from the classroom environment, but as students exit the building or move to a lunchroom or cafeteria, they enter a space where they yet again can encounter fat bullying. One participant regularly felt threatened at recess and as a result always tried to stay in view of a teacher, but still fell victim to her bullies and was disappointed that her teachers never intervened. Breaks to eat food were also unsafe for participants as food intake and body type were often commented on, regardless of what students were actually eating or not eating. Schools, like other spaces in our society, are embedded in and reinforce dieting cultures (Dohnt & Tiggemann, 2005) so it is no surprise that fat phobia would be present in the cafeteria. Further, the ways in which participants learned to self-monitor their food intake in a public setting like a cafeteria, for example, points to the way they internalized fat oppression.

Assigning Responsibility

Some have advocated fat shaming as a useful strategy to motivate fat people to change their apparently horrible lifestyles (Callahan, 2013). Similarly, Jacqueline Weinstock and Michelle Krehbiel (2009) observe that others have made arguments that bullying of fat youth would stop if they just lost weight, thereby implying that shaming and blaming the victim are helpful. My findings did indeed demonstrate that as victims of fat bullying, the participants internalized dominant obesity discourse and felt compelled to lose weight because of the bullying. Some participants did lose weight and later wondered whether fat bullying had indeed been helpful in the end by pressuring them to lose weight. What is important to note here is how each participant endured much emotional and physical stress. None of the participants came out of these experiences unscathed, so for them to restory the fat bullying as perhaps helpful is disturbing.

Participants held a number of people accountable for the fat bullying they endured, but none blamed the systemic forces at play. Instead, those who did the bullying were clearly blamed and so too were peers who did not intervene. Similarly, teachers and administrative staff were found accountable for not intervening immediately or for not doing so effectively enough to prevent further occurrences. With little help from others, all the participants seemed to blame themselves for the weight that prompted the bullying, internalizing the fat oppression.

Bullies and Other Peers

Participants felt that bullies were most responsible for their victimization but also felt some disappointment in not being helped by their peers. Rebecca Puhl, Joerg Luedicke, and Chelsea Heuer's (2011) study of weight-based teasing illustrated that peers were unlikely to intervene when it came to incidents of fat bullying, which certainly resonates with my own findings. Participants suspected that their peers did not know how to intervene effectively and also understood that they, too, might have been afraid of being bullied themselves. Further, this lack of intervention was modeled by teachers. Students are certainly aware of their teachers' actions; as Peterson et al. (2012) observed, "When teachers do not intervene in bullying situations, their students are also less likely to intervene" (p. 178).

Many of the participants reported turning into aggressors themselves as a way to release tension. One participant consistently teased a girl for being too skinny out of jealousy. Another explained how she found competitive pleasure in her bully gaining weight while she became thinner: "I started losing weight, and she, this is going to sound bad, and she continued to get fat. I wanted to get skinnier just because she bullied me because I was fat." Her bully's sudden weight gain was this participant's drive to lose more weight. As shown here, fat bullying led to retaliatory behaviors that perpetuated a vicious cycle.

Teachers

Two participants spoke about the difficulties of reporting to teachers. One hated feeling like a tattletale and therefore hoped the teacher would notice on her own. Another participant emotionally explained that "it actually hurt to repeat what was said to me. It was like being bullied all over again." What was clear was their need for teachers who did witness an event of fat bullying to act.

Instead of action, participants shared multiple examples of teachers neglecting to address, or ineffectively addressing, fat bullying and how that allowed the bullying to persist. One teacher punished a participant for physically confronting her bullies but did not discipline the bullies for the original behavior that prompted the participant's retaliation. The lesson that fat bullying is acceptable but responding to it is not was a sad one learned by that participant. Even when teachers do try to address bullying, they did so in a general way, neglecting to address the underlying fat phobia; as Gerald Walton (2005) observes, students hear generic anti-bullying messages all the time and if these do not get to the systemic roots of the problem, such as fat phobia, they are ineffective. Further, when teachers uncritically teach curriculum content that privileges the thin ideal or use activities such as fitness tests that mandate students comparing themselves with one another, they reproduce fat phobia.

Brady (2004) argued that social groups and social attitudes are first "constructed by students and reinforced by administrators and teaching staff" (p. 356), whereas in a number of stories my participants shared, it is evident that teachers were the ones who had set the example for students. To use one example from the data, peers picking teams that resulted in fat students always being picked last and teachers apparently nonchalantly supporting that method reinforced to participants that this was an appropriate practice. This clearly echoes Heather Sykes and Deborah McPhail's (2011) finding that the way teachers conduct their HPE classes can reproduce or disrupt negative stereotypes of fat students in ways that are very clear to all students. HPE teachers and coaches reinforcing fat phobia has been noted in other studies too (Peterson et al., 2012; Yager & O'Dea, 2005).

Administrative Staff

Changing teaching practices and the culture of schools certainly is part of the mandate of administrators. In the case of the participant who was disciplined for retaliating against her bullies, her principal ignored the fat bullying she was experiencing and focused instead on her own confrontational behavior. Walton (2010) remains critical of policies, and those who enforce such policies, that promote "regulation of student behaviour [because it] appears to provide order in schools, a key factor that relieves the pressure placed upon educational administrators to 'do something'" (p. 147). In this instance, the principal was able to appear as though he addressed the issue of physical violence in the class because he addressed the participant's behavior, but the fat bullying itself and the systemic forces that fostered the fat bullying were not addressed, thus school continued to be an oppressive environment for her and other fat students.

Participants shared few stories about their experiences with principals, but the ones who did felt unsupported. One participant said that her pain seemed invisible, saying, "No one ever engaged me." Another felt that her experience of bullying was unimportant, and another came to understand that she was perceived as a nuisance with her repetitive visits to the office. In these examples, administrators were too distant and set an example of tolerance for fat bullying by either refusing to investigate specific instances when reported or remaining unresponsive despite participants being adamant that the principals were aware of what was going on. The administrators described in these interviews appeared to be complicit in the fat bullying.

Blaming Oneself

Research has shown that women's body image is most defined by peer response (e.g., Sheldon, 2010) so it is not surprising that fat bullying led to participants focusing so much on their own bodies. One participant described how she would go home after an incident of fat bullying, look in the mirror, and stare at herself in agreement with what her bullies had said. Eleanor Mackey and Annette La Greca (2008) stipulated "that girls' own attitudes and their perceptions of peers' weight and appearance norms are pathways through which peer crowd identification may influence weight control behaviors" (p. 1099). Echoing the disturbing idea that fat shaming or bullying can motivate people to lose weight (Dohnt & Tiggemann, 2005; Mackey & La Greca, 2008; Li & Rukavina, 2012), the bullying seemed to reinforce participants' view that the body is a trainable machine and that they should be able to simply lose weight (Cameron et al., 2014). Their own lived experiences should have helped them challenge that idea given they were themselves unable to lose weight easily, but instead they described often feeling like failures.

Fat bullying thus led to participants internalizing fat phobia, which led them sometimes to engage in dangerous weight loss behaviors such as disordered eating and to disengage from physical activity. They absorbed the blame that society places on the fat individual who apparently lacks self-discipline (Cameron et al., 2014; Weinstock & Krehbiel, 2009). Other studies on fat bullying also noted how internalized fat phobia can lead to low self-esteem, eating disorders, and becoming a bully (Griffiths, Wolke, Page, & Horwood, 2005; Wojtowicz & von Ranson, 2012); each participant experienced one or more of these.

Their Future Students

When discussing how they might address fat bullying when they become teachers themselves, participants indicated that they did not yet feel adequately prepared to do so effectively. Their proposed interventions, all imaginative and involving either or both the bully and the bullied, tended to reflect what did or did not work in their own experiences, and thus were based on intuitive understandings rather than explicit techniques or approaches. Further, none of their proposed interventions involved peers even though they had discussed how they themselves had felt when their peers either did not intervene or were not able to so do effectively.

While I interviewed them early in their BEd program, the findings suggest that they were as yet unprepared to deal with bullying in general and they certainly were not prepared to deal with fat bullying specifically. Although most participants felt that their professors recognized how prevalent bullying was in schools and how important it was for them as pre-service teachers to be aware of it, superficial awareness alone cannot possibly address the problem, especially given that the systemic roots of and responses to bullying presumably take sustained effort and time (Walton, 2005). Ultimately, given such limited attention to bullying, I wonder whether the implicit curriculum is that bullying is still not a very big concern. Further, the implicit curriculum may also be that all bullying is similar and that the specific types of bullying are not important.

With these data and these problems in mind, I turn now to how this study offered a critique of both the current school system and pre-service teacher education and offer three recommendations for pre-service education.

Recommendations

Challenging the way school environments reproduce fat phobia is possible, and one place to start is through ensuring that we offer more critical teacher education. I thus offer some suggestions on how teacher education might respond to this problem more critically to help teachers develop skills to address fat bullying.

1. Offer a specific course, or part of a course, to pre-service teachers that tackles oppression and bullying from a systemic perspective. A course with critical pedagogy content could provide pre-service teachers with the tools to recognize privilege and oppressive social relations and pedagogical approaches that would enable them to critically and creatively reimagine both the explicit and implicit curriculum, including physical space. It should include critical approaches to bullying that make clear that the targets of bullying are usually those without the advantages of privilege (e.g., based on race, class, gender, sexuality, ability, body size) and that effective responses must address these systemic issues (Walton, 2005). Including fat bullying in the mix as well as critical information on fat phobia, fat acceptance, and Health At Every Size could be very enlightening. As such, a course like this could help BEd students build a foundation on which to confront all types of bullying, including the bullying of fat youth that is currently not merely tolerated but often actively encouraged (Weinstock & Krehbiel, 2009).

2. Ensure that fat pedagogy is infused throughout health and physical education courses. Some Canadian provinces, namely, Alberta and Prince Edward Island, have curriculum content that promotes inclusion of all body shapes and sizes; as such, the curriculum, at least in theory if not in practice, works to deconstruct thin privilege and create space for learning about the Health At Every Size movement (Robertson & Thomson, 2012). In contrast, the curriculum in Ontario and the other provinces is far less progressive (Cameron et al., 2014; Robertson & Thomson, 2012; Sykes & McPhail, 2011). Imagine what might occur if students learned about the inaccuracy and political construction of the Body Mass Index (Burkhauser & Cawley, 2008), about fat oppression and thin privilege (Bacon, 2009), how weight stigma negatively impacts one's health more than weight (Burgard, 2009; Schafer & Ferraro, 2011; Wann, 2009), and how fat children and youth are routinely excluded and bullied in physical education classes which often leads to avoidance of physical education altogether (Cameron et al., 2014; Russell, Cameron, Socha, & McNinch, 2013; Sykes & McPhail, 2011).

Peterson et al. (2012) found that, in particular, "physical educators (e.g., PE teachers, coaches, and students in training to become PE teachers or coaches) endorse negative beliefs about overweight individuals" (p. 178). This was echoed in my findings. These negative beliefs are based on common misconceptions about health and weight that evidently need to be deconstructed in teacher education in health and physical education. We need to disrupt dominant "obesity" and "healthy living" discourses that are so prevalent, and help foster in pre-service teachers the desire and ability to teach about health holistically, rather than teaching students a single formula for how to be healthy (Quennerstedt, Burrows, & Maivorsdotter, 2010). Teachers need to focus more on deconstructing contemporary understandings of health and create opportunities for students to investigate various ways of improving overall health (Gard, 2003). It is therefore integral for health and physical education professors to take a leadership role in ensuring that they disrupt fat oppression, including that embedded in healthy living discourse, and that they mentor future teachers on how to include *all* children and youth.

3. Offer workshops on fat bullying. As my findings demonstrated, participants were unsure of how specifically to address fat bullying. Walton (2005) argues that bullying cannot be addressed in general terms. As noted earlier, bullying is rooted in systemic forces of oppression that target specific individuals. Without addressing the underlying reason for the bullying, the behavior might be disciplined but the prejudice that led to the behavior remains unchanged. Pedagogical strategies that teach students to embrace, celebrate, and learn from the differences within student populations are important (Walton, 2005). While specific strategies for addressing fat bullying may not yet have been stated clearly in a single resource at this point, these certainly could be developed and there is much to be built on if the critical bullying literature and fat studies literature are brought together. In addition, further research on the lived experiences of those who have been fat bullied may result in useful ideas.

Conclusion

My research identified and explored participants' experiences with fat bullying and the potential impacts on their future profession as teachers. Through critical discourse analysis of interviews, the data illustrated that while participants would not tolerate fat bullying, they had nonetheless internalized fat phobia, which was unfortunately left undisrupted in their BEd. As stated in my recommendations, teacher education needs to be revamped by offering required courses in critical pedagogy to address the root causes of bullying, by seriously redesigning existing health and physical education courses, and by offering workshops on specific strategies for addressing fat bullying. As educators, it is our duty to create a safe space for students of all shapes and sizes. Being able to see fat through a critical lens will help to deconstruct the fat-phobic ideologies that contribute to the bullying of girls based on their body size. In doing so, we can proactively educate students about fat oppression, the dangers of fat phobia, and the potential for all bodies to be valued in our society.

References

Bacon, L. (2009). *Reflections on fat acceptance: Lessons learned from privilege.* Retrieved from http://www.lindabacon.org/Bacon_ThinPrivilege080109.pdf

Brady, P. (2004). Jocks, teckers, and nerds: The role of the adolescent peer group in the formation and maintenance of secondary school institutional culture. *Discourse: Studies in the Cultural Politics of Education, 25*(3), 351–364.

Burgard, D. (2009). What is Health At Every Size? In E. Rothblum & S. Solovay (Eds.), *The fat studies reader* (pp. 41–54). New York, NY: New York University Press.

Burkhauser, R., & Cawley, J. (2008). Beyond BMI: The value of more accurate measures of fatness and obesity in social science research. *Journal of Health Economics, 27,* 519–529.

Callahan, D. (2013). Obesity: Chasing an elusive epidemic. *Hastings Center Report, 43*(1), 34–40.

Cameron, E., Oakley, J., Walton, G., Russell, C., Chambers, L., & Socha, T. (2014). Moving beyond the injustices of the schooled healthy body. In I. Bogotch & C. Shields (Eds.), *International handbook of educational leadership and social (in)justice* (pp. 687–704). New York, NY: Springer.

Dohnt, H. K., & Tiggemann, M. (2005). Peer influences on body dissatisfaction and dieting awareness in young girls. *British Journal of Developmental Psychology, 23,* 103–116.

Freire, P. (1970). *Pedagogy of the oppressed.* New York, NY: Continuum.

Gard, M. (2003). Producing little decision makers and goal setters in the age of the obesity crisis. *Quest, 60*(4), 488–502.

Gesser-Edelsburg, A., & Endevelt, R. (2011). An entertainment-education study of stereotypes and prejudice against fat women: An evaluation of "Fat pig." *Health Education Journal, 70*(4), 374–382.

Griffiths, L., Wolke, D., Page, A., & Horwood, J. (2005). Obesity and bullying: Different effects for boys and girls. *Archives of Disease in Children, 91*, 121–125.

Li, W., & Rukavina, P. (2012). The nature, occurring contexts, and psychological implications of weight-related teasing in urban physical education programs. *Research Quarterly for Exercise and Sport, 83*(2), 308–317.

Mackey, E., & La Greca, A. (2008). Does this make me look fat? Peer crowd and peer contributions to adolescent girls' weight control behaviors. *Journal of Youth Adolescence, 37*, 1097–1110.

Peterson, J. L., Puhl, R. M., & Luedicke, J. (2012). An experimental investigation of physical education teachers' and coaches' reactions to weight-based victimization in youth. *Psychology of Sport and Exercise, 13*, 177–185.

Puhl, R. M., Luedicke, J., & Heuer, C. (2011). Weight-based victimization toward overweight adolescents: Observations and reaction of peers. *Journal of School Health, 81*(11), 696–703.

Quennerstedt, M., Burrows, L., & Maivorsdotter, L. (2010). From teaching young people to be healthy to learning health. *Utbilning & Demokrati, 19*(2), 97–112.

Robertson, L., & Thomson, D. (2012). "BE"ing a certain way: Seeking body image in Canadian health and physical education curriculum policies. *Canadian Journal of Education, 35*(2), 335–354.

Russell, C., Cameron, E., Socha, T., & McNinch, H. (2013). "Fatties cause global warming": Fat pedagogy and environmental education. *Canadian Journal of Environmental Education, 18*, 27–45.

Schafer, M., & Ferraro, K. (2011). The stigma of obesity: Does perceived weight discrimination affect identity and physical health? *Social Psychology Quarterly, 74*(1), 76–97.

Sheldon, P. (2010). Pressure to be perfect: Influences on college students' body esteem. *Southern Communication Journal, 75*(3), 277–298.

Sykes, H., & McPhail, D. (2011). Fatness: Unbearable lessons. In H. Sykes, *Queer bodies* (pp. 49–74). New York, NY: Peter Lang.

Taylor, N. L. (2011). "Guys, she's humongous!" Gender and weight-based teasing in adolescence. *Journal of Adolescent Research, 26*(2), 178–199.

Walton, G. (2005). The notion of bullying through the lens of Foucault and critical theory. *Journal of Educational Thought, 39*, 1, 55–73.

Walton, G. (2010). The problem trap: Implications of Policy Archeology Methodology for anti-bullying policies. *Journal of Education Policy, 25*(2), 135–150.

Wann, M. (2009). Foreword: Fat studies: An invitation to revolution. In E. Rothblum & S. Solovay (Eds.), *The fat studies reader* (pp. ix–xxvi). New York, NY: New York University Press.

Weinstock, J., & Krehbiel, M. (2009). Fat youth as common targets for bullying. In E. Rothblum & S. Solovay (Eds.), *The fat studies reader* (pp. 120–126). New York, NY: New York University Press.

Wojtowicz, E., & von Ranson, K. (2012). Weighing in on risk factors for body dissatisfaction: A one-year prospective study of middle-adolescent girls. *Body Image, 9*, 20–30.

Wykes, M., & Gunter, B. (2004). *The media and body image: If looks could kill.* Thousand Oaks, CA: Sage.

Yager, Z., & O'Dea, J. A. (2005). The role of teachers and other educators in the prevention of eating disorders and child obesity: What are the issues? *Eating Disorders, 13*, 261–278.

TWELVE

Critical Pedagogical Strategies to Disrupt Weight Bias in Schools

Richard Pringle and Darren Powell

The scientific knowledge about diet, fatness, and health is constantly changing and being challenged (Gard & Wright, 2005; Kirk, 2006). The validity of the Body Mass Index (BMI), for example, has fallen into disrepute (Ross, 2005), the food pyramid has had several rearrangements (Kinney, 2005), the alleged health benefits of a high carbohydrate/low fat diet are being challenged (Paoli, Rubini, Volek, & Grimaldi, 2013), and ideas about being "overweight" or "underweight" and their relationship to poor health have been turned on their head (Gard & Wright, 2005). Despite the scientific uncertainties concerning diet, body composition, and health, many teachers—particularly physical education teachers (e.g., Trost, 2006)—continue to believe that the world is in the grips of an "obesity epidemic" and it is their duty to promote the virtues of physical activity and the problems of fat. Although many of these teachers are well-intentioned, concern has been raised that the simplistic messages promoted in schools can act to position fat people as unhealthy and even, at times, as moral failures (Evans, Rich, & Davies, 2008).

Our concerns are not simply that these messages lack coherent evidence but that they can be damaging for many who believe they are fat, with respect to psychological (e.g., body disorder ailments, poor self-esteem, depression), social (e.g., disaffection, alienation, and marginalization), and physical dimensions (e.g., as associated with starvation, purging, bingeing, and the effects of excessive exercise). Paradoxically, therefore, the promotion of such "health knowledge" can act, in itself, to produce poor health (Campos, 2004). The American Academy of Pediatrics (2013) reports, for example, that children deemed to be fat are frequently teased and bullied at school to such an extent that they lose friends, suffer poor self-esteem, and eventually dread going to school. Some even drop out altogether as they accept it is better to fail in education than be the subject of ongoing ridicule.

In this chapter, given our concerns about weight bias and the body composition and health messages circulating in schools, we reveal strategies employed in the education of teachers at a tertiary institute that aim to disrupt mainstream understandings of the relationships between fatness and health. We do so with the intent of promoting a more respectful and nuanced way of teaching about bodies, fitness, physical activity, and health within schools. We begin by providing the results from an examination of two elementary schools that illustrate how children are taught about fatness and fitness and how they subsequently make meanings about bodies and health. It was primarily the results from this initial study that motivated our pedagogical strategies to disrupt weight bias in the education of teachers.

An Ethnography of Elementary Schools' Health and Physical Education Programs

The evidence we draw on in this section comes from an ethnographic research project that examined health and physical education (HPE) programs and teaching resources in two New Zealand elementary schools. This research, undertaken by Darren, included document analysis, observations, and interviews with teachers and students. To protect privacy, all names of schools and participants used are pseudonyms. These HPE programs and resources were funded, devised, and implemented by a range of public, private, and voluntary sector organizations, often working in partnership. They were typically promoted as "part of the solution" to childhood "obesity" through the assumption that they would "support students to develop healthy eating habits that contribute towards maintaining a healthy body weight" (Nestlé New Zealand, 2011, p. 14). While external providers of these HPE programs (i.e., not a classroom teacher, but an employee of an organization outside of the school), classroom teachers, and principals broadly understood these programs and resources as playing a role in ameliorating the "crisis" of childhood "obesity," there was still a degree of uncertainty about how successful they were. For instance, St. Saviour's School teacher Miss Black reported that these programs were "definitely needed and … must have an effect, even if it's just a very small one." Although program effectiveness was questioned, there was no doubt in teachers' minds that the "obesity epidemic" was a real crisis.

When discussing "obesity" and fatness, students and teachers frequently drew on the ideas of energy imbalance, physical inactivity, and overconsumption of junk food as the main causes of "obesity" (see also Burrows & Wright, 2004; Powell & Fitzpatrick, 2013). Dudley School teacher Mr. Spurlock, for instance, asserted that "five or six" of his students were "obese" as the result of playing "on the X-box" and because "they're not very active." He subsequently described their "skill in PE" as "awful." His colleague Mrs. Donna also blamed children's "lack of interest in physical activity" as part of the problem, especially for Pasifika children (i.e., children with ancestral and cultural ties to the Pacific Islands), who she claimed "are brought up not to be active," and eat too much "fast food," "processed food," and other "cheap nasty stuff."

For Leon, a 5-year-old student at Dudley School, the relationship between fatness, health, eating, and exercise was relatively straightforward: "If you eat heaps of not healthy things, I think you get fat!" When asked, "Why are fat people fat and skinny people skinny?" Leon replied: "If you [do] exercise you are skinny, and if you [don't] you might get fat." This was a similar response to 5-year-old Sita from St. Saviour's School who thought that "exercise makes you not fat." Eton, an 11-year-old student in Mr. Spurlock's class, also understood fatness in a simplified way: "If you eat lots of fatty foods you become really fat. If you eat really healthy, you stay healthy." By and large, there was little acknowledgment by these younger students of the complex relationships between eating, physical activity, health, body size, and other elements. Bodies and behaviors were reduced to simple binaries of good/bad, healthy/unhealthy, fat/healthy, and exercised/inactive.

The children's understandings about the problem of "obesity" were connected to the "pedagogical work" (Tinning, 2014, p. 208) in both school-based and public settings: pedagogies tended to link dominant discourses associated with health, inactivity, and "obesity" in a correlative manner. By drawing on the science of energy balance, official nutrition advice, and individualistic notions of health, an individual's body size, shape, and weight were inextricably linked with his/her (in)ability to make "healthy" choices. It was hardly surprising then that the proposed solutions to "obesity" were also centered on the science of energy balance and educating children to make the "correct" choices for health, lifestyles, eating, exercise, and, of course, fat avoidance.

Individual choice is a key pillar of neoliberalism and was regularly employed in elementary schools to teach children to be healthy and non-fat. A *Warrant of Fitness* workbook used with Years 7 and 8 (11- to 13-year-olds) with Dudley School students repeatedly emphasized the importance of informed choice: "To make great choices we need to be informed. When we are thinking about food choices, we need to be informed about what is in the food we eat" (Life Education Trust, n.d., p. 15). One common pedagogical device to "inform" children about what choices to make was through the ubiquitous use of food pyramid kinds of illustrations. The *Warrant of Fitness* workbook, for example, included two food pyramids, while the Year 1 students (aged 5) at Dudley School were informed about a traffic light system for categorizing different food (which included a cartoon of a fat man eating a hamburger and drinking a soft drink next to the "red light" foods of sugar, salt, and fat).

The promotion of informed choice as a key factor for healthy lifestyles and healthy body weight was joined to another strategy: teaching children to make the "right" decisions and eat the "right" foods while avoiding those that were "wrong." Children's knowledge of good/bad, right/wrong, wise/stupid choices in eating were (re)produced through various educational resources and games that simplified, categorized, and fused certain values to children's food choices. For instance, in a resource titled *Be Healthy, Be Active*, students were expected to learn about healthy choices from a "food plate" that was "designed to allow ... students to explore the many aspects of a balanced diet and wise food selection ... [and] the importance of sensible eating" (Nestlé New Zealand, 2011, p. 2).

The moral imperative for individuals to make wise or sensible choices (i.e., those choices that will not lead to being unhealthy or fat) conversely intimated that fat people made "unwise" choices. Darren spoke with Eton (aged 11) about a lesson that included a short fictional television news story featuring two characters: *Henrietta Hen*, a skinny bird who was an expert on matters of health and weight loss, and *Ham Trotter*, who according to Eton was a "fat" pig who was "eating burgers all the time":

Darren: Do you think that's fair to fat pigs or fat people that they are portrayed in that way, to be eating junk food all the time, because surely there's some people ...

Eton: No, it's their choice, isn't it?

Darren: It's their choice to be fat or to eat?
Eton: Well, to eat, but it's their choice to go to McDonald's every day of [their] life.

Rather than encouraging children to challenge the "façade" (Ayo, 2012, p. 104) of choice or the notion that fat people were fat simply because they ate too many hamburgers and did too little exercise, the HPE programs and resources were utilized as a tactic to direct "young people to behave in particular ways that align with contemporary governmental imperatives around weight and the body" (Leahy, 2009, p. 173). The pedagogies employed to teach children about fatness were, correspondingly, mostly *undisruptive* to dominant discourses of "obesity," health, and fatness. One such pedagogy was that of *silence*, which revolved around teacher unwilling-ness or inability to engage in discussions about the complexities of fatness. For instance, at Dudley School the Year 1 students participated in a lesson about sugar. Marion, the external provider for the *Life Education* program, asked the children: "Why don't we eat sugar?" Five-year-old Leon raised his hand and shouted out: "Because it makes you fat!" Marion looked at Leon, remained silent, and then turned back to the class and asked: "Anybody else?" This pedagogy of silence meant that a potential teaching opportunity to engage in a discussion around "what makes people fat" was ignored, and Leon's understanding of fatness and fat people remained undisrupted. The silence, as such, worked as a "shelter for power" (Foucault, 1978, p. 101).

This is not to say that all children were unwilling or unable to challenge the idea that be-ing fat was unhealthy, that all fat people were lazy, and that fatness was simply the cause of energy balance, bad choices, and personal irresponsibility. When Darren asked Leon: "Can fat people also be healthy?" he replied, "Yeah, they can, but if they eat too many lolly-things they won't be." Children were particularly adept at resisting stereotypes of the slothful and glutton-ous fat person when children reflected on themselves and family members. Eton, for instance, described himself as fat but said he was also very active, regularly taking his dogs for a walk on his bike or scooter. Nicole described her mother as "obese" but also healthy. Yet when talking about "others" who were deemed fat, the conversations veered back to notions of individual-ism, irresponsibility, and poor health.

The promotion of individual choice as a panacea to children's future health and fat-ness was inextricably interconnected to the assumption that once informed of the "correct" choices, children could, indeed *should*, take individual responsibility to make these choices (see Crawford, 1980). These individualistic notions of health were supported by key aspects of neoliberalism: free choice, autonomy, consumption, and self-responsibility. The *Warrant of Fitness* unit, for example, stated that its prime learning goal was to get students to learn to "take responsibility for … [their] own food choices" (Life Education Trust, 2011, p. 1), while the *Iron Brion* curriculum stated that students will "demonstrate increasing responsibility for what they eat" (New Zealand Beef and Lamb Marketing Bureau, n.d., p. 13). The focus on individual health, choice, and responsibility acted as a smokescreen to the multiple forces that constrained the choices an individual child was "able" to make.

One striking example of the broader social forces related to Natia, a 12-year-old Tongan girl at St. Saviour's School. A number of children and adults had talked about Natia and linked her fatness with poor food choices and irresponsibility. The school receptionist, for example, observed that Natia's lunch might consist entirely of a large bag of potato chips and that she would share this with her 5-year-old brother. Natia's classmates also noted her "habit" of bringing "junk" food to school, and some described her as unhealthy and fat, although by Natia's own account she was very active and enjoyed playing a range of sports at school, especially "rugby against the boys." The moralistic and corporeal positioning of Natia's assumed health (i.e., the assumption that because she was fat and ate processed food she was unhealthy) and its relationship to her "poor choices" belied powerful forces that shaped her ability to negotiate life and make the "correct" choices. During a conversation with Natia, for example, she revealed that her family had recently been evicted from their home and they were all currently living in a car. Natia's "wrong" choices, her fat body, and her irresponsibility were attributed to her failing as an individual, rather than a range of interlinking social forces, such as the failure of a political system to reduce poverty, provide adequate housing, and increase access to affordable and nutritional food.

This is not to suggest that children and adults were ignorant of the effects of political, cultural, economic, and environmental factors on children's lives. In fact, teachers and principals regularly discussed the broad range of forces that impinged on their students' *learning*. Mr. Woodward, principal of Dudley School, and Mrs. Sergeant, the principal of St. Saviour's School, both spoke at length about how socioeconomic factors—gambling, unemployment, lack of housing, crime, hunger, minimum wage—made it difficult for their students to learn, or even attend school. However, when the topic of conversation turned to children's health and fatness, the same forces were deemed to be less important than an individual's responsibility to make the "right" choices.

While there were a number of students, teachers, and principals who recognized some of the complexities around issues of fatness, and drew attention to notable contradictions between dominant discourses of fatness and their own knowledge of fat people (including themselves), there was an overwhelming reluctance for adults to "teach" children about these complexities and contradictions in any deep or meaningful manner. Rather than encouraging students to challenge "truths" about the relationship between fatness and health, the positioning of fat people as irresponsible, uninformed, or immoral, and the notion that fat is bad and something to be avoided, prevailed. The abject, fat, unhealthy "other" (Leahy, 2012) was reproduced via the dominant obesity discourse of this pedagogy of simplicity and silence. Children's and teachers' understandings about fatness and health, correspondingly, remained undisrupted.

Disrupting Fat Knowledge in the Education of Teachers

What Darren's research project did was provide us with concrete examples of how dominant obesity discourse and pedagogy were enacted in actual schools. This also helped to illuminate how these discourses and pedagogies interwove with children's and adult's understandings of fatness and health in ways that were, in a Foucauldian sense, "dangerous." As colleagues we have been able to reflect on and critique these (and other) discourses and pedagogies, and by doing so have assembled our own fat pedagogy that we hope will disrupt dominant obesity discourses. Given our concerns about the "obesity" messages circulating in schools, and the associated marginalization and victimization, we have carefully thought about how we teach education students at our tertiary institute so that they can offer a more respectful, healthful, and inclusive set of understandings to children. In this section, we discuss two such attempts—*deconstructing fat* and the employment of *differing rhetorical styles*—to illustrate how these critical pedagogical strategies have been used and what apparent impact they have on student understandings of "obesity."

Deconstructing Fat

Previously, Richard had attempted to disrupt university students' understandings of fatness by encouraging them to deconstruct competing forms of knowledge (see Pringle & Pringle, 2010). This critical strategy revolved around the implementation of a simplified version of Jacques Derrida's (1992) process of deconstruction. Derrida was concerned that the Western philosophical tradition was underpinned by a series of dualisms (e.g., masculinity/femininity, mind/body, nature/culture) that imposed a way of understanding reality that favored particular political perspectives. For instance, he was concerned that Western philosophy had promoted a broad way of "knowing" that privileged the masculine over the feminine and worked to produce a society that advantaged males over females. Derrida's aim in deconstructing seemingly clear-cut binaries (e.g., healthy/unhealthy, obese/thin, rational/irrational) was to challenge the broad authority of dualistic thinking by illustrating that the meanings between each binary category were not distinctly different. More specifically, he hoped to challenge the idea that one of the binaries was better than the other and correspondingly disrupt the associated hierarchies and sets of power relations (e.g., as associated with fat and thin people). Keith Jenkins (1999) clarified that "once clear-cut distinctions become blurred, their natural-ness is seen as being ultimately arbitrary and thus precisely 'unnatural'" (p. 47). In other words, the seemingly "natural" understanding that equates "obese" bodies with poor health and thin bodies with good health gets disturbed via deconstruction.

To encourage students to deconstruct the binaries associated with "obesity," Richard provided his university students with a range of competing readings associated with "obesity" and health. These readings illustrated that scholars held opposing views on similar topics. As examples, readings illustrated that scientists differed on their views of whether a high-fat diet was healthier than a low-fat diet, an "obesity epidemic" existed, dieting was effective for losing weight, and so-called "overweight" people could be healthier than the "underweight." The students were then asked to draw on this conflicting set of readings and undertake an assignment to discuss whether schools should be used as a site to challenge the "obesity epidemic" via the monitoring of student physical activity levels, diet, and body compositions.

The aim in setting this assignment was to provide the students with an opportunity to grapple with uncertainty and "undecidability" and experience the associated confusion of doing deconstruction. Derrida had theorized that experiencing such confusion would promote a more humble and nuanced way of knowing the social world, so that individuals could understand issues from multiple perspectives and be less dogmatic in promoting set "solutions" to various issues. In this particular case, Richard hoped that the students would gain an understanding that the differences between fat and thin, good and bad food, and healthy and unhealthy were not clear cut and, as such, they would be less inclined to believe that fatness was a "health" problem.

Class discussions revealed that some of the students found the assignment difficult, as they could not ascertain the "correct" answer. In other words, they believed that a "correct" answer existed and either more research was needed or that some of the existing research was currently incorrect. For these students, unfortunately, the point of doing deconstruction had been missed as they had not learned "to live with uncertainty" (Schwandt, 1996, p. 59). Other students, however, recognized that competing points of view about "obesity" existed and, as such, they were less certain that fatness was a health problem and less inclined to believe that teachers should aim to combat the alleged "obesity epidemic."

Richard subsequently acknowledged that although there was value in encouraging the students to deconstruct fat knowledge, that as a strategy to disrupt "obesity" knowledge it was only modestly successful. He was particularly concerned that by focusing selectively on competing forms of scientific knowledge that he had missed an opportunity to present other ways of knowing "fat" that might potentially be more disruptive of dominant obesity discourses. Hence, he now employs a pedagogical approach, adopted from Richard Tinning (2002), which employs the use of "differing rhetorical styles."

Modest Pedagogy via the Use of Differing Rhetorical Styles

Tinning (2002) recognized that critical pedagogical attempts to challenge student views typically have only limited impact. Through examining how critical pedagogues teach, he realized that they are often overly reliant on presenting scientific knowledge with an expectation that the "truths" of science will subsequently produce certain emancipatory outcomes. Yet, of course, many people know the scientific truths about various "social ills" (e.g., global warming, alcohol and cigarette consumption), but do not always amend lifestyle habits accordingly. In this way, Tinning accepted "the limits of rationality as a catalyst for change" (p. 236). However, in recognizing that people can be motivated to enact change or fight injustices through exposure to a mixture of differing voices or rhetorical styles—such as the use of biographical narratives, philosophical arguments, film, literature, or the findings of science—Tinning accepted the value in adopting a teaching style that drew on multiple forms of knowledge. He specifically drew from Dennis Carlson's (1998) reading of Plato's *dialogues* to suggest that critical pedagogues could interweave different teaching voices in order to better achieve political goals. Carlson suggested that Plato distinguished between three prime rhetorical styles:

> *logos*, an analytic voice of critique associated with the truth games of science and philosophy; *thymos*, a voice of rage at injustice from the perspective and position of the disempowered, the disenfranchised, and the marginalized; and *mythos*, a personal voice of story-telling, cultural mythology, autobiography, and literature. (p. 543)

Carlson reported that Plato's mission, and possibly even the broader mission of philosophy, has been to disaggregate these three voices while simultaneously privileging the voice of logos (the "objective" voice of science). Carlson suggested that the postmodern project had more recently worked to reveal "voices" that had been marginalized in the modern academy and to encourage a blurring between different rhetorical styles. He added:

> The new postmodern academic voice is a hybrid voice that crosses borders, one that interweaves voices of *logos*, *thymos*, and *mythos* and that shifts back and forth from analysis to anecdote, from theory to personal story-telling, from principled talk of social justice to personal and positioned expressions of outrage at injustice. (p. 543)

In adopting the differing rhetorical styles approach, Richard now teaches critically about fatness using multiple voices. He still draws on the rhetorical style of *logos* by presenting competing scientific knowledges to illustrate that the truths about fatness and health are debated, but he also interweaves research on the problems of weight discrimination and stigmatizing, such as Rebecca Puhl and Chelsea Heuer's (2009) epidemiological work on the stigma of "obesity." With respect to *mythos*, he draws on narratives that reveal individuals' stories of fat prejudice and bullying and on the use of video clips from films such as *Hairspray*, which connects racism with body discrimination, specifically, prejudice against fatness. The voice of *thymos* (rage) is reflected upon in drawing from the work of fat activists (e.g., National Association to Advance Fat Acceptance or the Obesity Action Coalition) and associated blogs. The voice of rage is clearly evident, for example, in Sleepydumpling's (2012) blog, where she reports:

> When it comes to social justice, which is what fat activism is a form of, anger is a completely understandable emotion to feel, and to see from social justice activists. Because really, we're talking about injustices here. We're talking about the oppression of people based on their size. We're talking about the open hatred of people because of their weight. We're talking about social and medical discrimination of human beings. We're talking physical, emotional and social abuse of a whole swath of people, simply because their bodies don't fit into a narrow, arbitrary measure of "acceptable." I say there's something wrong with you if you're not getting angry about this. In fact, I get angry about ALL forms of social injustice, be they based on gender, size, race, sexuality, spiritual beliefs, physical ability, economic status or beyond. I get angry at the marginalisation and oppression of human beings for any arbitrary reason. *Because it's fucking wrong!* (para. 4.; emphasis in original)

In comparison to the deconstructive pedagogical strategy, the employment of differing rhetorical styles has had more apparent impact in disrupting dominant understandings about "obesity." The students become aware that scientific understandings of fat are subject to change and challenge and that much uncertainty and confusion exist. Yet they also become aware, via research findings, of how fat discourses can stigmatize, harm individuals, and produce ill health. In addition, through the use of various biographical narratives, film clips, and blogs, they gain a sense of empathy and concern with respect to how messages about fatness circulate within schools. And for some, they develop a sense of rage and subsequent desire to disrupt this circulation. As such, we are hopeful that some of our trainee teachers will eventually act as change agents in their future teaching.

Final Words

Scientific understandings about the interconnections between health, diet, fatness, and fitness have changed markedly since the 1950s. Yet dominant discourses still circulate in schools to simplistically position "obesity" as a health problem—a problem, however, that can be allegedly solved if individuals learn to make the "right" choices about diet and physical activity. This pedagogy of individualism contributes to the discursive construction of fat people as irresponsible, weak-willed, unhealthy, and immoral. Such discourses, we argue, inadvertently act to legitimize the stigmatization, marginalization, and abuse of fat children in schools: abuse that in itself causes health problems. To disrupt the circulation of problematic "obesity" discourses in schools, this chapter illustrated how critical pedagogical techniques revolving around the *deconstruction* of "obesity" knowledge and the use of *multiple rhetorical styles* can be employed in the training of teachers. Although we acknowledge that it is difficult to socially engineer understandings of bodies, health, weight, and fatness, we have illustrated that these pedagogies show promise in disrupting problematic understandings of "obesity" and can work to blur associated binaries (e.g., good/bad food, good/poor choices, fat is unhealthy/thin is healthy). We accordingly hope that this chapter works to challenge weight bias and encourages teachers and students to problematize the simplistic "obesity" and health messages that circulate in schools.

References

American Academy of Pediatrics. (2013). *Teasing and bullying of obese and overweight children: How parents can help*. Retrieved from http://www.healthychildren.org/English/healthissues/conditions/obesity/Pages/Teasing-and-Bullying.aspx

Ayo, N. (2012). Understanding health promotion in a neoliberal climate and the making of health conscious citizens. *Critical Public Health, 22*(1), 99–105.

Burrows, L., & Wright, J. (2004). The good life: New Zealand children's perspectives on health and self. *Sport, Education and Society, 9*(2), 193–205.

Campos, P. (2004). *The obesity myth: Why America's obsession with weight is dangerous to your health*. New York, NY: Gotham.

Carlson, D. (1998). Finding a voice, and losing our way? *Educational Theory, 48*(4), 541–554.

Crawford, R. (1980). Healthism and the medicalization of everyday life. *International Journal of Health Services, 10*, 365–388.

Derrida, J. (1992). Force of law: The "mystical foundation of authority." In D. Cornell, M. Rosenfeld, & D. Carlson (Eds.), *Deconstruction and the possibility of justice* (pp. 3–67). New York, NY: Routledge.

Evans, J., Rich, E., & Davies, B. (2008). Health education or weight management in schools? *Physical Education Matters, 3*(1), 28–32.

Foucault, M. (1978). *The history of sexuality: Vol. 1. The will to knowledge*. London, England: Penguin.

Gard, M., & Wright, J. (2005). *The obesity epidemic: Science, morality, and ideology*. New York, NY: Routledge.

Jenkins, K. (1999). *Why history? Ethics and postmodernity*. London, England: Routledge.

Kinney, J. M. (2005). Challenges to rebuilding the US food pyramid. *Current Opinion in Clinical Nutrition & Metabolic Care, 8*(1), 1–7.

Kirk, D. (2006). The "obesity crisis" and school physical education. *Sport, Education and Society, 11*(2), 121–133.

Leahy, D. (2009). Disgusting pedagogies. In J. Wright & V. Harwood (Eds.), *Biopolitics and the obesity epidemic: Governing bodies* (pp. 172–182). New York, NY: Routledge.

Leahy, D. (2012). *Assembling a health[y] subject* (Doctoral dissertation). Deakin University, Melbourne, Australia.

Life Education Trust. (n.d.). *Warrant of fitness*. Wellington, New Zealand: Author.

Life Education Trust. (2011). *Warrant of fitness*. Retrieved from http://www.lifeeducation.org.nz/schools/The+Life+Education+Programme/Warrant+of+Fitness+Year+7++8.html

Nestlé New Zealand. (2011). *Be healthy, be active: Teachers' resource*. Wellington, New Zealand: Learning Media.

New Zealand Beef and Lamb Marketing Bureau. (n.d.). *Iron Brion's hunt for gold resource kit*. Auckland, New Zealand: Author.

Paoli, A., Rubini, A., Volek, J. S., & Grimaldi, K. A. (2013). Beyond weight loss: A review of the therapeutic uses of very-low-carbohydrate (ketogenic) diets. *European Journal of Clinical Nutrition, 67*(8), 789–796.

Powell, D., & Fitzpatrick, K. (2013). "Getting fit basically just means, like, nonfat": Children's lessons in fitness and fatness. *Sport, Education and Society, 20*(4), 463–484.

Pringle, R., & Pringle, D. (2012). Competing obesity discourses and critical challenges for physical educators. *Sport, Education and Society, 17*(2), 143–162.

Puhl, R., & Heuer, C. (2009). Weight bias: A review and update. *Obesity, 17*(5), 941–964.

Ross, B. (2005). Fat or fiction: Weighing the "obesity epidemic." In M. Gard & J. Wright (Eds.), *The obesity epidemic: Science, morality and ideology* (pp. 86–106). London, England: Routledge.

Schwandt, T. A. (1996). Farewell to criteriology. *Qualitative Inquiry, 2*(1), 58–72.

Sleepydumpling. (2012, February 8). Rage against injustice. Retrieved from http://fattheffalump.wordpress.com/2012/02/08/rage-against-injustice/

Tinning, R. (2002). Toward a "modest pedagogy": Reflections on the problematics of critical pedagogy. *Quest, 54*, 224–240.

Tinning, R. (2014). Getting *which* message across? The (H)PE teacher as health educator. In K. Fitzpatrick & R. Tinning (Eds.), *Health education: Critical perspectives* (pp. 204–219). Oxford, England: Routledge.

Trost, S. (2006). Public health and physical education. In D. Kirk, D. Macdonald, & M. O'Sullivan (Eds.), *Handbook of physical education* (pp. 163–188). London, England: Sage.

THIRTEEN

Recognizing and Representing Bodies of Difference Through Art Education

Lori Don Levan

Since children form their opinions about the world through multiple experiences, it is important to remember that many types of influences will shape their attitudes. If those influences are numerous and go unchallenged, they can begin to form the basis for developing stereotypes. Those stereotypes might include negative characteristics that pertain to gender, race, and ethnicity, for instance. Fatness is one kind of human characteristic that has acquired social negativity as represented through various stereotypes (Levan, 2004). If children never encounter fat people in their life experiences and/or never encounter positive examples of fatness, then the stereotype will begin to stand in for the "real thing" and the negative attitudes and bias that support those stereotypes can be perpetuated throughout that child's lifetime (Bergen, 2001). For fat children, the stereotype might serve as a point of comparison that could work against them through the process of internalization.

As a fat studies scholar and art educator, part of what I am concerned with is how fatness is portrayed in the visual arts and visual culture and how prejudice against fatness might be affecting my students and their artistic practice. I have worked with students ranging in age from preschool through adult. As part of my doctoral studies at Teachers College, Columbia University, I worked with children aged 4 through 16 by asking them to draw what they think fat people look like. What I discovered is that there was a great reluctance among children and adolescents to represent fatness in their image making. This chapter is primarily concerned with how fat stigma might be negatively affecting children and adolescents as they develop opinions about themselves and their own body image as well as that of other people, and how that affects what they choose to represent or not in their art. My discussion is focused through the lens of art education where visual representation is considered a process of meaning-making. I also discuss how what I learned has affected my current teaching practice at the college level.

Representing Bodies of Difference

If children can be influenced by visual representations of the human body that exist in the world around us, how do they process this information? In the field of art education, much research has been conducted on childhood development and visual representation (Burrill, 2005; Burton, 2000, 2009; Campbell, Simmons, & National Art Education Association, 2012; Chapman, 1978; Day & Hurwitz, 2011; Gaitskell & Gaitskell, 1954; Kindler & Wilson, 1997; Lowenfeld, 1952). While it is not within the scope of this chapter to present a full discussion of this research, I provide a brief discussion of how childhood development has been linked to drawing the human figure in order to provide context.

Childhood Development and Drawing

Individual development follows a sequence that combines cognitive, emotional, and creative growth (Lowenfeld, 1952). Growth can manifest itself in different ways; language acquisition, the ability to solve problems, independent decision-making, and physical changes are just a few. Through visual imaging children and adults alike can express themselves in ways that are unavailable to them through other types of expression, such as writing poetry, for instance. The drawing activity of children and adolescents, and people of all ages, for that matter, can provide a way for them to better understand the world they experience. Drawings leave a record that can be used to communicate or simply be used as a way to work out an interest or problem at hand. Drawings also reflect the internalization of socially dictated norms. This is different from what artists do when they draw for artistic expression.

Developmental psychologists and art educators who study child development through visual imaging often look at how the human body is represented through stage theory modeled after Piaget (1954, 1959). Stage theory suggests that cognitive development follows a certain path as a child grows. This path is divided into predictable stages that depend on each other for further growth to take place. Children's drawings can provide documents that record visually where they are developmentally. Over time, the developmental stages that a child is going through will emerge in the sequence of drawings produced by that child. A well-known example of stage theory in art education comes from Viktor Lowenfeld's *Creative and Mental Growth* (1952). His stages focus on the time between approximately 2 and 13 years of age. According to Lowenfeld, recognizable representations of the human figure begin at about 4 or 5 years when the child develops a need to satisfy "a desire to establish a relationship between his drawing and reality" (p. 26). The first figural images generally start with some sort of enclosure, such as a circle, that represents the head and body. Lines may be drawn to represent limbs and sometimes oddly placed facial features will be present within the enclosure. As children develop, they begin to expand their figural representations based on new experiences, greater conceptual awareness of the body, and continued creative and mental growth. By the time they reach about 13 years of age, children reach an intermediate "crisis" stage in which they realize that their current methods of expression are no longer appropriate and they may regress or abandon image-making altogether if they do not get helpful guidance.

Passage through these stages depends on children's use of their active knowledge and their ability to use it when creating visual images. The teacher's role in a child-centered approach is to help children connect with their active knowledge. Art educators who use this type of approach see drawing as an activity that reflects children's relationships to the world around them

(Lansing, 1976). It is considered a meaning-making process rather than an artistic process; however, it can lead to and can be used towards artistic practice as the child matures. Drawings are often used in order to discover the ways in which children make meaning in their world. The process is the most important part of the activity and the drawing is merely an end product. Dialogue is very important to this process, so children are encouraged to share their experiences with their teachers and others while they draw to understand what their thinking process is at the moment.

My early training as an art educator was heavily influenced by this developmental theory and resulting pedagogy. Since then I have had the opportunity to teach art at many levels that range from kindergarten to adult education, and in many settings including public schools and colleges. Eventually, I came to a point in my teaching practice where I started to ask myself questions about my younger students that I had not asked before. I started to wonder whether children actually did draw a diverse range of body types, including fat ones. Many additional questions arose. How often do children represent different body types, if they do at all? How can we identify these body types? What would happen if we asked children directly to draw different types of bodies? How are different bodies defined and/or (re)presented by children? How much do social perceptions determine what children do and do not draw? Are children editing themselves as they develop a greater understanding of what is "good" and "bad"? Do children stereotype their body schema according to their own socialized prejudices about the human body? If so, could we say that children do not always draw what they know, but what they have been conditioned to (re)present?

Fat and Skinny

I decided to try to answer some of these questions. To do so I developed and implemented a pilot study and collected children's drawings between 1997 and 2000. Three teachers in the New York City area helped me collect the drawings and reported on their students' reactions. What follows is a brief discussion of the study and what I found out about what happens when children are specifically asked to draw a fat person.

Draw Me a Picture

Three teachers volunteered to collect drawings in their art classes in the New York City area in the first two rounds and I collected one round of data in my own art classroom in Harlem. Children from different backgrounds and ethnicities were present in the classroom environments. The ages of the children ranged from about 6 to 13 years old and included boys and girls. Of the children who participated in the study, only three were identified by their teachers as fat. For this reason, the study did not include special attention to them as a sub-group. The drawings were gathered in three rounds with a few minor procedural adjustments made between the first and second round and again in the third round. Approximately 600 drawings were collected through this process, including the drawings I collected in my own classroom.

No discussion of body diversity was conducted before the exercise so that the students would not be influenced by it. In the first two rounds, the students were asked to make three drawings. The first drawing was to be a picture of the student with a friend or friends doing something to determine a baseline for their drawing style, to make some visual connections between the drawings and what the children looked like, and to give them a comfortable way to begin the series. For the second drawing, the children were asked to draw a picture of a skinny person whom they knew doing something, because I wanted the drawings to be active. For the third drawing, the children were asked to draw a picture of a fat person in the same manner. I planned to use the words "fat" and "skinny" for all age groups in the study, but the teachers and my supervisor felt that "heavier than" and "lighter than" would be more appropriate for the older students in one of the schools. I did not agree with this need to change the terms since we planned to use them with the younger students, but I did compromise so that I still would be able to gather the drawings. I also suspected that the request to change the terms reflected more the discomfort of the adults than concern for the children's feelings.

You Want Me to Do What?!

What initially had seemed like a pretty straightforward request for drawings turned out to be quite a challenge in all three rounds of data collection. In rounds one and two, the students were receptive to making drawings about themselves with a friend and of a skinny person, but almost across the board there was a definite reluctance to draw the fat (or "heavier than") person. As reported by the teachers in the first two rounds, protests included a range of negative reactions from the students. Many of the children felt that they should not have to draw a fat person as it would be an insult to the person they were drawing, they did not want to use the word "fat," they thought that the request was prejudiced, and/or they chose to represent cartoon characters and, in the case of some boys, WWF wrestlers. All three teachers had to coax many of the students to make their fat person drawings; still, in the end, with a few exceptions some kind of drawing was made. For the older students, who readily translated "heavier than" as fat, a need to identify themselves as "normal" emerged in the comments that they made about themselves in the context of doing the drawings. To me, this reflected reluctance on their part to possibly identify themselves as fat people, despite the adults' attempts to somehow make them feel more comfortable with the subject matter by using a substitute for the word "fat."

For the third round, I was able to collect the drawings myself. I asked students to make a different series of drawings in this round to avoid some of the confusion that unfolded in the earlier rounds. Some of the younger children in the first two rounds seemed to interpret the word "fat" to mean "big." This would make sense, since children are small in relation to most adults. I wondered, then, if "fat" and "big" might be represented in similar ways, especially when it came to representing adults. To find out if this overlap would still emerge, I asked the children to draw big and fat as two different people. In this round, the children were given a larger sheet of paper than they had been given in the first two and told that they would be drawing several people standing next to each other. A game emerged as the children were asked first to draw themselves, then a small person, a big person, a skinny person, and a fat person. The children got to guess what the next person would be as they went along. When it came to drawing the fat person (who was last in the sequence), the same kinds of protests emerged as in the previous two rounds although the children did continue with encouragement from me and most produced a drawing that showed all of the body types.

When it came time to draw a big person, all of the students made drawings without difficulty and none of them represented a fat person. As with the first two rounds, however, many stereotypes emerged in the fat person drawing. The fat person usually did not have any kind of identity (lacked details and was not named or associated with any real person as most of the other drawings were). Since I facilitated this round of data collection myself, I wondered how my own fat body type might influence what the students wanted to draw since the three teachers who participated in the first two rounds would not be considered fat by conventional standards. My own size did not seem to be an issue though and, interestingly, the children never chose to use me as the example of a fat person. I did monitor the children's drawing process and asked many of them to tell me something about their work. In one case, I noticed that a 4-year-old girl who had been drawing happily as we went along seemed to stop when I asked the group to draw a fat person. So I circulated to her seat and asked her a few questions about the people she had been drawing. When I asked her where the fat person was, she didn't answer my question. When I asked her whether she was okay, she said she was, and so I asked why the fat person was missing. She looked up at me and said that she hated all fat people and that she was not going to make that drawing. I am not sure whether she meant for that to be directed at me, her fat teacher, since she was only four years old; nonetheless, I took it as a sobering illustration of how prejudices can develop at a very early age (Bergen, 2001).

More Questions

When a child makes a drawing, is she always representing what she knows? How much do attitudes and prejudices play a role in what a child will or will not represent? If a child is asked to draw something that is uncomfortable, then attitudes towards the subject itself might determine how it is represented. A child is asked to draw a fat person. That child has been socialized to think that fat and fat people are bad in some way. She might be concerned about fat being an insult. To call someone fat and/or to draw someone who is fat might mean you are making fun of that person. The child may not want to insult anyone or may have hostile feelings towards the concept of fatness. Therefore, the child may choose not to draw at all or might produce extreme stereotyped images.

Children may not be able to deal with extremes beyond their own experiences but we also know that they can be very imaginative. If a child can depict in great detail his grandmother as a giant dragon that has to be defeated by him and his father and his uncle dressed as ninjas (something that actually happened in a class I was teaching), why might he have trouble drawing a picture of a fat person based on imagination if not recollection? Conflicted feelings about the subject matter and the perception of children's own body image and where they fit in might be rendering them unable to represent fatness. In this study, many of the children depicted fat people as having to choose between eating and losing weight, as inactive, and in a negative light. For instance, fat people were portrayed as lazy, out of control, and alone.

And how did this play out for fat kids? There were only three fat children identified in the study I have described. One of those children chose to draw herself ice skating with her dad, and she did depict herself as appearing heavier than the other children whom she included in her set of drawings. She was one of the few children to depict a positive and active image of fatness.

Children also might be censoring themselves. They may not always be drawing what they know even if they themselves are fat or have seen fat people around them in different settings. They might be drawing what they feel safe drawing given internalized ideals. What did they *not* draw, and why, became fascinating questions for me to consider. Perhaps children aren't drawing fat people because they have learned that fat people are bad. Fat people have been socially marginalized, demonized, and rendered invisible. Children observe how other children and adults treat fat people: name-calling, rejection from social groups, nice to your face but making fun behind your back, unsolicited advice about health and looks; for girls, "you have such a pretty face, if only…", for boys, correlating big with aggressive or if not, considered wimps (Brumberg, 1997; Pope, Phillips, & Olivardia, 2000). Combine these behaviors with constant visual reminders in magazines, TV, social media, and advertising, and the result may indeed be a dangerous mix likely resulting in confusion and moral conflict.

Implications for My Teaching Practice

In the years since I conducted that study, I have used what I learned to actively engage my college students in activities that bring a sense of social consciousness around body diversity to my classroom. My original study was partially grounded in the assumption that fat phobia and fat oppression exist and many people have written about this in the years since the pilot study was conducted (e.g., Farrell, 2011; Gard & Wright, 2005; Rothblum & Solovay, 2009). While the study was conducted 15 years ago, I think that the results remain relevant to this day. In general, fat phobia continues to act as a policing agent that affects all people through attempted regulation of the body. Specifically, fat phobia polices women and serves to subordinate their power in a patriarchal context (Bordo, 1993; Wolf, 1991). Chela Sandoval in *Methodology of the Oppressed* (2000) proposes "a method of oppositional consciousness" (pp. xii, 2) that applies specifically to oppression occurring in the United States and the so-called Third World, and that offers a plan of action for people of color. I have been inspired by her work as well as that of Paulo Freire (1990), Michel Foucault (1977), and others who hold that liberation from oppression is possible but can only occur through education and social action. By exposing and disrupting the visualizing language of oppression that surrounds fat phobia and fat oppression, and examining the images that emerge in visual culture, an argument can be made that the system of oppression that attempts to regulate fatness links to systems of oppression towards difference in general. Understanding where these systems intersect and how they may be resisted will provide a direction for social action that redirects attention to fat phobia and fat discrimination.

What Can Happen in the Classroom?

Images from magazines reinforce self-monitoring by promoting and advertising products a person might need to improve a "flawed" self (Levan, 2014). Constant help and maintenance are needed to make sure no one else discovers these flaws. Weight Watchers, Jenny Craig, Curves, and the like also market themselves more often to women than to men, sometimes exclusively so. Excessive attention paid to diet and activity is masked by a concern for health when the reality is that the products these companies are selling are designed to have consumers obsessively monitor and sculpt their bodies, carefully molding them into a social ideal that is impossible to achieve for most. It saddened me to see the need to lose weight surfacing in some of the children's drawings with fat people depicted as having to choose between eating and losing weight.

Wanting to pursue this work further, I decided that I would design activities in some of my college courses to uncover weight bias in visual culture. To that end, I used collage as a visualizing activity for a women's studies class I was teaching. The course was an advanced undergraduate class focused on women in the arts, so we began our studies with the Guerrilla

Girls and their text on art history (1998) and on female stereotypes (2003). Once we had discussed key concepts in the texts and the politics of the Guerrilla Girls, I asked the students to participate in a collage activity. Students were asked to construct a person using magazine images that fit a certain body type. The body types they used were written on slips of paper that were pulled out of a hat. On the slips of paper were written four descriptive words that were to be used to guide their image-making. For example, they might get the description "tall, fat, female, old" or "short, average, male, young." To make the collage, they were told to use the magazine images to construct their person. They could not just cut out an image of a person that fit the description; rather, they had to actually construct that person using body parts that could be modified as necessary. I explained that the result would be a creative and interesting image that reflected the level of difficulty that the descriptive words created for that person. Once the images were completed, the students were asked to write a short introduction to their person and name him or her. Then they answered a series of questions that highlighted the different concepts that were raised in our discussion of the activity as it related to the texts that we had been studying.

I was always pleasantly surprised at how receptive my students were to this activity. Unlike the young students in my pilot study, I never observed anyone who could not or did not want to participate based on the body type on his or her slip of paper. Through our discussions about the activity, the students observed that magazine images of people were very restricted to certain types of bodies and unless the magazine was aimed at a specific market in which diverse body types might be ghettoized, diverse bodies were not represented in them. We were able to examine our own assumptions about body diversity and how those assumptions might have been developed over time. Some students were able to propose action plans for breaking stereotypes, sometimes on campus through the Women's Center or other venues as well as in their own lives. The catalyst for this call to action was the art-making activity that gave the students a concrete way to explore the ideas we had been dealing with on a theoretical level and put them into a living context. It offered a chance for the students to engage in reflective and critical thought concerning their own ideas about diverse body types and where they fit into the greater social systems that promote negative stereotypes.

I also have used this collage activity in college workshops dealing with body image. Usually for a mix of undergraduate and graduate women, the focus of the workshops has been on stereotyping and the media. Many observations and questions have come out of the discussions and the participants are often surprised to find how restrictive the media images that we were using seemed to be. I have also used this activity with art teachers in conference situations during which the subject of the workshop was diversity and inclusiveness in the art classroom. I use the collage activity not only to help the teachers see what kinds of stereotypes are present in visual media but also to help them understand their own prejudices as teachers. Most of the teachers who participated in these workshops were very receptive to ensuing discussions concerning body diversity, although several teachers were not. Of those who resisted, it appeared that much of their resistance centered on their own discomfort with fat bodies and their unwillingness at that point to confront their own prejudices about fatness. While it is not within the scope of this chapter to discuss the workshops in greater detail, I have included their mention here to show that art-making and dialogue together can help learners engage in critical reflection and help them to confront internalized biases that might be affecting their teaching.

Conclusion

Attitudes towards fatness are shaped in intricate ways, often with moral judgment at the center; visual images can support and reinforce fat phobia. As children begin to solidify their own ideas and become socialized to prevailing attitudes, their actions will reflect what they have come to believe is true. The child who says, "All fat people are ugly, I hate them!" is expressing a socially perpetuated stereotype that reflects the anxieties and fears that we all face concerning our weight. How might we find ways to develop a more inclusive aesthetic that reflects diverse bodies? For those of us who choose to challenge these stereotypes, part of the process is helping others understand that our concerns have merit. As an educator, I have taken on the challenge because it means that at least some of my students will become thoughtful people who are willing to examine their own beliefs about body size critically. Using art-making as a tool can be a very powerful path towards enlightenment.

References

Bergen, T. J. (2001). The development of prejudice in children. *Education, 122*(1), 154–162.

Bordo, S. (1993). *Unbearable weight: Feminism, Western culture, and the body.* Berkeley, CA: University of California Press.

Brumberg, J. (1997). *The body project: An intimate history of American girls.* New York, NY: Vintage.

Burrill, R. R. (2005). Natural biology vs. cultural structures: Art and child development in education. *Teaching Artist Journal, 3*(1), 31–40.

Burton, J. M. (2000). The configuration of meaning: Learner-centered art education revisited. *Studies in Art Education, 41*(4), 330–345.

Burton, J. M. (2009). Creative intelligence, creative practice: Lowenfeld redux. *Studies in Art Education, 50*(4), 323–337.

Campbell, L. H., Simmons, S., & National Art Education Association. (2012). *The heart of art education: Holistic approaches to creativity, integration, and transformation.* Reston, VA: National Art Education Association.

Chapman, L. (1978). *Approaches to art in education.* New York, NY: Harcourt Brace Jovanovich.

Day, M., & Hurwitz, A. (2011). *Children and their art: Art education for elementary and middle schools* (9th ed.). Boston, MA: Wadsworth Cengage Learning.

Farrell, A. E. (2011). *Fat shame: Stigma and the fat body in American culture.* New York, NY: New York University Press.

Freire, P. (1990). *Pedagogy of the oppressed.* New York, NY: Continuum.

Foucault, M. (1977). *Discipline and punish: The birth of the prison.* New York, NY: Vintage.

Gaitskell, C. D., & Gaitskell, M. R. (1954). *Art education during adolescence.* Toronto, ON, Canada: Ryerson Press.

Gard, M., & Wright, J. (2005). *The obesity epidemic: Science, morality and ideology.* New York, NY: Routledge.

Guerrilla Girls. (1998). *The Guerrilla Girls' bedside companion to the history of Western art.* New York, NY: Penguin.

Guerrilla Girls. (2003). *Bitches, bimbos, and ballbreakers: The Guerrilla Girls' illustrated guide to female stereotypes.* New York, NY: Penguin.

Kindler, A. M., & Wilson, B. (1997). *Child development in art.* Reston, VA: National Art Education Association.

Lansing, K. M. (1976). *Art, artists and art education.* Dubuque, IA: Kendall/Hunt.

Levan, L. (2004). *Fat beauty: Giving voice to the lived experience of fat women through a search for and creation of sites of resistance* (Doctoral dissertation). Teachers College, Columbia University, New York.

Levan, L. (2014). Fat bodies in space: Controlling fatness through anthropometric measurement, corporeal conformity, and visual representation. *Fat Studies, 3*(2), 119–129.

Lowenfeld, V. (1952). *Creative and mental growth.* New York, NY: Macmillan.

Piaget, J. (1954). *The child's construction of reality.* London, England: Routledge.

Piaget, J. (1959). *The psychology of intelligence.* London, England: Routledge.

Pope, H., Phillips, K., & Olivardia, R. (2000). *The Adonis complex: How to identify, treat and prevent body obsession in men and boys.* New York, NY: Simon & Schuster.

Rothblum, E., & Solovay, S. (2009). *The fat studies reader.* New York, NY: New York University Press.

Sandoval, C. (2000). *Methodology of the oppressed.* Minneapolis, MN: University of Minnesota Press.

Wolf, N. (1991). *The beauty myth: How images of beauty are used against women.* New York, NY: Anchor Books.

FOURTEEN

Moving Beyond Body Image: A Socio-Critical Approach to Teaching About Health and Body Size

Jan Wright and Deana Leahy

Concerns about young people's (read, young women's) body dissatisfaction in schools have resulted in the introduction of programs promoting positive body image in an effort to reduce eating disorders. These programs, informed by psychological or socio-psychological notions of the relations between self and bodies, seem to have considerable credibility in schools and in the academic literature because of their authoritative underpinnings. In this chapter, we want to examine the ways in which such programs engage with discourses around bodies, fat, and size. For example, do they challenge discourses of weight-based oppression, create safe spaces for learning about weight and size, and/or (re)produce normative notions of individual responsibility and health?

The term "body image" has come to be used widely in the academic world, clinical practice, schools, and popular culture to signify a range of meanings, but mostly these days, meanings associated with body weight and shape. The body image programs we examine in this chapter are firmly embedded in a psychological tradition founded on the view that an individual's own subjective experience of their appearance, which may not be the same as the social "reality" of their appearance (Cash, 2004), impacts how they interact with the world. For Thomas Cash, this "inside view" is what underpins psychological research on body image, the "multifaceted psychological experience of embodiment" or "one's body-related self-perceptions and self-attitudes" (p. 1). From Cash's perspective, body-related perceptions are not only related to appearance; he points to an increasing emphasis on clinical and psychiatric research focusing on eating disorders among young women. This focus has been criticized as reinforcing the notion that body image only concerns girls and young women, and is primarily about body weight and shape (Cash, 2004; Pruzinsky & Cash, 2002).

Body image's genesis in psychology means that it has inherited certain understandings of the individual and ways of understanding how individuals think and behave. Research on body image is dominated by psychological scales of body (dis)satisfaction and self-esteem that have and continue to inform how interventions are imagined and enacted. In her paper assessing the contribution of psychological theory and research to understanding women's pervasive body image discontent, Linda Wolszon (1998) points to the "*individualistic* moral outlook and a narrowly instrumental view of human action and personality" (p. 543, emphasis in original) that underpins body image research. She argues that body image researchers and, as we argue later in this chapter, body image interventions, assume individuals who can separate themselves from the social pressures and constraints of life, individuals who can abstract themselves from their lived body experiences. This is not to say that body image proponents do not acknowledge cultural expectations about appearance but such attention is often tokenistic without a theoretical explanation of the relationship between the social and the individual. Their focus rather is on "self-determination and the power of personal effort" (Wolszon, 1998, p. 549) in resisting social and cultural messages. We would argue that this is particularly evident in contemporary school programs that assume knowing how media images of women are manipulated to make them appear more attractive is sufficient to diminish their effect.

Wolszon (1998) argues that such an approach also assumes women are "'cultural dopes' (Davis, 1995) who have blindly and stupidly colluded with irrational cultural practices" (p. 549). She goes on to say that "such a perspective is ultimately demeaning and overlooks women's creative participation, negotiation and resistance to cultural narratives concerning what a woman should do and be" (p. 553). This is not to say that there is an absence of feminist writing in the field of body image research. Indeed, feminist concerns about widespread reporting of women's unhappiness with their appearance have influenced the turn to eating disorder research and interventions. For example, in her contribution to the book *Body Image*, Nita McKinley (2002) draws on social constructivist feminist writing to draw attention to how "women's normative body dissatisfaction is not a function of individual pathology but a systematic social phenomenon" (p. 55). Women and girls are constituted as objects of the gaze, to "be watched and evaluated in terms of how their bodies fit cultural standards" (p. 56). According to McKinley, they learn from an early age to watch themselves and to objectify their own bodies in order to avoid approbation and to attract approval. On the basis of this logic, McKinley developed a measure of "objectified body consciousness" (OBC) to "study the internalization of social constructions of women's bodies" (p. 56). Items in the OBC include measures of body surveillance, body shame, and appearance control beliefs. The psychological context of this work means that a more sophisticated view of the social impacts on bodily experiences is again reduced to measurable internal individualized states that are assumed to predict the likelihood of eating disorders.

Body Image Interventions

The association of body image dissatisfaction with eating disorders has led inevitably to the proliferation of interventions. These have targeted children and young people perceived to be "at risk" of eating disorders and, perhaps more problematically, the general student population of schools. Most of these interventions have been directed at girls and young women, but increasingly interventions have included boys and young men as the eating disorder literature has pointed to the growing "risks" for the male population subjected to "ideal" images of masculinity in the media and elsewhere (Vandenbosch & Eggermont, 2013).

The most widely used approach in these interventions is a "psychoeducation" approach designed to "teach specific strategies for changing participants' social and personal environments, thoughts, attitudes, and behaviours" (Pruzinsky & Cash, 2002, p. 488). School-based programs taking this approach are underpinned by social learning theory and behavior therapy (Levine & Smolak, 2002). These programs usually take 6 to 12 weeks and are presented by specialists (i.e., psychologists or body image researchers) and/or teachers.

In a review of programs, Michael Levine and Linda Smolak (2002) suggest that results vary considerably; while there seems to be some positive effect on self-esteem and eating behaviors, they are usually short term. They note that it is surprising, given the importance of sociocultural influences in shaping negative body image and disordered eating, that so many interventions focus on "students as individuals and not on changing the physical and social environments that frame negative body image" (p. 498). They thus argue that psychoeducation programs are insufficient to "foster critical understanding of the body-in-context and to effect healthy changes in relationships, norms [and] values" (p. 498). As alternatives to psychoeducation programs, Levine and Smolak point to activist and ecological approaches to the prevention of eating disorders, including what they call "a relational empowerment model" that builds on feminist theory, media literacy, and a Health Promoting Schools (HPS) model. They provide several examples of relational empowerment models that draw on feminist theory to construct programs that work with the participants' shared meanings of the contextual factors that "shape participants' body image feelings and actions" (p. 498).

Levine and Smolak also describe Niva Piran's work with an elite residential ballet company with program goals "derived from dialogue with the group, not from quantitative research generated by experts seeking to apply general psychosocial principles" (p. 499). Piran's program goes well beyond individual body perceptions:

> The active processes of describing and then critically evaluating "lived experiences" of racism, harassment, and gender inequity help participants transform the private feelings of shame, concealment, and frustration inherent in body dissatisfaction into a shared public understanding. Permitting girls to voice the truths in their own lives sets the stage for the construction of alternative healthier norms and practices within the group, and from there to individual and group actions that change environments outside the group. (p. 499)

Finally, Levine and Smolak turn their attention to Health Promoting Schools as a model that directly addresses the school and community environment where "students, staff, teachers, parent and community resources share the responsibility for constructing healthier school environments" (p. 501). The turn to HPS is not a surprising one given that it has held significant currency and appeal in the schools and health literature. Despite attempting to address the broader social and environmental aspects of schooling, however, the kinds of aspirations inherent in the HPS model are precarious to say the least. For example, the idea that students, staff, parents, and the community share responsibility for constructing healthier school environments assumes that there is a consensus among people around any health issue, in this case body image, given the HPS approach advocates that health messages be consistent across what is being taught, all teachers in the school, their resources, and parents. Consistency is difficult in a context in which efforts to encourage feeling positive about one's body come up against "obesity" prevention initiatives that use shame and disgust to demonize "overweight" bodies

(Leahy, 2009). In fact, we would suggest that while teaching for positive body image has always been difficult, the dominant "obesity" discourse in contemporary times makes this work even more difficult, if not impossible.

A Closer Look at School-Based Body Image Programs

As Levine and Smolak (2002) illustrate, on the one hand the psychoeducation body image approach is one usually designed and administered by mental health professionals or academics for an identified "at risk" group. School-based body image programs, on the other hand, target whole school or year group populations, not a small group identified as "at risk" of eating disorders. The school programs, however, often draw on the same strategies and activities. Both kinds of programs seem to work on the assumption that girls and young women are "unrealistically" unhappy with their potentially "normal" bodies and that they are making unrealistic estimations of their body size. This raises questions about what happens when these programs are used in schools. How do they take account of the realistic feelings of shame and alienation at least partially generated by messages in their health and physical education and other classes that frame "obesity" and "overweight" as health problems and as moral problems where individuals are assumed to be irresponsible, indulgent, and lazy (Leahy 2009)? This becomes particularly interesting when programs claim to address simultaneously issues of "obesity" and eating disorders (e.g., O'Dea, 2007).

In the following analysis, we describe a number of programs currently being used in schools and ask how these programs engage with discourses around bodies, fat, and size. Do they challenge discourses of weight-based oppression, create safe spaces for learning about weight and size, or (re)produce normative notions of individual responsibility and health?

What the Programs Have in Common

The conflation of body image with eating disorders already sets up a clinical relation between self and body, and health and behaviors. This is evident particularly in the assumption underpinning many of the programs that suggest improving self-esteem will mitigate the risk of disordered eating/poor health behaviors and that self-esteem can be improved by activities designed to encourage a positive body image, self-acceptance, and an understanding that "everyone is different." In programs that also target "obesity," the assumption seems to be that improving self-esteem will not only mitigate against disordered eating, but also help prevent "obesity" (e.g., O'Dea, 2007). Most recent interventions also include or have as their main component a section on media literacy, designed again to persuade participants in the program that they are being duped by the media into accepting unrealistic ideal images.

The simple relationships and implicitly moralistic positions underpinning many of the body image programs are exemplified in the Australian Government's (2012) *Body Image Information Sheets*. In these sheets, the normative body is not *any* body but a body that falls within particular parameters, i.e., not "unrealistically thin," or for boys, too muscular (Information Sheet 3), and there is a moral position on how a person should be—"people with a positive body image love their bodies for what they are" (Information Sheet 3), and we should and are all capable of developing better feelings about our bodies through self-discipline. This last directive seems to involve closely monitoring what we watch, read, and listen to as well as taking responsibility for how we are feeling:

Our body image is not set in stone; it is very susceptible to change by the influences around us. This means that we may improve our body image by minimising all the things we see, watch, read, and listen to that have a negative effect on our body image. It also means that we have the power to change the way we see, feel and think about our bodies! (Information Sheet 1)

In Information Sheet 5, we are also incited to "think and feel" happy: "try saying something positive to yourself everyday (i.e. 'I love my body'), you may just start believing it."

Through a series of imperatives, readers are ordered to take charge of their lives, to closely monitor everyday behavior, and govern their everyday thoughts and feelings. Given the ubiquity of images of slim and attractive bodies in all forms of media, together with the fat hate and shame evident in these same media, to realize these directives might necessitate withdrawing from normal life! The degree of power that one is assumed to have over one's actions, one's environment, and one's thinking is so extreme as to be absurd. However, these messages of individual rationality, autonomy, and capacity to change the way one thinks and feels, while not expressed quite so explicitly, are evident in other body image programs.

Happy Being Me

Happy Being Me is a school-based body image intervention program, usually presented by a trained facilitator (Richardson & Paxton, 2010). It consists of three sessions. The first targets media literacy and the reduction of "the internalization of the cultural appearance ideal." Content covers techniques used to manipulate media images and concepts such as "appearance does not equal how valuable you are" and "the "ideal body" differs across time and between cultures" (p. 115). The second session focuses on "fat talk" and teaches ways of handling fat talk directed at self and others. The third targets "body comparison," teaches about negative consequences of body comparisons, and explores strategies to deal with body comparison. Learning processes include didactic presentations, worksheets, role-plays, and class discussions prompted by film clips.

The program has been evaluated in Australia (with girls in their first year of high school) (Richardson & Paxton, 2010) and the U.K. (boys and girls between 10 and 11 years) (Bird, Halliwell, Diedrichs, & Harcourt, 2013). Assessment instruments used for the evaluation included tests of topic knowledge and questionnaire items on risk factors for eating disorders such as body (dis)satisfaction, attitudes towards appearance, appearance conversation (or talk about body appearance and size), weight teasing, dietary restraint, bulimic propensities, and self-esteem. On the basis of these measures, the Australian implementation is claimed to have had a positive impact post-intervention and at follow-up after a 3-month period. The program, according to the measures, did not have the desired impact on teasing about appearance directed towards peers. The U.K. program was less successful on the same measures, particularly over the longer term. Emma Bird and her colleagues (Bird, Halliwell, Diedrichs, & Harcourt, 2013) explain the failure of enduring effects in a number of ways, including the following:

> Children are regularly exposed to appearance-related pressures … and therefore, it may be that providing three 50 min sessions is insufficient to counter the socially normative behavior described by Jones and colleagues as an "appearance culture." (p. 323)

This seems, at best, a serious understatement and other explanations for the failure of such programs to have lasting effects on children and young people's feelings about themselves are suggested at the end of this section.

Everybody Is Different

Everybody's Different is a program developed by Australian dietician, health, and nutrition researcher Dr. Jenny O'Dea (2007) and published as a weighty 326-page book and as an online resource. Although part of its rationale is the prevention of eating disorders, it claims a broader focus: "A positive approach to teaching about health, puberty, body image, nutrition, self-esteem and obesity prevention." This program is interesting particularly because of its claim to address both eating disorders and "obesity" prevention. It is well-intentioned and great efforts are made to follow O'Dea's own dictum, "do no harm" (p. 47). For example, in the section "Weighty Issues and Child Obesity Prevention," she urges teachers to consider how "obesity" prevention activities may "inadvertently create or worsen body image concerns among students" (p. 227) and provides case studies on "the adverse effects of the well meaning preventive intentions" (p. 240). But the bottom line of the program is that it continues to address body dissatisfaction through improving self-esteem and encouraging "healthy eating and physical activity amongst children and adolescents" (p. 228). O'Dea argues that such an approach will address the prevention of both "obesity" and eating disorders "because the two issues are inextricably intertwined" (p. 228). This is achieved through activities that develop self-esteem through teaching that "everybody's different" and through education about the benefits of sound nutrition, growth and development lessons, and through lessons on media literacy.

O'Dea makes the claim, relatively unjustified we would argue (see Levine & Smolak, 2002), that "[m]edia literacy and media advocacy interventions are effective in the promotion of a positive body image" (p. 98). The main purpose of media literacy lessons in this context "is to encourage self-acceptance and help to reduce the internalisation of the thin ideal and the pervasive body image norms" in the context of "an overall self-esteem building approach" (p. 98). Like many similar programs, the focus of activities is on how particular stereotypes are used to sell products. For example, O'Dea writes that "one of the most salient lessons of media literacy is that virtually all media messages are linked to marketing activities which have commercial aims" and we "need to be aware of how media operates to create messages and 'sell' ideas and products" (p. 99). Like most of the media literacy components in other body image programs, *Everybody's Different* focuses narrowly on an ideal body constituted in advertisements and completely ignores other messages about fat bodies, including those promoted by government health campaigns and policies, reality TV programs such as *The Biggest Loser*, and regular commentary on the "obesity epidemic" on talk shows and so on.

Media Smart

The focus on media is central to another program called *Media Smart*, an eight-lesson media literacy program for girls and boys in late primary school or early high school, designed by psychologists from Flinders University. Like other media literacy interventions in the body image field, it assumes that the media play a major role in children's and young people's negative body image. Like other programs, its approach, therefore, is to demonstrate how the media manipulate images and to provide strategies for analyzing and challenging media messages. It is a program intended to be integrated into various areas of the curriculum or to student welfare programs.

Media Smart does seem to go further than other body image media literacy programs as it provides more time to develop content and emphasizes the importance of teaching the program in an interactive way and "not talking about eating disorders" (Wilksch & Wade,

2010a, p. 6). However, like other programs, it skirts around the social stigmatization of fat, and continues to reproduce health and medical notions of "overweight." For example, in a list of "don'ts," the program advises not to "comment on other people's appearance or weight" nor to "encourage weight as the *only* measure of health" (Wilksch & Wade, 2010b, p. 3, emphasis in original). This still suggests that weight should be a measure of health and does not allow for any critical engagement with that idea. As well, in a section on stereotypes, students are encouraged to think about "any people who do not fit the stereotypes in our society" (p. 5). The suggested examples for "females who might not fit the thin-ideal" are Kim from *Kath and Kim* and Kate Winslet. Kath and Kim are the lead female characters in an Australian situational comedy, and while Kath's body certainly does not conform to a thin ideal, it is telling that the fat character, Sharon (played by the Australian comedian Magda Szubanski), is not featured. We are not invited to like or admire Sharon or to examine how particular stereotypes about fatness are played out with her character. The choice of Kate Winslet also sends some very ambiguous messages. While she may not conform to the thin ideal (and, really, how thin does the ideal have to be?), her body is clearly not far outside normative social ideals. Does this mean that you can be round so long as you are also beautiful? All of this suggests that the designers of the program are not comfortable with directly addressing the stereotyping of the fat body, or in engaging with media messages about fatness.

The Problem With Body Image Programs

First, we want to be clear that we recognize that the programs are well-meaning; proponents have assessed a risk and seek to address that risk through programs informed by evidence from psychology and social psychology. This grounding, however, seems to us to be a major part of the problem. The programs are limited by a psychological view of individual change and validity associated with measurable outcomes based on psychological scales. The programs are designed with a very specific phenomenon, eating disorders, in mind and are administered to children and young people in educational contexts as broader health interventions.

Second, the programs are very narrow in their focus and assume a rational child or young person who can, through sheer will, control the way he or she thinks and feels. As unlikely as it seems, there are parallels here with some fat activist approaches to empowerment that call for simply rejecting social norms and instead loving one's fat body. Sam Murray's (2008) critique of fat activism is useful in considering the limitations of these body image programs. Drawing on Merleau-Ponty's theories of the body-subject, she argues that "the individualistic premise of fat activism that offers agency and emancipation through the privileging of the mind over the body is … mythic, as it discounts the culturally and historically specific discourses [and aesthetics] that … mobilise particular ways of seeing" (p. 170). She argues that "the dominant discourses that have marked and inscribed [a woman's] 'fatness' over the course of her life, and that have indeed formed her own corporal schema and mode of being-in-the-world" (p. 174) make reinscribing the meanings of fatness an immensely difficult task. Body image programs ask children and young people to engage in a similar reinscription of their body, to simply ignore and/or reject cultural messages that they have learned from an early age and are continually negotiating in their everyday lives. The responsibility is placed firmly on the children to change their way of being-in-the-world, without acknowledging the intersubjective nature of their everyday existence.

Third, the body image programs do not engage with the complexity of the discourses shaping body ideas, but rather skirt around the edges. The programs claim to be dealing with cultural stereotypes but in the name of challenging the thin ideal, they reproduce normative notions of the acceptable body. They do not engage at all with stereotyping and stigmatization of fat bodies, nor do they engage with the multiple and authoritative messages from governments and popular media that fat bodies are not acceptable, and indeed at times even reinforce this idea. In the school context, body image programs are likely to run alongside health education programs that educate about preventing "overweight" and "obesity" through healthy eating and activity. Research with children and young people makes it clear that many associate "healthy lifestyle" practices with avoiding becoming fat (Wright & Burrows, 2004). These ideas are left untouched in the programs we examined.

What Would We Argue for in Relation to Fat Pedagogies?

On the one hand, we argue that the primary purpose of schools is not to address public health issues per se but to educate (see also Gard & Pluim, 2014; St. Leger, 2006). This is not to say that schools are not responsible for enhancing children's health by providing safe environments where every child is treated with respect. When a whole school or HPS approach that addresses the school culture is taken—that is, one that addresses body-based teasing, body comments, bullying by teachers and students, school policies around uniforms, and so on—there is a chance of a useful contribution to young people's health and well-being. However, as we have pointed out and as is reiterated in the literature, such an approach is a considerable challenge for a school and requires a commitment that is rarely in evidence.

On the other hand, we would argue that there are a number of places in the school curriculum where pedagogies addressing body stigmatization and the nature and effects of social and cultural ideas about the body and shape could be addressed educationally using a socio-critical approach (see Leahy, O'Flynn, & Wright, 2013). We draw on a quote from a paper intended to guide the design of the Australian national curriculum in Health and Physical Education to explain what this might mean:

> The Health and Physical Education curriculum will draw on its multi-disciplinary base with students learning to question the social, cultural and political factors that influence health and well-being. In doing so students will explore matters such as inclusiveness, power inequalities, taken-for-granted assumptions, diversity and social justice, and develop strategies to improve their own and others' health and wellbeing. (ACARA, 2012, quoted in Leahy et al., 2013, p. 179)

In the context of a socio-critical approach, we suggest there is some value in media literacy around social body norms and that this should be embedded in a broader media literacy program. Such a media literacy program would start with the assumption that choices in language (or images, frames, or camera angles) are not neutral but are motivated, not necessarily consciously, but certainly by particular social values or ways of thinking about the world; that is, meaning-making needs to be understood as a social practice (see Wright, 2004). The tools of textual analysis developed within the areas of critical literacy, critical discourse analysis, media literacy, and cultural studies provide the means of critically analyzing media texts to help make more visible the work they do in constructing social and cultural values.

It is rarely useful to tell or show students how media texts work to construct particular social values, particularly in the many cases where these social values are very similar to those that they themselves hold. To see the world differently, as in most cases of critical inquiry, the students need to become "active researchers in their worlds" (Wright, 2004, p. 187), interrogators of the taken-for-granted. In the case of media texts, they need to be helped to collect, explain, interpret, and present their own data about media texts (see Wright, 2004).

There are many other approaches to fat pedagogy, as illustrated by the many chapters in the *Fat Pedagogy Reader*. Here we argue for the end of interventions such as those described here that, despite their good intentions, serve to reproduce fat prejudice and instead propose a socio-critical approach as one possible fat pedagogy that addresses the issues of body weight and size more broadly, indirectly, and educatively.

References

Australian Government. (2012). *Body information sheets.* Retrieved from http://www.youth.gov.au/sites/Youth/bodyImage/informationsheets

Bird, E. L., Halliwell, E., Diedrichs, P. C., & Harcourt, D. (2013). Happy Being Me in the UK: A controlled evaluation of a school-based body image intervention with pre-adolescent children. *Body Image, 10,* 326–334.

Cash, T. F. (2004). Body image: Past, present and future. *Body Image, 1,* 1–5.

Davis, K. (1995). *Reshaping the female body: The dilemma of cosmetic surgery.* New York, NY: Routledge.

Gard, M., & Pluim, C. (2014). *Schools and public health: Past, present and future.* Lanham, MD: Lexington.

Leahy, D. (2009). Disgusting pedagogies. In J. Wright & V. Harwood (Eds.), *Biopolitics of the "obesity epidemic": Governing the body* (pp. 172–182). New York, NY: Routledge.

Leahy, D., O'Flynn, G., & Wright, J. (2013). A critical "critical inquiry" proposition in Health and Physical Education. *Asia-Pacific Journal of Health, Sport and Physical Education, 4*(2), 175–187.

Levine, M. P., & Smolak, L. (2002). Ecological and activism approaches to the prevention and changing of body image problems. In T. F. Cash & T. Pruzinsky (Eds.), *Body image: A handbook of theory, research and clinical practice* (pp. 497–505). New York, NY: Guilford Press.

McKinley, N. M. (2002). Feminist perspectives and objectified body consciousness. In T. F. Cash & T. Pruzinsky (Eds.), *Body image: A handbook of theory, research and clinical practice* (pp. 55–62). New York, NY: Guilford Press.

Murray, S. (2008). *The 'fat' female body.* Basingstoke, Hampshire, England: Palgrave Macmillan.

O'Dea, J. (2007). *Everybody's different: A positive approach to teaching about health, puberty, body image, nutrition, self-esteem and obesity prevention.* Camberwell, Australia: Australian Council for Educational Research.

Pruzinsky, T., & Cash, T. F. (2002). Understanding body images: Historical and contemporary perspectives. In T. F. Cash & T. Pruzinsky (Eds.), *Body image: A handbook of theory, research and clinical practice* (pp. 3–12). New York, NY: Guilford Press.

Richardson, S. M., & Paxton, S. J. (2010). An evaluation of a body image intervention based on risk factors for body dissatisfaction: A controlled study with adolescent girls. *International Journal of Eating Disorders, 43,* 112–122.

St. Leger, L. (2006). *Health promotion and health education in schools: Trends, effectiveness and possibilities.* Melbourne, Australia: Royal Automobile Club of Victoria.

Vandenbosch, L., & Eggermont, S. (2013). Sexualization of adolescent boys: Media exposure and boys' internalization of appearance ideals, self-objectification, and body surveillance. *Men and Masculinities, 16,* 283–306.

Wilksch, S., & Wade, T. (2010a). *Media smart: Eating disorder and body image information for presenters.* Content prepared for Monash University, Melbourne, Australia.

Wilksch, S., & Wade, T. (2010b). *Media smart: Eating disorder and body image presenter lesson plans.* Content prepared for Monash University, Melbourne, Australia.

Wolszon, L. R. (1998). Women's body image theory and research: A hermeneutic critique. *American Behavioral Scientist, 41*(4), 542–557.

Wright, J. (2004). Analysing sportsmedia texts: Developing resistant reading positions. In J. Wright, D. Macdonald, & L. Burrows (Eds.), *Critical inquiry and problem-solving in physical education* (pp. 183–196). London, England: Routledge.

Wright, J., & Burrows, L. (2004). "Being healthy": The discursive construction of health in New Zealand children's responses to the National Education Monitoring Project. *Discourse, 25,* 211–230.

Fifteen

Promoting Physical Activity for All Shapes and Sizes

Angela S. Alberga and Shelly Russell-Mayhew

"Obesity" has amassed considerable scientific, political, and media attention and has been framed as a public health concern (Ebbeling, Pawlak, & Ludwig, 2002). The focus on the physiological health consequences of "obesity" (Diaz-Melean et al., 2013) has led to a "fat panic" (McPhail, 2009) that has had negative outcomes including body weight preoccupation, body dissatisfaction, and weight bias. Children and youths are growing up in a culture that vilifies fat and idolizes thin. At the same time, physical activity has been categorized as something only "the athletes" do, and is often promoted as a way to manage, control, or manipulate body weight. There is evidence to suggest that students will avoid physical activity if they experience weight-based teasing in physical education class (Jensen, Cushing, & Elledge, 2014), yet physical education in schools plays an important role in promoting (or discouraging) physical activity throughout the life span.

Participation in different types of physical activities confers health benefits above and beyond any connection to weight and should be promoted to children and youths of all shapes and sizes. The notion of physical activity has been hijacked by dominant weight-centric discourses that position physical activity as a virtuous activity for individuals to undertake to control their weight or for weight loss (Monaghan, Colls, & Evans, 2013). In line with Louise Mansfield and Emma Rich (2013), we argue that it is time for all bodies to reclaim the right to physical activity and that, particularly for children, we need to promote physical activity without focusing on body weight.

The weight-focused approach to defining health has contributed to increasing frequency and intensity of fat bias (Latner & Stunkard, 2003), defined as "negative weight-related attitudes, beliefs, assumptions and judgments towards individuals who are overweight and obese" (Washington, 2011, p. 1). Fat bias can be subtle or overt, and can occur verbally (e.g., name-calling, derogatory remarks, teasing), physically (e.g., bullying or aggression by hitting, kicking, pushing, shoving), or through relational victimization (e.g., social exclusion, being ignored or avoided, the target of rumors) (Puhl & Brownell, 2007). There is a common belief that shaming people who live in larger bodies will motivate behavior change, which rests on the assumption that someone living in a larger body could not practice healthy behaviors already (Puhl, Peterson, & Luedicke, 2013). Experiencing fat bias can have psychosocial effects such as vulnerability to depression, stress, anxiety, low self-esteem, body dissatisfaction, and social isolation (Major, Eliezer, & Rieck, 2012; Puhl & Heuer, 2009) as well as impacts on health behaviors (Puhl et al., 2013).

Fat bias has been observed among teachers, physical educators, and administrators in educational settings (Greenleaf & Weiller, 2005). It has also been shown that education professionals exert more anti-fat attitudes than the general public (Puhl & Heuer, 2009). Being on the receiving end of fat bias can have several long-lasting negative consequences for children and youths. We begin this chapter by discussing the prevalence and negative implications of fat bias in physical education settings in schools. Next, we discuss the overall health benefits of physical activity for children and adolescents of varying weight. Finally, we explore current pedagogical approaches used to reduce fat bias in physical education settings and effective ways to promote physical activity for overall health of all children and youths in schools.

Fat Bias in Physical Education Settings

Students who were picked last for a team often remain last when it comes to physical activity participation. (Cardinal, Yan, & Cardinal, 2013, p. 49)

Adolescents have reported that stigmatization related to weight occurs more often in the school setting than in any other setting (Neumark-Sztainer, Story, & Faibisch, 1998). Many studies have reported fat bias is experienced among students in schools (Puhl & Luedicke, 2012), and there is also evidence to show that physical educators and coaches are culprits of fat bias against their students (Greenleaf & Weiller, 2005). Teachers' fat bias is often shown through expressing lower expectations (O'Brien, Hunter, & Banks, 2007), and/or attributing to them negative characteristics such as being untidy, more emotional, less likely to succeed, and more likely to have family problems compared with children and adolescents at "normal" weights (Neumark-Sztainer, Story, & Harris, 1999). Fat bias shown by educators can negatively impact students' body image, well-being, and participation in physical activity in schools (Haines & Neumark-Stzainer, 2009). Compared with adolescents who were not teased, adolescents who were teased about their weight experienced lower levels of psychological well-being (e.g., lower levels of self-esteem and higher levels of depression) (Greenleaf et al., 2014), which cannot help but impact their comfort with organized physical activity opportunities at the school.

Children and youths experiencing fat bias are more likely than adults (Puhl & Brownell, 2006) to resort to unhealthy coping strategies such as negative self-talk, avoidance, eating more, and dieting (Salvy et al., 2011). Bad experiences such as being ostracized in physical education settings might negatively affect physical activity participation in the short term (Barkley, Salvy, & Roemmich, 2012) as well as into adulthood (Cardinal et al., 2013). For example, Bradley Cardinal, Zi Yan, and Marita Cardinal (2013) found that undergraduate students who had been chosen last for a team in their school-age days participated in one less mild and one less moderate exercise session per week in adulthood compared with their peers who did not report such a negative experience.

Heather Sykes and Deborah McPhail (2008) described the "unbearable" experiences in physical education of 15 North American adults who once identified as fat or overweight. The interviews revealed that fat phobia in physical education "is oppressive and makes it extremely difficult for most students to develop positive fat subjectivities" and that "fat phobia created extremely difficult situations that demanded constant psychic/emotional work, provided pitiful opportunities for learning, and numerous alienating and traumatic movement experiences" (pp. 66–68). Many interviewees recalled feelings of humiliation, vulnerability, or incompetence in physical education that one could imagine negatively impacting both physical and mental well-being over the long term.

Children and Physical Inactivity in Canada

Active Healthy Kids Canada releases an annual Report Card on the most current and comprehensive assessment of the physical activity of children and youths in Canada. Canada's overall physical activity levels got a "D-" grade, which means children need to be more active both within and outside the school environment (Active Healthy Kids Canada, 2014). The Canadian Society for Exercise Physiology (2013) recommends that children and youths aged 5 to 17 years should accumulate at least 60 minutes of moderate to vigorous physical activity every day for measurable health benefits. However, only 7 percent of Canadian children met those guidelines at ages 5 to 11 and only 4 percent met guidelines at ages 12 to 17 (Colley et al., 2011).

Active Healthy Kids Canada (2014) also clearly outlines indicators that affect physical activity participation in children, including government and non-government "strategies and investments" and "settings and sources of influence" such as school, family and peers, community, and the built environment. These larger systemic indicators largely influence four behaviors that contribute to overall physical activity, namely, organized sports, active transportation, active play, and sedentary behaviors such as screen time in front of a TV, video game, or computer, and/or doing things that do not require movement such as sitting in class at school. Their schema illustrates how larger systemic influences and social determinants of health play a role in overall physical activity participation in children and youths.

It is clear that we need to find innovative ways to engage children in physically active lifestyles. Organized sport reaches only a small portion of children and youths but physical activity should not be just for those who "are good at it" or can afford it. Although physical activity often declines as children become adolescents (Nader, Bradley, Houts, McRitchie, & O'Brien, 2008), younger children generally are naturally active beings if they are in environments that support movement and play. We argue that physical activity should be promoted to children and youths of all shapes and sizes and with a range of skills and abilities to help form positive associations with being active in different settings, whether that might be organized sport participation, active transportation, or active play. Fat is not an attribute that should inhibit participation in movement as children and youths of all shapes and sizes benefit from physical activity. That a child would be excluded from or discouraged to participate in physical activity because of his or her weight only serves to devalue that child.

Benefits of Physical Activity

Although there is strong evidence supporting both the physical and mental health benefits of regular physical activity, the supposed physical benefits of increased energy expenditure (i.e., for weight loss) have been overemphasized through weight-centric approaches to promoting physical activity. Many school-based physical activity interventions have been devised to reduce the prevalence of "obesity" in children and youths. However, the dominant discourse about "moving more" to fight the "war on obesity" does not stand up to scrutiny. Some school interventions aimed at reducing students' Body Mass Index (BMI), a crude marker of body composition that is not a valid indicator of health status, by increasing physical activity participation have been unsuccessful and indeed harmful to students' well-being. For example, Lee, Lee, Pathy, and Chan (2005) uncovered the unintended consequence of a mandatory after-school "trim and fit" nutrition and physical activity program for children who were identified as "obese." The program was initially considered a success because "obesity" rates decreased from 13.1 percent to 9.4 percent in the first year of the program. However, a later examination of hospitalization records for children with anorexia nervosa found that 11 percent had participated in this "trim and fit" program. Of those, almost half indicated that being chosen for the program was a factor in the development of their eating disorder (Lee et al., 2005). The unintended iatrogenic effects related to body dissatisfaction, unhealthy weight change behaviors, and mental illness associated with BMI measurement and attempted manipulation are fundamental as we consider our discourses about, and practices in, physical activity. Promoting physical activity for overall health and wellness of all students rather than focusing on weight reduction or maintenance is the best course of action in school settings. It is imperative that we create friendly cultures and environments to develop positive associations between activity and bodies of all shapes and sizes (Sykes & McPhail, 2008).

Physical activity interventions have shown improvements in students' physical health (cardiovascular and muscular fitness, sleep, motor skill development, and physical literacy) and mental health (improved academic performance, happiness and self-confidence, and decreased stress). There is strong evidence to support that physical activity and physical fitness provide health benefits regardless of an individual's weight status (Lee, Blair, & Jackson, 1999). As well, physical activity can and should be promoted for reasons unrelated to weight, such as improving quality of life, promoting camaraderie, working as a team, building friendships, and appreciating nature and the environment. Physical activity can also be viewed as a social venue that can help foster friendships and connections.

Current Approaches Aimed to Reduce Fat Bias in Education Settings

The role that physical educators and schools play in promoting physical activity and health has been highlighted in recent years. Given the complexity of health and wellness issues that children are facing in schools, we urgently need innovative and coordinated strategies to create school environments that promote the health of all learners without focusing on weight-related outcomes. Efforts are needed to "facilitate physical educators to design a caring environment and a relevant curriculum that is connected and inclusive to overweight or obese students" (Li & Rukavina, 2009, p. 94). We must create environments that are less threatening and more size accepting, and that emphasize health and wellness rather than focus on efforts to attain a socially constructed aesthetic appearance ideal to increase motivation for movement. We also need much more research in this area to help determine what works and what does not in particular contexts.

Perhaps counterintuitively, in addition to the evidence of anti-fat attitudes of some physical educators (Greenleaf & Weiller, 2005), there is also research that indicates that physical education teachers are themselves at an increased risk of experiencing body dissatisfaction, dieting, and disordered eating (Yager & O'Dea, 2009). Further, most teachers in one pilot study in Canada reported feeling uncomfortable and unprepared to address weight-related issues in schools, and were seeking changes in training and practice that could lead to improved knowledge and efficacy (Russell-Mayhew, Ireland, & Peat, 2012). In another study designed to determine the needs of teachers responsible for health education, Sandra Vamos and Mingming Zhou (2009) found that both pre-service and in-service teachers reported barriers to teaching about, and discomfort with, health-related education. It appears that many teachers "find it difficult to make the fundamental connections between health and education and, therefore, the importance of this in their future role as health promoters" (Speller et al., 2010, p. 504).

There is some evidence that suggests that supplementary professional development possibly could reduce teachers' anti-fat attitudes. For example, it has been shown that a full-day workshop on raising awareness of fat bias decreased anti-fat attitudes, the internalization of thin-ideal stereotypes, and weight and shape preoccupation among public health professionals (McVey et al., 2013). In a related vein, teachers who receive health promotion training tend to be more frequently invested in health-related projects and have a more comprehensive understanding of health in schools (Bryne, Almond, Grace, & Memon, 2012). Although these are promising results, more research is needed to evaluate the effects of professional development programs in fat bias reduction among teachers and administrators in education settings (Russell-Mayhew et al., 2012). Beyond such programs, Sykes and McPhail (2008) argue that in addition to improving attitudes and behaviors of educators and administrators, larger systemic changes to curriculum and physical education pedagogies are needed if we are to eliminate oppression in physical education settings.

This underlines a need for university teacher training programs to address the preparation of teachers in the area of school health. Effectively addressing wellness in schools requires a multimethod approach that tailors interventions with the goal of maximizing system-wide change. To make this work, collaboration between universities, professional institutions, and communities is needed (Greenberg et al., 2003), especially given the demonstrated lack of quality and quantity of health education in university pre-service teacher training (Smith, 2005). This "upstream" approach, addressing the need for curriculum change in teacher education in health, acknowledges not only the growing complexity of the role of the teacher but also the potential to positively influence both the university environments pre-service teachers are in and the future school environments they will later find themselves in. However, research is needed to elucidate the best ways to educate teachers in health-related curriculum and school-based health promotion.

Effective Ways to Promote Physical Activity for Overall Health

There are many different strategies that can be implemented in physical education settings to target the reduction of fat bias, increase physical activity levels, and promote overall health. It is clear from the evidence presented here that physical educators and school environments play important roles in the development and continuation of attitudes and behaviors towards physical activity. To eliminate humiliating and marginalizing experiences for students, educators and schools must make use of best practices grounded in research that demonstrate utmost sensitivity to all chidren's needs if we are to inspire and foster lifelong physical activity.

Despite research showing the difficulties associated with designing, implementing, and adhering to physical activity interventions for children and youths, some practical strategies have been proposed. There is strong evidence showing that there are many factors that influence physical activity participation in youths (Sallis, Prochaska, & Taylor, 2000). Angela Alberga and her colleagues (2013) published a paper offering practical evidence-based advice on how to increase physical activity in children and youths. They suggest that (a) one must carefully consider the physical activity setting since context is important; (b) the choice of fitness trainer matters (i.e., someone knowledgeable about the complexity of weight and who would not demonstrate fat bias); (c) physical activities should be varied and fun; (d) the role of the parent or guardian should be considered; (e) individual physical and psychosocial characteristics should be accounted for; (f) realistic goals not focused on weight should be set; (g) regular reminders of the benefits of physical activity without focusing on weight should be offered; (h) a multidisciplinary approach should be taken; (i) barriers should be identified early and a plan to overcome them developed; and (j) the focus should be on the children and youths and clearly articulate what is in it for them.

These recommendations highlight the importance of creating a warm, welcoming environment that offers children varied options for being active according to their interests, preferences, skills, and comfort level. Children and youths can encounter multiple social, familial, biological, behavioral, and environmental barriers to physical activity. It becomes important, then, for physical education teachers to tailor physical activity to both the physical characteristics and psychosocial characteristics (e.g., personality traits, autonomy, perceptions of physical activity) of children to mitigate these barriers. Children and youths of all shapes and sizes need guidance, structure, and variety as well as motivational role models who consider the context and the whole person in order to engage in physical activity on a consistent basis.

Other organizations have evaluated school-based approaches to improve physical activity participation. The World Health Organization (1986) recommends that schools use a comprehensive approach to health promotion. In Canada, Comprehensive School Health (CSH) is used as a multifaceted approach to health promotion in which a "broad health education curriculum is supported by the environment and ethos of the school" (Lee, 2009, p. 11). CSH is an internationally recognized and empirically supported approach to creating healthy school communities (Veugelers & Schwartz, 2010). The aim of the CSH approach is to support the wellness of all members of the school community (students, parents, teachers, and staff), thereby improving education outcomes for children and youths (Mohammadi, Rowling, & Nutbeam, 2010). CSH has shown effectiveness in increasing physical activity levels of children both inside and outside the school environment (Vander Ploeg, McGavock, Maximova, & Veugelers, 2014) and has been recognized nationally as best practice (Comprehensive School Health, 2007). The

Pan-Canadian Joint Consortium for School Health is a partnership of 25 Ministries of Health and Education across Canada working to promote a CSH approach to student wellness, well-being, achievement, and success for all children and youths; they offer many resources for parents and educators to effectively promote CSH in the school environment.

The University of Connecticut Rudd Center for Food Policy and Obesity (previously known as the Yale Rudd Center) under the leadership of Marlene Schwartz and Rebecca Puhl has also played a pivotal role in fat bias reduction through research projects, media appearances, development of policy statements, and publicly accessible resources (e.g., documents, videos, toolkits, presentations) that describe the negative implications of fat bias and offer practical strategies for its reduction in various settings. For example, the Rudd Center's "Weight Bias & Stigma Tools for Schools and Educators" includes resources and handouts on how to effectively reduce weight bias in the classroom. Another organization, Operation Respect, has developed "Don't Laugh at Me" programs for Grades 2 through 5 and 6 through 8 as well as programs for summer camps and after-school settings, and has various free resources available for parents, children, and educators alike. The article by Mansfield and Rich (2013) offers insights into Physical Activity at Every Size (PAES) that is in line with Health in Every Respect and Health at Every Size (HAES) approaches (Aphramor & Gingras, 2011).

Synthesizing the various interventions described earlier, we offer the following practical advice for teachers on key factors that help reduce fat bias in educational settings:

- Question your own assumptions about weight and health
- Understand the complexities of body weight
- Emphasize physical activity benefits such as improvements in mental health and quality of life rather than weight
- Adapt physical actvities for all abilities and skills
- Emphasize the importance of effort and participation, not "winning"
- Seek to eliminate fat bias messages in environmental surroundings; for example, avoid the use of stigmatizing images in teaching and learning resources, stop laughing at fat jokes, include size-friendly furniture, ensure accessible buildings and hallways, and offer gym clothes for students of all shapes and sizes
- Include weight-based teasing as part of policies on bullying and discrimination
- Remember that children can choose behaviors but cannot choose their weight

Conclusion

Fat bias is widely prevalent in physical education settings and has several adverse consequences including embarrassment, stress, anxiety, shame, low self-esteem, and depression, all of which can lead to unhealthy behaviors. Canadian children and youths are not meeting physical activity recommendations despite the well-known health benefits including improvements in both physical and mental health. The school setting is the ideal location to expose children and youths of all shapes and sizes to a variety of ways to move, participate, challenge, and care for their physical bodies. Physical activity should neither be exclusive to particular groups of students nor promoted in relation to weight but instead encouraged for overall health. Physical activity is for every body.

References

Active Healthy Kids Canada. (2014). *Is Canada in the running? The 2014 Active Healthy Kids Canada Report Card on physical activity for children and youth.* Toronto, ON, Canada: Author.

Alberga, A. S., Medd, E. R., Adamo, K. B., Goldfield, G. S., Prud'homme, D., Kenny, G. P., & Sigal, R. J. (2013). Top 10 practical lessons learned from physical activity interventions in overweight and obese children and adolescents. *Applied Physiology Nutrition & Metabolism, 38,* 249–258.

Aphramor, L., & Gingras, J. (2011). Helping people change: Promoting politicised practice in the healthcare professions. In E. Rich, L. Monaghan, & L. Aphramor (Eds.), *Debating obesity: Critical perspectives* (pp. 192–218). London, England: Palgrave.

Barkley, J. E., Salvy, S. J., & Roemmich, J. N. (2012). The effect of simulated ostracism on physical activity behavior in children. *Pediatrics, 129,* e659–e666.

Bryne, J., Almond, P., Grace, M., & Memon, A. (2012). Health promotion in pre-service teacher education: Effects of a pilot inter-professional curriculum change. *Health Education, 112,* 525–542.

Canadian Society for Exercise Physiology. (2013). *Canadian physical activity and Canadian sedentary behaviour Guidelines.* Ottawa, ON, Canada: Author.

Cardinal, B. J., Yan, Z., & Cardinal, M. K. (2013). Negative experiences in physical education and sport: How much do they affect physical activity participation later in life? *Journal of Physical Education, Recreation and Dance, 84,* 49–53.

Colley, R. C., Garriguet, D., Janssen, I., Craig, C. L., Clarke, J., & Tremblay, M. S. (2011). Physical activity of Canadian children and youth: Accelerometer results from the 2007 to 2009 Canadian Health Measures Survey. *Health Reports, 22*(1), 15–23.

Comprehensive School Health. (2007). *Canadian consensus statement: Schools and communities working in partnership to create and foster health-promoting schools.* Surrey, BC, Canada: Author.

Diaz-Melean, C. M., Somers, V. K., Rodriguez-Escudero, J. P., Singh, P., Sochor, O., Llano, E. M., & Lopez-Jimenez, F. (2013). Mechanisms of adverse cardiometabolic consequences of obesity. *Current Atherosclerosis Reports, 15,* 364.

Ebbeling, C. B., Pawlak, D. B., & Ludwig, D. S. (2002). Childhood obesity: Public-health crisis, common sense cure. *Lancet, 360,* 473–482.

Greenberg, M. T., Weissberg, R. P., O'Brien, M. U., Zins, J. E., Fredericks, L., Resnik, H., & Elias, M. J. (2003). Enhancing school-based prevention and youth development through coordinated social, emotional, and academic learning. *American Psychologist, 58,* 466–474.

Greenleaf, C., Petrie, T. A., & Martin, S. B. (2014). Relationship of weight-based teasing and adolescents' psychological well-being and physical health. *Journal of School Health, 84,* 49–55.

Greenleaf, C., & Weiller, K. (2005). Perceptions of youth obesity among physical educators. *Social Psychology of Education, 8,* 407–423.

Haines, J., & Neumark-Sztainer, D. (2009). Psychosocial consequences of obesity and weight bias: Implications for interventions. In L. Heinberg & J. K. Thompson (Eds.), *Obesity in youth* (pp. 79–95). Washington, DC: American Psychological Association.

Jensen, C. D., Cushing, C. C., & Elledge, A. R. (2014). Associations between teasing, quality of life, and physical activity among preadolescent children. *Journal of Pediatric Psychology, 39,* 65–73.

Latner, J. D., & Stunkard, A. J. (2003). Getting worse: The stigmatization of obese children. *Obesity Research, 11,* 452–456.

Lee, A. (2009). Health-promoting schools: Evidence for a holistic approach to promoting health and improving health literacy. *Applied Health Economics and Health Policy, 7,* 11–17.

Lee, C. D., Blair, S. N., & Jackson, A. S. (1999). Cardiorespiratory fitness, body composition, and all-cause and cardiovascular disease mortality in men. *American Journal of Clinical Nutrition, 69*(3), 373–380.

Lee, H. Y., Lee, E. L., Pathy, P., & Chan, Y. H. (2005). Anorexia nervosa in Singapore: An eight-year retrospective study. *Singapore Medical Journal, 46*(6), 275–281.

Li, W., & Rukavina, P. (2009). A review on coping mechanisms against obesity bias in physical activity/education settings. *Obesity Reviews, 10,* 87–95.

Major, B., Eliezer, D., & Rieck, H. (2012). The psychological weight of weight stigma. *Social Psychological and Personality Science, 3,* 651–658.

Mansfield, L., & Rich, E. (2013). Public health pedagogy, border crossings and physical activity at every size. *Critical Public Health, 23,* 356–370.

McPhail, D. (2009). What to do with "The Tubby Hubby"? "Obesity," the crisis of masculinity, and the reification of the nuclear family in early Cold War Canada. *Antipode, 41,* 1021–1050.

McVey, G. L., Walker, K. S., Beyers, J., Harrison, H. L., Simkins, S. W., & Russell-Mayhew, S. (2013). Integrating weight bias awareness and mental health promotion into obesity prevention delivery: A public health pilot study. *Preventing Chronic Disease, 10*, E46.

Mohammadi, N. K., Rowling, L., & Nutbeam, D. (2010). Acknowledging educational perspectives on health promoting schools. *Health Education, 110*, 240–251.

Monaghan, L. F., Colls, R., & Evans, B. (2013). Obesity discourse and fat politics: Research, critique and interventions. *Critical Public Health, 23*, 249–262.

Nader, P. R., Bradley, R. H., Houts, R. M., McRitchie, S. L., & O'Brien, M. (2008). Moderate-to-vigorous physical activity from ages 9 to 15 years. *Journal of the American Medical Association, 300*, 295–305.

Neumark-Sztainer, D., Story, M., & Faibisch, L. (1998). Perceived stigmatization among overweight African-American and Caucasian adolescent girls. *Journal of Adolescent Health, 23*, 264–270.

Neumark-Sztainer, D., Story, M., & Harris, T. (1999). Beliefs and attitudes about obesity among teachers and school health care providers working with adolescents. *Journal of Nutrition Education, 31*, 3–9.

O'Brien, K. S., Hunter, J. A., & Banks, M. (2007). Implicit anti-fat bias in physical educators: Physical attributes, ideology and socialization. *International Journal of Obesity (London), 31*, 308–314.

Puhl, R. M., & Brownell, K. D. (2006). Confronting and coping with weight stigma: An investigation of overweight and obese adults. *Obesity (Silver Spring), 14*, 1802–1815.

Puhl, R. M., & Brownell, K. D. (2007). *Weight bias in health care settings.* New Haven, CT: Rudd Center for Food Policy and Obesity, Yale University. Retrieved from http://biastoolkit.uconnruddcenter.org/toolkit/Module-3/3–03a-Overview-Slides.pdf

Puhl, R. M., & Heuer, C. A. (2009). The stigma of obesity: A review and update. *Obesity (Silver Spring), 17*, 941–964.

Puhl, R. M., & Luedicke, J. (2012). Weight-based victimization among adolescents in the school setting: Emotional reactions and coping behaviors. *Journal of Youth and Adolescence, 41*, 27–40.

Puhl, R. M., Peterson, J. L., & Luedicke, J. (2013). Motivating or stigmatizing? Public perceptions of weight-related language used by health providers. *International Journal of Obesity (London), 37*, 612–619.

Russell-Mayhew, S., Ireland, A., & Peat, G. (2012). The impact of professional development about weight-related issues for pre-service teachers: A pilot study. *Alberta Journal of Educational Research, 58*(3), 314–329.

Sallis, J. F., Prochaska, J. J., & Taylor, W. C. (2000). A review of correlates of physical activity of children and adolescents. *Medicine & Science in Sports & Exercise, 32*, 963–975.

Salvy, S. J., Bowker, J. C., Nitecki, L. A., Kluczynski, M. A., Germeroth, L. J., & Roemmich, J. N. (2011). Impact of simulated ostracism on overweight and normal-weight youths' motivation to eat and food intake. *Appetite, 56*, 39–45.

Smith, B. J. (2005). Challenges in teacher for school health education and promotion. *Global Health Promotion, 12*, 162–164.

Speller, V., Byrne, J., Dewhirst, S., Almond, P., Mohebati, L., Norman, M., … Roderick, P. (2010). Developing trainee school teachers' expertise as health promoters. *Health Education, 110*, 490–507.

Sykes, H., & McPhail, D. (2008). Unbearable lessons: Contesting fat phobia in physical education. *Sociology of Sport, 25*(1), 66–96.

Vamos, S., & Zhou, M. (2009). Using focus group research to assess health education needs of pre-service and in-service teachers. *American Journal of Health Education, 40*, 196–206.

Vander Ploeg, K. A., McGavock, J., Maximova, K., & Veugelers, P. J. (2014). School-based health promotion and physical activity during and after school hours. *Pediatrics, 133*, e371–e378.

Veugelers, P. J., & Schwartz, M. E. (2010). Comprehensive school health in Canada. *Canadian Journal of Public Health, 101*(Suppl. 2), S5–S8.

Washington, R. L. (2011). Childhood obesity: Issues of weight bias. *Preventing Chronic Disease, 8*. Retrieved from http://www.cdc.gov/pcd/issues/2011/sep/10_0281.htm

World Health Organization. (1986). *Ottawa Charter for Health Promotion: A discussion document on the concepts and principles.* Geneva, Switzerland: Author.

Yager, Z., & O'Dea, J. (2009). Body image, dieting and disordered eating and activity practices among teacher trainees: Implications for school-based health education and obesity prevention programs. *Health Education Research, 24*, 472–482.

SIXTEEN

Inclusion of Fat Studies in a Difference, Power, and Discrimination Curriculum

Patti Lou Watkins

Until recently, bias based on body weight, shape, and size has received little attention in diversity discussions. Indeed, weight bias is an underrecognized and oft overlooked social justice issue (Cardinal, Whitney, Narimatsu, Hubert, & Souza, 2014). Stephanie Jones and Hilary Hughes-Decatur (2012) note that it is suspiciously absent in social justice curricula as well as in education research. Traditional education, particularly in the health sciences, seems to reinforce bias via weight-centric curricula (Watkins & Concepcion, 2014). As such, stigmatizing beliefs about fat tend to be the status quo among contemporary college students (Ambwani, Thomas, Hopwood, Moss, & Grilo, 2014).

Weight bias has increased exponentially over the past decade (Andreyeva, Puhl, & Brownell, 2008), coincidentally in conjunction with the so-called "obesity epidemic" that has permeated both public discourse and higher education. Furthermore, it intersects with bias based on other areas of difference. Consequently, scholars have begun to recognize weightism as a social justice issue on par with racism (Puhl, Andreyeva, & Brownell, 2008). A growing number of college courses now incorporate lessons on weightism, with several focused solely on this topic (Watkins, Farrell, & Hugmeyer, 2012). These courses reflect the emergent, interdisciplinary field of fat studies, which is akin to women's studies (WS) and fields of inquiry based on race that evolved from grassroots activism and political movements to resist discrimination. Like queer studies, fat studies reclaims the historically pejorative word "fat" as a form of resistance to inequities perpetrated around this category of difference. In this chapter, I describe the evolution of a fat studies course in terms of its content as well as the process by which it is taught. Throughout this account, I rely abundantly on student voices via their class assignments to illustrate the impact of this particular pedagogical approach.

In the early 1990s, Oregon State University (OSU) instituted a Difference, Power, and Discrimination (DPD) requirement within its Baccalaureate Core. DPD classes were charged with facilitating students' critical thinking around socially constructed categories of difference. Specifically, they were to "provide historical and contemporary examples of difference, power, and discrimination across cultural, economic, social, and political institutions and illustrations of ways in which the interactions of social categories, such as race, ethnicity, social class, gender, religion, sexual orientation, disability, and age, are related to difference, power, and discrimination in the United States." Notably missing from this array is discrimination based on body size. Constance Russell, Erin Cameron, Teresa Socha, and Hannah McNinch (2013) strongly advocate for the inclusion of fat oppression in such intersectional analyses. In line with this recommendation, the DPD curriculum now includes a fat studies course that acknowledges weight as a category of difference subject to oppression.

I am a clinical psychologist who developed and teaches fat studies at OSU. I have held faculty positions in both psychology and WS. The course is cross-listed between these disciplines, although most students have majored in psychology or other behavioral health fields. Teaching such a cross-listed course can be a challenge on many levels. First, while diversity is the cornerstone of WS classes, Guy Boysen (2011) decries the overall lack of diversity education in psychology. Similarly, undergraduate psychology education largely reflects a pedagogy that emphasizes content over process, with formal mastery of material prioritized over the development knowledge. In this model, the instructor is considered expert and expected to deliver content primarily through lecture. Logical positivism and objectivity are central to this model, with personal experience and affect devalued and considered irrelevant to the learning process (Sincacore, Healy, & Justin, 2002).

As the course evolved from my time in WS, in contrast to the norms of psychology, it is based on feminist pedagogy that values collaboration and multiple ways of knowing including personal experience. There is an effort to minimize hierarchies; thus, I describe myself as a "point guard," disseminating the material to the class and expecting them to run with it. This is a novel approach to most psychology students who are accustomed to sitting silently during lectures, memorizing material, and demonstrating their mastery on multiple choice exams. My fat studies course has no exams. Instead, grades are based on class participation and completion of written assignments that require students to reflect on personal experience as it relates to the academic material provided throughout the course. Thus it represents a mixture of experiential and analytic ways of knowing (MacDonald, 2002). As such, it may take several class sessions for students to warm up to the idea that they are active participants in the learning environment and that their voices, and emotions, are welcome and necessary parts of the learning process. As Jan McArthur (2011, p. 583) explains, traditionally educated students tend to exile themselves to "Siberia," sitting silently in the far reaches of the classroom. Such students, therefore, need to learn how to participate in different kinds of public space, something that does not happen automatically.

Finally, while WS regularly delves into the social construction of knowledge, psychology has positioned itself as a science that uses "objective" research methods to generate knowledge. Ryan King-White, Joshua Newman, and Michael Giardina (2013) critique the "Evidenced Based Research (EBR) paradigm that dominates obesity science," calling it "dishonest in that it does not acknowledge that knowledge, evidence, and indeed, truth, is socially constructed—largely by the context from which it emerges" (p. 83). They describe the neoliberal environment in which "obesity" researchers operate, where tangible rewards are predicated upon perpetuating the mainstream dogma around weight and health. For example, "so-called evidence based researchers fail to take into account the various ways that corporate influences drive and benefit from the general public's fear of fat" (p. 95). Consistent with this contention, Nir Menachemi et al. (2013) observed that "obesity" researchers often overstate results from their studies, for instance conflating causation with correlation. Psychology and other behavioral health sciences have been loathe to acknowledge that the conceptualization, conduct, generation, dissemination, and application of research occur in a social context subject to bias, especially when it comes to matters of weight. Maureen McHugh and Ashley Kasardo (2012) describe how psychology promotes weight bias in its educational practices by presenting weight-based paradigms in teaching materials to the exclusion of contradictory evidence that weight is a poor predictor of health and evidence that weight loss interventions are ineffective.

Given this backdrop, many students enrolling in fat studies understandably enter the class harboring these ideas despite the following course description:

> This course examines body weight, shape, and size as an area of human difference subject to privilege and discrimination that intersects with other systems of oppression based on gender, race, class, age, sexual orientation, and ability. It employs a multi-disciplinary approach spanning the social-behavioral sciences and humanities. The course frames weight-based oppression as a social justice issue, exploring forms of activism used to counter weightism perpetuated throughout various societal institutions. Consistent with the university's Strategic Plan and its signature area, Improving Human Health & Wellness, this course presents a "holistic approach to health by preparing students to empathize with the sufferings of others, reflect critically on medical knowledge and discourse, create new representations of the medical experience, and confront moral, psychological and ethical dilemmas."

For instance, students recounted, "When I first signed up for this course, I honestly thought it was a class teaching people how to eat healthier to avoid getting fat" and "I thought going into this class we were going to learn about what goes on in a fat person's head, why they're fat, why they eat too much, and the disease that many have that I thought was obesity."

Course content included readings designed to shift students' thinking about fat from a pathologized perspective to thinking about it simply as a form of human difference that, like gender, race, and sexual orientation, has historically been subject to discrimination. The primary resource in the course is *The Fat Studies Reader* (Rothblum & Solovay, 2009), an interdisciplinary anthology organized into six sections (history, health and medicine, social inequality, popular culture and literature, embodying and embracing fat, and political activism). Particularly salient given my professional background and the makeup of the class is the second section that introduces the Health At Every Size (HAES) paradigm as a means of pursuing holistic health via intuitive eating, joyful movement, and body acceptance regardless of size and without the goal of weight loss (Burgard, 2009). Students are required to read each chapter of the text, producing a written reaction in which they articulate three main points of the reading, identify a quote or passage they found most striking, and discuss how the reading relates to their personal and professional lives.

I supplement *The Fat Studies Reader* with journal articles, many based on quantitative research published in psychology and other behavioral health or medical journals. I endeavor to incorporate such readings because some students tend to discount readings based on qualitative methods, narrative reports, case studies, and writings from the humanities or persons operating outside of academia. For instance, students attempted to discredit Ariane Prohaska and Jeannine Gailey's (2009) chapter on sexual violence against fat women based on the small sample in this qualitative study because their major instills the supremacy of quantitative experimental design. I also make a point of highlighting the source of various readings and the professional background of the authors so that students recognize that there *are* voices and findings within their own behavioral health fields that counter the weight-based paradigm. This strategy helps to diffuse comments such as "This class is an attack on my profession!" made early on by one public health major.

Assigning readings of various styles seems to work well, as one student stated: "I think the most important aspect of fat studies is the inclusion of personal narratives supported by scientific research. This allows, as it did for me, the attention of the viewer to be grabbed and hopefully educated by the scientific support." Students from science-based majors reiterated the salience of empirical support, explaining that being able to cite data boosted their believability in conversations with peers and professors: "I have told several people about this information, many replying with hesitation. I am now able to provide them with resources, research, and statistics to prove my point without my audience considering my discussion an emotional one." Another student explained: "Before this class I felt like I could have an alright conversation with people about the implications of fat bias, but that conversation was always limited because I didn't have much quantitative information, but rather just my own personal experiences. I really feel like I can talk about fat in a number of ways now."

A further feature of fat studies is inclusion of the voices of fat people themselves. A number of authors in *The Fat Studies Reader* identify as fat, such as Bianca Wilson (2009) who also speaks of her affiliation with Black, lesbian, and bisexual communities. A teachable moment arose during discussion of this chapter when an undergraduate psychology major adamantly challenged Wilson's credibility despite the fact that she is identified as having a doctoral degree and a faculty position in psychology. Such challenges are not uncommon when teaching about difference, as Ada Sinacore, Patricia Healy, and Monica Justin (2002) found in their survey of feminist psychology educators. Russell et al. (2013) advise that educators be prepared to negotiate these affective responses to facilitate insight rather than ignore such displays. In this vein, I prompted the class to consider these comments in the context of the research on gender and race bias with which they were familiar from introductory psychology classes, examining whether the same message from a "normal" weight, white heterosexual male would similarly be dismissed. The class was receptive to such self-examination. In fact, it represented an "aha moment" in the term.

Linda Bacon's (2009) article on thin privilege, which I assign the first week of class, is an invaluable resource for framing such conversations. In this paper, Bacon adeptly draws comparisons between thin privilege and white privilege. Overwhelmingly, students find this article useful in understanding weight bias as a social justice issue. As a thin person, Bacon presents herself as an ally, a role that many of the thinner students embraced.

> I really related to this article because it made me realize how fat oppression happens to all people in such an unknowing manner. I never consciously think about how much I have internalized about this topic, or how much invisible privilege I have. It made me think about how I can alter my own ways of thinking, learning, and interacting with others to help stop fat oppression.

> This article is a good eye opener and will help me grow as a person. Realizing that because of my weight I am sometimes privileged can help me better control how I act in certain situations. I can also start informing others of ways to create more of a neutral weight society rather than target fat people.

> I have witnessed thin privilege, I understand the advantages that are available simply because I am a certain size. I never have to worry about the size of a seat or if the clothing store carries my size of clothing. These are just little things people have to worry about, bigger issues like health care I still do not have to worry about but others do. By being thin privileged I am better suited to be able to help the fat studies community.

Apart from the readings, I endeavor to provide positive visual representations of fat people to help combat the ubiquitous "headless fatties" and other derogatory portrayals of fat people in mainstream media. Films such as *Weightless* and *The Fat Body (In)Visible*, reviewed in *Fat Studies: An Interdisciplinary Journal of Body, Weight, and Society* (Ellison, 2012; Watkins & Rochat, 2013), help to humanize fat people, depicting them as whole persons with intellect, skills, personality, emotions, and physical capabilities. I have also shown *Dieting: At War With Our Bodies*, a film that follows a group of women on their journey from weight loss programs to a program based on HAES principles. Additional film resources are in the making including *The Student Body* (http://thestudentbodyfilm.com/) and *Fattitude: A Body Positive Documentary* (https://www.kickstarter.com/projects/319256879/fattitude-a-body-positive-documentary).

In addition to the reading reactions, students completed activities such as reviewing websites (e.g., https://www.sizediversityandhealth.org/), interviewing peers about topics covered in class, and critically analyzing body-related messages communicated via magazines, music videos, and other forms of media. Finally, students completed a group activism project of their own design. Thus far, students have created a "Stop-Fat-Hate" Facebook page, held a scale-smashing event, broadcast a fat-positive radio show, posted fat-positive messages around campus, published an article on HAES in the student newspaper, designed fat-positive T-shirts, held a body-positive photo shoot, and led discussions with both college and high school audiences. Jan McArthur (2010) stresses the importance in social justice pedagogy to move from mere critique to action, creating an active exchange between ideas and practice. The group activism projects prompted students to do just that, imbuing them with the sense that they can indeed be agents of change. Interestingly, students also reported informal types of activism, disseminating class concepts to others beyond the dictates of assignments.

> Recently, I have had a number of friends posting on Facebook about their summer weight loss goals. I am currently working on a message that introduces HAES and highlights the need to live in the now and not solely focus on weight.

> Being in this class has made me more vocal toward people who are worried about their self and body image. I hear a lot of my friends talking about looks and weight. Before this class I didn't think much of it. I now catch myself telling my friends they need to stop focusing on their weight and constantly trying to lose weight. Before I just kind of let it slide and thought it was more normal. Now I see myself actively trying to explain to friends about how weight doesn't matter; as long as they live a healthy life they shouldn't be concerned with their looks. Their body is their body and they should start accepting it more.

> This class was so special to me that I involved my family in it. I have taken so many of the readings and websites that we have looked at and shared them with family members.

Feminist pedagogy generally encourages students to connect personal experiences to course content; however, the value of this approach in teaching fat studies remains in question. Although some fat studies instructors allow for self-disclosure in written assignments, they have explicitly discouraged discussion of personal experiences in the classroom, citing concerns that such conversation might reinforce traditional body discourses or result in emotional distress that they are ill-equipped to handle (Watkins et al., 2012). In our review of fat studies pedagogy, I along with Amy Farrell and Andrea Doyle Hugmeyer (2012) also consider the issue of instructor self-disclosure regarding the body. Jones and Hughes-Decatur (2012) assert that "the teacher's body *is* pedagogy" (p. 54, emphasis in original) and rightly constitutes a topic for discussion. I choose to self-disclose that I am "obese" by BMI standards, have experienced weight bias, and have a history of dieting and eating disorders. At the same time, I attempt to model my current state of body acceptance and personal engagement with the HAES paradigm. That is, I present myself as a coping model, someone with struggles similar to many students, but who has dealt with these issues in a relatively healthy manner.

Similarly, I encourage students to scrutinize their own life experiences both on paper and in classroom discussions to create an understanding about systems of oppression through personal testimony. Self-disclosure in class is not a requirement, but I have found most students are eager to relate their experiences with weight bias, dieting, media messages, and the like to course material. Although my fat studies classes have been primarily comprised of young, white women, Jones and Hughes-Decatur (2012) attest that their students across gender, race, ethnicity, and sexual orientation have all been "wounded by discourses around the body and body image" (p. 53). McArthur (2011) observes that the production of knowledge in higher education can be both painful and disturbing. As an example, one larger student disclosed that upon visiting the campus recreation center, a thin woman gave her the once-over and exclaimed, "Why even bother? It's too late for you!" Obviously, this was a painful experience for the student, and the collective gasp from her classmates indicated that they shared her pain. This incident resonates with McArthur's (2011) contention that the oppressed and oppressor need to work together, with higher education serving as a place "where people can share, consider and feel the pain of others." She continues, "For without this, there can be no social justice" (p. 585).

According to Jones and Hughes-Decatur (2012), when students engage with their own bodies, these can become sites of self-transformation. Students can learn to "move, speak, and interact differently and produce new social spaces—perhaps spaces of inclusion, value, acceptance, and power" (p. 53). This transformative pedagogy seemingly assisted my students in resisting hegemonic discourse, empowering those whose bodies have been marginalized, and creating allies among those whose bodies have been conferred privilege. Specifically, students related gaining greater body acceptance as well as greater awareness and sensitivity to others' experiences of weight bias. Changes in behavior included less frequent weighing, less dieting and restrictive eating, and engaging in different types of physical activity, shifting the motivation from weight loss to health and enjoyment.

> Health At Every Size has changed my life. I used to wake up every morning and weigh myself and get so angry when I didn't see the number I wanted to see. I used to work out hardcore just to lose weight. I wasn't really happy with my body or my life. I no longer exercise because I feel I have to. I exercise now to make me feel good. Working out doesn't have to be going to the gym. Working out can be snowboarding, hiking, playing basketball. I have stopped weighing

myself every morning. I put the scale in the storage closet so I don't have to look at it. I even encouraged my roommate to stop weighing herself too. I will never go on another diet. The material in this class has taught me I can be happy with my body just the way it is.

I used to always be worried about counting calories and making sure to exercise every day for a certain amount of time. This class made me realize I should be happy, and counting calories was not making me happy. I now still make smart food choices, but I never obsess over how many calories I've eaten that day, and if I can't make it to the gym, it isn't the end of the world.

I think I can now confidently say, I will never diet again! I also now understand one of the biggest reasons I hate the gym. I will never be a waif, but I will be proud of my strong and larger than model size body. I can understand that my bigger thighs probably help me bike and swim faster and that my normal weight is A-OK.

Thanks to this class, I know I can have pizza without freaking out about the calories I put in my body. Before this class, eating that pizza would make me feel terrible and would cause me to want to work out for hours to burn the calories, but I now know that I am human and I should never stop eating the things I love because of a number that is attached to it.

Through this class, I came to recognize that I was actually internalizing the stereotypical messages that I was being hounded with. I immediately made an appointment with a counselor and with her help as well as the information I was receiving in class, I was able to begin better recognizing and tearing down that prejudice.

As Sinacore et al. (2002) suggest, this pedagogy also can help students in privileged positions, those of "normal" weight in this case, to change their worldviews. As an example, one student stated, "Before taking this class, I was not aware as to how much discrimination fatter individuals face." At the same time it validated the worldviews of those in oppressed positions. Fat students seemed appreciative that their experiences of weight bias were reframed as affronts to social justice rather than seen as deserved treatment for personal failure. Additionally, students seemed able to move from mere intellectual critique of dominant discourse to actually living with their bodies differently as Jones and Hughes-Decatur (2012) describe; these authors relate that their students also connected their newfound knowledge to professional aspirations. Similarly, many fat studies students vowed to conduct their future careers in ways that counteract weightism.

This class has changed my entire outlook on the world. My graduate field of study has a social justice focus. I can't recall very much said about weight. This term I have written about weight bias in my counseling course and even touched on space accessibility with my internship supervisor when planning an event.

As a teacher, I plan to incorporate discussion on size diversity and how this should be addressed within the world of general and adapted physical education.

Since I am working toward being a clinical psychologist, I think this reading was a great reminder that even the best intentions can sometimes be flawed. I don't want to have a client who is pursuing weight loss and then blindly believe that they need to lose weight. I'd rather be of the mindset that every person is unique, and that there are other markers of health.

In sum, teaching fat studies as part of a DPD curriculum has been challenging as well as rewarding. Among the challenges of feminist pedagogy, Sinacore et al. (2002) describe students denying the legitimacy of the material and practices, refusing to complete assignments, and stating that they have no inherent interest in the class but are simply taking it for the required credit. I have experienced all of the above, with one student boldly proclaiming that she finds fat people to be disgusting and that she was only in the class because she needed the credits to graduate. McArthur (2010) describes engaging with people and beliefs with which one disagrees as an essential part of critical pedagogy. Amie MacDonald (2002) finds that in these situations, the faculty member is seldom alone as other students chime in on the issue at hand. Feminist educators in Sinacore et al.'s study report comparable experiences, one noting that as the term progresses students take more ownership of the classroom climate. I too have found this to be the case. For instance, when a petite gymnast reported seeing no problem with public weigh-ins, even before I could reply classmates engaged her in a discussion of thin privilege. Despite the challenges, Sinacore et al.'s participants also elucidated benefits associated with feminist pedagogy, foremost of which are enhancing students' development and promulgating social justice in the process. Comments extracted from assignments, some of which have been presented here, seem to support these outcomes for students in my fat studies classes.

Because fat studies is a relatively new field of academic inquiry, efforts to integrate these concepts into higher education are as yet limited. In an effort to facilitate the infusion of fat studies into social justice curricula, this chapter has delineated resources and described strategies for doing so, relying on student voices to illustrate the impact of this pedagogy. Although fraught with challenges, fat studies pedagogy has its rewards in helping students think, feel, and behave in healthier and more socially conscious ways with respect to weight.

References

Ambwani, S., Thomas, K. M., Hopwood, C. J., Moss, S. A., & Grilo, C. M. (2014). Obesity stigmatization as the status quo: Structural considerations and prevalence among young adults in the U.S. *Eating Behaviors, 15,* 366–370.

Andreyeva, T., Puhl, R. M., & Brownell, K. D. (2008). Changes in perceived weight discrimination among Americans, 1995–1996 through 2004–2006. *Obesity, 16,* 1129–1134.

Bacon, L. (2009). *Reflections on fat acceptance: Lessons learned from thin privilege.* Retrieved from http://www.lindabacon.org/Bacon_ThinPrivilege080109.pdf

Boysen, G. A. (2011). Diversity topics covered in a teaching of psychology course. *Teaching of Psychology, 38,* 89–93.

Burgard, D. (2009). What is "Health At Every Size"? In E. Rothblum & S. Solovay (Eds.), *The fat studies reader* (pp. 41–53). New York, NY: New York University Press.

Cardinal, B. J., Whitney, A. R., Narimatsu, M., Hubert, N., & Souza, B. J. (2014). Obesity bias in the gym: An under-recognized social justice, diversity, and inclusivity issue. *Journal of Physical Education, Recreation, and Dance, 85,* 3–6.

Ellison, J. (2012). Exercise for every body. *Fat Studies, 1,* 134–137.

Jones, S., & Hughes-Decatur, H. (2012). Speaking of bodies in justice-oriented feminist teacher education. *Journal of Teacher Education, 63,* 51–61.

King-White, R., Newman, J. I., & Giardina, M. D. (2013). Articulating fatness: Obesity and the scientific tautologies of bodily accumulation in neoliberal times. *Review of Education, Pedagogy, and Cultural Studies, 35,* 79–102.

Kristjansson, M. (Director). (2011). *The fat body (in)visible* [DVD]. New York, NY: Women Make Movies.

MacDonald, A. A. (2002). Feminist pedagogy and the appeal to epistemic privilege. In A. A. Macdonald & S. Sanchez-Casal (Eds.), *Twenty-first-century feminist classrooms* (pp. 111–133). New York, NY: Palgrave Macmillan.

McArthur, J. (2010). Exile, sanctuary and diaspora: Meditations between higher education and society. *Teaching in Higher Education, 16,* 579–589.

McArthur, J. (2011). Achieving social justice within and through higher education: The challenge for critical pedagogy. *Teaching in Higher Education, 15,* 493–504.

McHugh, M. C., & Kasardo, A. E. (2012). Anti-fat prejudice: The role of psychology in explication, education, and eradication. *Sex Roles, 66,* 617–627.

McNabb, C., & Finley, A. (Producers). (2006). *Dieting: At war with our bodies* [DVD]. Toronto, ON, Canada: National Eating Disorder Information Centre.

Menachemi, N., Tajeu, G., Sen, B., Ferdinand, A. O., Singleton, C., Utley, J., … Allison, D. B. (2013). Overstatement of results in the nutrition and obesity peer-reviewed literature. *American Journal of Preventive Medicine, 45*, 615–621.

Pennick, F. (Director). (2010). *Weightless* [DVD]. Brooklyn, NY: Organized Chaos Mediaworks.

Prohaska, A., & Gailey, J. (2009). Fat women as "easy targets": Achieving masculinity through hogging. In E. Rothblum & S. Solovay (Eds.), *The fat studies reader* (pp. 158–166). New York, NY: New York University Press.

Puhl, R. M., Andreyeva, T., & Brownell, K. D. (2008). Perceptions of weight discrimination: Prevalence and comparison to race and gender discrimination in America. *International Journal of Obesity, 32*, 992–1000.

Rothblum, E., & Solovay, S. (2009). *The fat studies reader.* New York, NY: New York University Press.

Russell, C., Cameron, E., Socha, T., & McNinch, H. (2013). "Fatties cause global warming": Fat pedagogy and environmental education. *Canadian Journal of Environmental Education, 18*, 27–45.

Sinacore, A. L., Healy, P., & Justin, M. (2002). A qualitative analysis of the experiences of feminist psychology educators: The classroom. *Feminism and Psychology, 12*, 339–362.

Watkins, P. L., & Concepcion, R. Y. (2014). Teaching Health At Every Size to health care professionals and students. In E. Glovsky (Ed.), *Wellness not weight: Motivational interviewing and Health At Every Size* (pp. 159–169). San Diego, CA: Cognella Academic.

Watkins, P. L., Farrell, A. E., & Hugmeyer, A. D. (2012). Teaching fat studies: From conception to reception. *Fat Studies, 1*, 180–194.

Watkins, P. L., & Rochat, M. (2013). Fat acceptance on film. *Fat Studies, 2*, 216–219.

Wilson, B. D. M. (2009). Widening the dialogue to narrow the gap in health disparities: Approaches to fat black lesbian and bisexual women's health promotion. In E. Rothblum & S. Solovay (Eds.), *The fat studies reader* (pp. 54–64). New York, NY: New York University Press.

SEVENTEEN

Learning to Teach Every Body: Exploring the Emergence of a Critical "Obesity" Pedagogy

Erin Cameron

I was thrilled. My proposal to develop and teach a graduate course on Obesity Discourses in Society, Education, and Healthcare in the Masters of Public Health program at Lakehead University had been accepted. But I was also nervous. Given that my previous experiences challenging dominant discourses at a postsecondary institution had resulted in overt resistance from students (Cameron, 2014a), I worried about how public health students would respond to a course that challenged the biomedical approach to "obesity" that equates weight with health and reinforces a culture of blame and shame for bodies outside normative ideals (Leahy, 2009; Rich & Evans, 2009). Would the students be open to learning new ways of thinking, approaching, and framing "obesity"? Would the students be able to move beyond weight-biased attitudes and a weight-based health paradigm towards a paradigm that supports the idea that healthy bodies can come in many shapes and sizes? While these questions were at the front of my mind as I prepared for the course, I also knew that I could not predict students' reactions to the course. So instead, I just got down to it. I decided to focus on developing a pedagogical approach that I called "critical obesity pedagogy," which I hoped would support students in being open to ideas that they likely would not have encountered elsewhere in the program or professionally.

I used self-study to reflect on my developing critical "obesity" pedagogy. Self-study is a research method that invites educators to consider how contexts—social, political, and cultural—inform educational practice (Hamilton & Pinnegar, 1998). It enables educators "to uncover, critique, and celebrate the less explicit, yet significant, aspects of professional practice" (Wilcox, Watson, & Paterson, 2004, p. 307), and allows educators to reflect on their curriculum and pedagogy in order to understand "the values, beliefs, and assumptions that inform their educative decisions and actions" (Brown, 2004, p. 520) in a process of stepping back to reveal influences on thoughts and actions in the classroom with an end goal of improving teaching practices (Pithouse, Mitchell, & Weber, 2009).

In this self-study, I drew upon field notes and engaged in reflective journaling. I also conducted semi-structured interviews with four students after the course was completed to explore the following question: what pedagogical strategies support students to think critically about "obesity"? The interviews lasted between 45 minutes and 1 hour and were transcribed verbatim. To respect confidentiality, pseudonyms were selected by the students. After verifying the transcripts with the students to ensure that they were comfortable with what was transcribed, I engaged in two rounds of successive coding and a thematic analysis of the data with the use of the qualitative data analysis software ATLAS.ti 7.0.

In this chapter, I highlight the context that contributed to my developing a critical obesity pedagogy, identify the key themes highlighted by the students, and outline some of the ways in which my teaching practice has benefited from this form of inquiry.

The Context: A Developing Critical Obesity Pedagogy

As I developed the course, I drew from "critical obesity" scholarship, which is an umbrella term for various labels and field descriptors, such as critical obesity studies, critical weight studies, critical geographies of body size, and fat studies. While there are differences in these respective approaches, "all of [the subfields] offer important *critical* perspectives on the dominant view of obesity and are united in their refusal to simply reproduce/legitimate/endorse biomedical narratives that would have us 'tackle' this putative problem" (Monaghan, Colls, & Evans, 2013, p. 251, emphasis in original). Immersed in this scholarship, I became very aware of the growing evidence on how weight-biased attitudes are negatively impacting teaching and learning in postsecondary institutions (e.g., Brown, 2012; Fisanick, 2006; Wann, 2009). Moreover, I became interested in how efforts to deconstruct "obesity" rhetoric, emphasize the biopolitics of "obesity," address the intersectionality of weight-based oppression, and explore the sociocultural origins of "obesity" are consistently met with resistance from students (Boling, 2011; Cameron et al., 2014; Escalera, 2009; Fisanick, 2007; Guthman, 2009; Russell, Cameron, Socha, & McNinch, 2013; Tirosh, 2006; Watkins & Concepcion, 2014; Watkins & Doyle Hugmeyer, 2013; Watkins, Farrell, & Doyle Hugmeyer, 2012).

In fact, a number of scholars have written about their "fledgling efforts, misgivings, and breakthroughs" (Boling, 2011, p. 110) to challenge obesity discourse and how efforts to destabilize contemporary obesity discourses in postsecondary institutions can provoke overt resistance, including strong negative emotional reactions in students (Guthman, 2009). While this emerging work has indeed contributed to our understanding of pedagogical approaches that help to challenge obesity discourse and reduce weight-biased attitudes, as I have argued elsewhere, there is a need for more research in this area and "pedagogy needs to take a more central role in critical fat scholarship" (Cameron, 2014b, p. 179). This chapter, in concert with all the other chapters in *The Fat Pedagogy Reader*, seeks to address this gap.

At the same time that I was immersed in developing and teaching this course, I was collecting data for my doctoral research examining the pedagogical approaches of faculty members teaching critical obesity scholarship and fat studies in postsecondary institutions (Cameron, 2015a, 2015b). Thus, my developing critical obesity pedagogy was informed not only by reading the literature but also by my interviews with faculty with teaching experiences in the area.

While I did not complete data analysis of these interviews until much later, the conversations drew my attention to those issues that I needed to pay attention to prior to the course, including: (a) how I could frame the course in order to create an inclusive, safe space; (b) how I could acknowledge where the students were at in terms of thinking about "obesity" while also introducing them to critical approaches; (c) how theory and research could support students' learning; and (d) content that I could use in my teaching, given the ever-expanding literature focused on critical obesity scholarship.

It was also helpful that I had an academic background in education; I had a BEd and was working on my PhD in educational studies. Therefore, I was well-versed in constructivist and student-centered approaches to education as well as in feminist pedagogy, critical pedagogy, and social justice pedagogy. I had been inspired by Michael Apple, Henry Giroux, Maxine Greene, bell hooks, and Peter McLaren, all scholars who argue that classrooms are not separate from, but instead extensions of, a society fraught by hierarchies, power, and privilege. Nonetheless, I still was finding that while concerns about oppression related to gender, race, class, sexuality, and ability figured prominently in critical pedagogy, there was little to no attention paid to body size as a social justice concern (Cameron et al., 2014).

Before turning to my study, I also think it is important to acknowledge my thin privilege. While I have experienced body oppression and been subjected to body policing, particularly within elite sport contexts, I acknowledge that I approach critical obesity pedagogy as a relatively thin, heterosexual, white, able-bodied female. For this reason, like Patricia Boling (2011), I have worried about standpoint epistemology while trying not to let this stop my work as a thin ally. As Boling argues:

> I think being thin is a problematic vantage point from which to address issues related to being fat. But I don't regard that as a sufficient reason for refusing to address the issues that face fat people, like stereotyping, fat bigotry, legal and social discrimination, and self-hatred. Standpoint theorists tell us that there is a problem with speaking for others … but there is also a problem with *not* speaking for others. (p. 119, emphasis in original)

Teaching Every Body: Paying Attention to Pedagogy

In preparing for the course, I carefully reflected upon my pedagogical approach. In previous courses I had taught, I had been clear about my stance as a critical pedagogue and had encountered a great deal of resistance. Upon reflection, I came to realize how much I tended to focus on teaching a course rather than on creating a community of learners. Given this, I decided to employ Richard Tinning's (2002, 2011) "modest pedagogy," an approach that combines and interweaves analytic voices of critique and truth, voices of rage over injustices, and personal voices of lived stories and culture. To me, this approach highlighted the importance of embracing diversity, relationality, and contextuality within one's teaching while working to advance a more socially just world. Given my own experiences and reading about student resistance experienced by others teaching fat studies (Guthman, 2009), I was wary of starting too strong, worried that my passion for disrupting weight-based oppression would override my compassion for where the students were on their journeys of learning about "obesity." What this meant for me was that I needed to determine, and then start, where the students themselves were at.

I began by acknowledging the dominant discourse, that "obesity" is often framed as a biomedical problem in need of addressing. I then endeavored to gently introduce other paradigms or frameworks, using readings to ground the discussions. I also engaged a multimedia approach using not only lectures but also videos, storytelling, and guest speakers to try to make the different paradigms come to life. I assigned weekly reading responses not only to ensure that students were reading the materials but also to facilitate them connecting the materials to their own professional and personal experiences. Unlike some (e.g., Tirosh, 2006), I invited students to bring their lived experiences to class discussions and assignments. I recognize doing this may be more difficult in undergraduate courses, but given my course was for graduate students, all of whom would be mature students working full-time in various health care professions (e.g., nursing, health promotion, public health, mental health), I felt comfortable inviting them to use their own experiences as one foundation.

Student Reflections: The (Un)learning Process

While self-study was vital to enabling critical reflection on my own pedagogies and practices, I also found it very helpful to deepen this reflection by explicitly seeking out student perspectives on the course upon its completion. When asked to describe their perspectives towards "obesity" prior to the course, students articulated that they had believed that "obesity" was an illness, a disease, something bad, something unattractive, and something to be policed. They talked about the influence of culture and society on their own perspectives of bodies, weight, beauty, and health. For example, Alexandria stated:

> We've been so conditioned to think that people that are overweight or obese are not attractive or not beautiful and I still feel that way because I've been so conditioned that way. That's why when you're overweight or obese, or you see someone that is, it's hard to see them as beautiful because you get bombarded with all these messages in society and it's just horrible to think that. There's nothing wrong with an obese body and we try to think: what is wrong with it? Why is it ugly? It's because the rest of the world has been hammering that thought into your head since you were born, so if you're naturally or genetically predisposed to being heavier set than how are you ever supposed to love yourself or learn to love yourself or naturally love yourself when all of these negative messages are being hammered into your head from birth? It's really sad when you think about it.

The students also talked about how their schooling in various health care professions had been instrumental in promoting a weight-based health paradigm that links weight to health and is built on harmful assumptions about individual responsibility, risk, and health behaviors. Deborah described it this way:

> It's something that my friends talk about a lot, I guess, because we're all in health care and I believe our education before taking this course has been [that] obesity is bad. It's costing the health care system money and it's fat people's fault that they're fat. I don't know if we are all necessarily to blame for having those opinions because that's what we've always been taught.

The students also freely shared how they initially felt frustrated, angry, and confused by the course content. As I reflected later in my journal, "How could they not? It was so different than what they had previously learned." Student resistance has often been described in school contexts as a manifestation of oppositional or anti-school behaviors, but this approach has been challenged because it fails to acknowledge student agency (Zine, 2010). Instead, resistance can be seen as a productive tool for learning, perhaps best articulated through Michalinos Zem-bylas and Megan Boler's (2002) concept of the "pedagogy of discomfort" that acknowledges that learning is not only about cognition, but also about evoking feeling and emotion (see also Boler, 2004a, 2004b). Such feelings of discomfort are well-articulated by Cleopatra:

> I remember just the first week's readings and just wanting to throw them against the wall be-cause they just challenged what I thought I knew about obesity and letting that go. It started from the first week. So I had just never considered that there was an alternative to what I had been taught or the information that had been shared with me. That was mind-blowing. I described it to someone else [that it was like] when I started reading Harry Potter, I just kept throwing it against the wall because I didn't understand it and I couldn't get into it and then something triggered and I loved it. You just have to change your mindset and that's a hard thing to do, I guess. I wasn't expecting to have to do that in the course.

Despite this discomfort, students reported that the course gave them the space and time to work through their resistance. By meeting them where they were and scaffolding the infor-mation by starting with the dominant discourse of "obesity" as a problem, then moving into different ways of reframing "obesity," students were able to slowly engage with the material at the same time that they were building trust with each other and with me as the instructor. The importance of starting where they were at was emphasized by Deborah:

> The first week we started talking about BMI [Body Mass Index] and I needed all that to kind of set a baseline before I was going to think about shifting my own paradigm. … I feel like the gradual process that you did the first couple of weeks was something that I needed and that they would need as well.

This sentiment was also shared by Cleopatra:

> You respected the fact that people were coming at the topic from different perspectives and people were working in different environments and people have different beliefs. So, I'm not saying, "No, that's wrong how could you possibly think that way? Didn't you read the reading or have you not been paying attention?" You brought us along slowly and not calling us out if we were taking our time coming along.

Students also articulated how the assigned readings helped them to work through their resis-tance. For example, Deborah articulated how the readings helped her think critically about "obesity":

> The first week I was kind of, like, oh my gosh. I couldn't think that way. I think it was about the BMI and Health At Every Size that just blew my mind because I was so conditioned to think that being fat equals unhealthy and that BMI is the predictor of all. So I think the read-ings for those weeks, I think the first two weeks of readings, is really what changed things for me. I needed to see the research. I needed to see the paper. Like, somebody just telling me about Health At Every Size and just talking about it wasn't enough. I had to read the journal articles. I think that's similar for people in Public Health and in health care. They need to see the research.

Students also discussed the assignments and articulated how the weekly reading responses, in which they had to summarize and connect the learning to their own lives, helped to make the content relevant and meaningful. For Lynne, it was what helped her engage in the course: "The reading responses were tough but they helped me to engage at a deeper level." For Alexandria, the reading responses made the learning more meaningful: "Throughout the course I was very engaged. I like how personal it was, which made it more relevant and meaningful."

Finally, students discussed how the course had changed them and what learning they found to be their most important "take-aways." Many of them talked about feeling an increased level of empathy for, and sense of empowerment in, working with patients. This is captured in an example given by Alexandria of how the course had changed her professional practice:

> In our clinic, I'm trained to do pelvic examinations and pap tests. There was a woman who came in who would, I guess, medically be classified as morbidly obese and I just took way more time with her. And while we don't typically help people undress before an exam, I knew that she needed help and I just made it very light. It wasn't a big issue that she needed help to remove her clothing or to get on the examination table and I just tried really hard to not make her feel bad about herself or her weight and I think I was really successful at that. I think just learning from the course more about how people feel helped me to be that much more conscientious about how difficult it is to be overweight, especially in the medical profession where people are just using your weight as an excuse for all your health problems when that's not even really the case.

Students also clearly described a shift in how they had conceptualized bodies, health, and weight prior to and after the course. Cleopatra, for example, said:

> I no longer believe that it is something that has to be changed for somebody to be healthy. I think on a personal level I try to be friendlier and smile more at people of different sizes and be more accepting of myself and of the people around me and that size is not an indicator of health.

Similarly, Deborah stated:

> Probably at the grocery store. Historically if I went to the grocery store and I saw someone overweight buying chips, I would usually think, "Oh my gosh, why are you buying chips if you're clearly overweight? You must want to lose weight if you're overweight so why are you buying chips?" So definitely when I go to the grocery store I think of that.

Interviewing these students about their experiences in the course, I learned that dominant obesity discourse can indeed be unlearned if one plans for resistance and understands it not as an obstacle but as an important part of the unlearning process. The students also helped me to see that while it can be challenging to consider new "obesity" paradigms, the benefits of doing so can be transformative and empowering both personally and professionally. These students fully supported the idea that a modest pedagogy, which embraced diversity, relationality, and contextuality, was effective.

Future Directions: A Developing Critical Obesity Pedagogy

While the course was a success on many fronts, as a result of this self-study and the interviews with the students, my course objectives would now look quite different were I to teach a similar course in the future. I now see the importance of not only focusing on *what* the students will learn (i.e., the curriculum), but also *how* they learn, (i.e., the learning process). It is in this focus on the pedagogical encounter (Leach & Moon, 1999), that moment where a teacher seeks to support a learner where they are at, that I now see the most potential for a critical obesity pedagogy. In other words, instead of expecting students (or any audience, for that matter) to do critical work by themselves, it is imperative that critical obesity scholars scaffold learning and engage disparate areas of knowledge across disciplines and sub-disciplines to effectively support students in learning the complexities and constructions of bodies, health, and weight. Implicit in this is a reversal of the prevailing pedagogical approach wherein content is identified first and leads the educational process; instead, the needs of individual students are put first (Armour & Harris, 2014). Shaping curriculum around a pedagogical model that takes the learner as the starting point is, I have found, a particularly effective approach when teaching students immersed in health-related professional programs in which resistance may be most high. Had I not engaged in this self-study prior to teaching this course and taken the time to reflect deeply about my pedagogical approach, I might have missed an opportunity to support students through their discomfort towards new ways of thinking personally and professionally about bodies, weight, and health.

References

Armour, K., & Harris, J. (2013). Making the case for developing new PE-for-Health pedagogies. *Quest, 65*, 201–219.

Boler, M. (2004a). *Feeling power: Emotions and education*. New York, NY: Routledge.

Boler, M. (2004b). Teaching for hope: The ethics of shattering world views. In D. Liston & J. Garrison (Eds.), *Teaching, learning, and loving: Reclaiming passion in educational practice* (pp. 117–131). New York, NY: Routledge Falmer.

Boling, P. (2011). On learning to teach fat feminism. *Feminist Teacher, 21*(2), 110–123.

Brown, E. (2004). The significance of race and social class for self-study and the professional knowledge base of teacher education. In J. Loughran, M. Hamilton, V. LaBoskey, & T. Russell (Eds.), *International handbook of self-study of teaching and teacher education practices* (pp. 517–574). Dordrecht, the Netherlands: Kluwer.

Brown, H. (2012). *Fashioning a self from which to thrive: Negotiating size privilege as a fat woman learner at a small liberal arts college in the Midwest* (Doctoral dissertation). Northern Illinois University, DeKalb, IL.

Cameron, E. (2014a). A journey of critical scholarship in Physical Education Teacher Education (PETE). In A. Ovens & T. Fletcher (Eds.), *Self-study in physical education: Exploring the interplay of practice and scholarship* (pp. 99–116). New York, NY: Springer.

Cameron, E. (2014b). *Throwing their weight around: A critical examination of faculty experiences with challenging dominant obesity discourse in post-secondary education* (Doctoral dissertation). Lakehead University, Thunder Bay, ON, Canada.

Cameron, E. (2015a). Teaching resources for post-secondary educators who challenge dominant "obesity" discourse. *Fat Studies, 4*(2), 212–226.

Cameron, E. (2015b). Toward a fat pedagogy: A study of pedagogical approaches aimed at challenging obesity discourse in post-secondary education. *Fat Studies, 4*(1), 28–45.

Cameron, E., Oakley, J., Walton, G., Russell, C., Chambers, L., & Socha, T. (2014). Moving beyond the injustices of the schooled healthy body. In I. Bogotch & C. Shields (Eds.), *The international handbook of social justice and educational leadership* (pp. 687–704). New York, NY: Springer.

Escalera, E. A. (2009). Stigma threat and the fat professor: Reducing student prejudice in the classroom. In E. Rothblum & S. Solovay (Eds.), *The fat studies reader* (pp. 213–220). New York, NY: New York University Press.

Fisanick, C. (2006). Evaluating the absent presence: The professor's body at tenure and promotion. *Review of Education, Pedagogy, and Cultural Studies, 28*(3–4), 325–338.

Fisanick, C. (2007). "They are weighted with authority": Fat female professors in academic and popular cultures. *Feminist Teacher, 17*(3), 237–255.

Guthman, J. (2009). Teaching the politics of obesity: Insights into neoliberal embodiment and contemporary biopolitics. *Antipode, 41*(5), 1110–1133.

Hamilton, M., & Pinnegar, S. (1998). Conclusion: The value and the promise of self-study. In M. Hamilton, S. Pinnegar, T. Russell, J. Loughran, & V. LaBoskey (Eds.), *Reconceptualizing teacher practice: Self-study in teacher education* (pp. 235–246). London, England: Falmer.

Leach, J., & Moon, B. (1999). *Learners and pedagogy.* London, England: Paul Chapman.

Leahy, D. (2009). Disgusting pedagogies. In J. Wright & V. Harwood (Eds.), *Biopolitics and the "obesity epidemic"* (pp. 172–182). New York, NY: Routledge.

Monaghan, L., Colls, R., & Evans, B. (2013). Obesity discourse and fat politics: Research, critique and interventions. *Critical Public Health, 23*(3), 249–262.

Pithouse, K., Mitchell, C., & Weber, S. (2009). Self-study in teaching and teacher development: A call to action. *Educational Action Research, 17*(1), 42–62.

Rich, E., & Evans, J. (2009). Performative health in schools: Welfare policy, neoliberalism and social regulation? In J. Wright & V. Harwood (Eds.), *Biopolitics and the "obesity epidemic"* (pp. 157–171). New York, NY: Routledge.

Russell, C., Cameron, E., Socha, T., & McNinch, H. (2013). "Fatties cause global warming": Fat pedagogy and environmental education. *Canadian Journal of Environmental Education, 18,* 27–45.

Tinning, R. (2002). Toward a "modest pedagogy": Reflections on the problematics of critical pedagogy. *Quest, 54*(3), 224–240.

Tinning, R. (2011, April). *A reflexive account of knowledge and discourse in physical education research (aka sport pedagogy).* Scholar's lecture, American Educational Research Association annual conference, New Orleans, LA.

Tirosh, Y. (2006). Weighty speech: Addressing body size in the classroom. *Review of Education, Pedagogy, and Cultural Studies, 28*(3–4), 267–279.

Wann, M. (2009). Foreword: Fat studies: An invitation to revolution. In E. Rothblum & S. Solovay (Eds.), *The fat studies reader* (pp. ix–xxv). New York, NY: New York University Press.

Watkins, P. L., & Concepcion, R. Y. (2014). Teaching Health At Every Size to health care professionals and students. In E. Glovsky (Ed.), *Wellness not weight: Motivational interviewing and Health At Every Size* (pp. 159–169). San Diego, CA: Cognella Academic.

Watkins, P. L., & Doyle Hugmeyer, D. (2013). Teaching about eating disorders from a fat studies perspective. *Transformations: The Journal of Inclusive Scholarship and Pedagogy, 23*(2), 177–188.

Watkins, P. L., Farrell, A., & Doyle Hugmeyer, A. (2012). Teaching fat studies: From conception to reception. *Fat Studies, 1*(2), 180–194.

Wilcox, S., Watson, J., & Paterson, M. (2004). Self-study in professional practice. In J. Loughran, M. Hamilton, V. LaBoskey, & T. Russell (Eds.), *International handbook of self-study of teaching and teacher education practices* (pp. 273–312). Dordrecht, the Netherlands: Kluwer.

Zembylas, M., & Boler, M. (2002). On the spirit of patriotism: Challenges of a "pedagogy of discomfort." *Teachers College Record.* Retrieved from http://www.tcrecord.org/library/abstract.asp?contentid=11007

Zine, J. (2010). Redefining resistance: Towards an Islamic subculture in schools. *Race, Ethnicity and Education, 13*(3), 293–316.

EIGHTEEN

An "Intervention" Into Public Health Interventions: Questioning the Weight-Based Paradigm

Krishna Bhagat and Shannon Jette

University students pursuing public health studies should be equipped with skills to promote health in safe, efficacious, and holistic ways. This includes identifying and confronting gaps, inconsistencies, or generalizations in commonly used public health frameworks, such as the weight-based paradigm. The weight-based paradigm is underpinned by a number of assertions, including: adiposity poses significant mortality and morbidity risk; anyone who is determined can lose weight and keep it off through appropriate diet and exercise; and the pursuit of weight loss is a practical and positive goal (Bacon & Aphramor, 2011). While the weight-based paradigm is a cornerstone of many public health pedagogies and informs a range of health policies (O'Reilly & Sixsmith, 2012), not all practitioners agree on its effectiveness or its safety, arguing that it can lead to food and body preoccupation, repeated cycles of weight loss and regain, distraction from wider health determinants, reduced self-esteem, eating disorders, and weight stigmatization (e.g., Bacon, 2010; Daníelsdóttir, Burgard, & Oliver-Pyatt, 2009; Neumark-Sztainer, 2009; O'Reilly & Sixsmith, 2012).

In this chapter, we present a pedagogical approach used to encourage kinesiology students to critically engage with the weight-based paradigm and its implications. Our approach was informed by a poststructuralist perspective that allows for an understanding of subjectivity (i.e., a person's identity) as not "fixed" but rather as fluid and, moreover, constructed through the already gendered, heterosexualized, and racialized discourses to which one has access (Rail, 2002; Weedon, 1997; Wright, 2001). Michel Foucault's conceptualization of discourses as historically and culturally situated systems of meaning that shape what can be "said" and "known" in a society—as ways of constituting knowledge—are central to a poststructuralist approach (Weedon, 1997). In this view, the "body" does not have meaning outside of its discursive articulation, and the ways in which discourses constitute the bodies of individuals are recognized as always being a part of a wider network of power relations, often with institutional bases.

Examined through a poststructuralist lens, the weight-based health paradigm that centers on dominant discourses of "obesity" is culturally produced and has the power to shape the way young people think about their bodies and the bodies of others (Rail, 2009). Therefore, our pedagogical approach entailed treating the weight-based paradigm not as objective "fact" but rather as something that is imbued with power and should be deconstructed through an examination of the knowledge(s) underpinning it, how it is mobilized (disseminated) in public health campaigns, and, finally, if, and how, it works to shape the embodied subjectivities of the young people who are the focus of such campaigns. In order to accomplish these three inter-related goals, we had students engage with and discuss Glenn Gaesser's (2003) article "Is It Necessary to Be Thin to Be Healthy?" that questioned some of the assumptions underpinning the weight-based paradigm. To provide an example of how the weight-based paradigm is dis-seminated, we presented materials from *Let's Move!* (Michelle Obama's public health initiative dedicated to solving the problem of "childhood obesity") and critiqued some of its arguments. Finally, to illustrate how the weight-based paradigm shapes individuals' subjectivity, we shared findings from two case studies that explored how young people appear to understand the link between health and body weight.

In what follows, we further describe the elements of our pedagogical approach and then move on to an evaluation and discussion of our efforts as informed by our observations of stu-dent discussions, transcriptions of the digital recording of the session, and results from a short evaluation administered after the module. Guided by a poststructuralist viewpoint of subjec-tivity as shifting and open to change, we viewed our lesson as an "intervention" to disrupt the weight-based paradigm of typical public health interventions, which seem to constitute the majority of the undergraduate curricula in the field. We wished to present an alternative lens on health and the body to the students in the hope of offering a different version of reality that might inform their own subjective positions, even if just for the duration of the class.

Pedagogical Approach

We presented our module during a single 75-minute class session of Foundations of Public Health in Kinesiology, a course for third- and fourth-year undergraduate students. The broad goal of the kinesiology course is to investigate the various determinants of physical (in)activ-ity across populations, while also considering the wider set of social, political, and economic conditions that influence health more generally. A social justice philosophy underpins the course, and as such a great deal of attention is given to health disparities—systematic and plausibly avoidable differences in health that disproportionately impact socially disadvantaged populations (Braveman et al., 2011). We explore how various "isms" (e.g., racism, classism, sexism) play a central role in the creation of health disparities, and challenge a view of health as something that can be reduced to lifestyle or genetics. As scholars who seek to challenge the common practice of equating body size with health as well as morality, we sought to address the issue of sizeism through the module discussed in this chapter. Thus, while this was the only class in which mainstream ideas about "obesity" (including the weight-based paradigm) were discussed, the course itself is a practice of critical engagement with questions around health inequity and stigmatization of particular types of bodies. Shannon is the lead instructor of the course but during this particular session, she and Krishna, who served as a guest lecturer for the day, took turns leading the module. Thirty-five students were enrolled in the class and 30 participated in the session on the day of the module.

Reading and Reflection Assignment

In preparation for this session, students read Gaesser's (2003) article. Although we find other, more critical readings that deconstruct healthist discourse more inspiring (for example, Linda Bacon and Lucy Aphramor's [2011] "Weight Science: Evaluating the Evidence for a Paradigm Shift" or Caitlin O'Reilly and Judith Sixsmith's [2012] "From Theory to Policy: Reducing Harms Associated With the Weight-Centered Health Paradigm"), we used Gaesser's article because he is an exercise physiologist and, as such, we felt that kinesiology students might better relate to him and to his article. Gaesser discusses how dieting has had little, if any, impact on "obesity" and can actually *perpetuate* it. He argues that a major problem with the argument that "fat people should lose weight because 'obesity' 'kills'" is the lack of evidence to substantiate it (p. 41). He presents evidence on how several health problems that are often considered weight related, such as high blood pressure, insulin resistance, and glucose intolerance, can be improved independently of weight loss. As an alternative to the weight-focused approach, Gaesser suggests that the Health At Every Size paradigm allows for a more compassionate view of body weight and has significantly more positive effects on public health.

Students were instructed to complete a Triple Entry Notebook (TEN) homework assignment on Gaesser's article. In the first entry, students summarized the reading. In the second entry, they responded to reflection questions such as: "Do you agree/disagree with the author? On what basis?"; "How does this fit in with your formulating theory and conceptions of health and physical activity?"; and "Where have your ideas changed/been confirmed?" Based on the presentation and conversation during the module, students completed their third entry in class by adding comments in the margins of their first and second entries.

The Ethics of Fighting "Obesity" Teaching Module

Because of the recent media attention and concern in response to high estimates and predictions of childhood "obesity" specifically, we felt focusing on childhood rather than adult "obesity" would be more conducive to a class discussion. Moreover, both the *Let's Move!* campaign and the two case studies were specific to childhood obesity. Prior to sharing any other information, we began class that day by asking students: "What have you heard about childhood 'obesity'?" Students gave verbal responses such as: "obesity increases the risk for diabetes"; "it can be related to the mother's health, like, when she was pregnant, her eating habits and obesity"; and "when, after the child is born, the lifestyles that the parents live can greatly affect the child." After this, we shared PowerPoint slides with examples of information we found on the Internet regarding "obesity," including a news story discussing the prevalence of "obesity" and a *Time* magazine cover story about overcoming "obesity" in America. Next, we asked students what they had heard about the *Let's Move!* campaign. One student shared the following:

> The *Let's Move!* campaign is Michelle Obama's initiative that she's taken since Barack took office. Basically it's to promote healthy eating and a better lifestyle and one of the biggest subcategories under it is to promote physical activity and meeting the minimum daily requirement for physical activity because basically if you go to the Learn the Facts section, I was just on the website the other day, it says that childhood obesity is on the rise, kids are eating worse, food in

> America is getting less and less healthy, and they're trying to take the initiative to prevent this concern. They say that at the rate we're going right now, diabetes and all these common health issues are going to be dangerously prevalent more than they are already.

We acknowledged with this student that he had a fairly comprehensive understanding of what the campaign entailed and summarized briefly that the campaign was indeed launched by the First Lady in 2010 to address the "childhood obesity epidemic." Next, we presented the learning objectives for the day: (a) to examine the assertions within the traditional weight-based paradigm (i.e., questioning the dominant discourse); (b) to explore how the *Let's Move!* campaign is rooted in the weight-based paradigm and how this may be problematic (i.e., how the dominant discourse is disseminated); and (c) to employ case studies to illustrate how young people interact with the weight-based paradigm (i.e., how the dominant discourse shapes subjectivity). The following is a summary of the discussion and activities that addressed each learning objective.

Pedagogy in Action

Questioning the Dominant Discourse

As previously mentioned, there are many questionable assertions underpinning the weight-based paradigm (Bacon & Aphramor, 2011), but we focused our discussion on critically evaluating the following three assumptions: "obesity" directly contributes to health problems; weight loss through measured food and activity choices will lead to better health; and "obesity" is a question of individual control over lifestyle. We began by asking students: "Would you say that these statements are 'common sense'?" There was general agreement that the first and third assumptions are common sense, but there were mixed feelings about whether weight loss through measured food and activity choices would lead to better health.

Next, we had the students examine these three assumptions in the context of Gaesser's article. They gathered in small groups to discuss and comment on their summaries and reflections from their TEN assignments. After some time, we began the large group discussion by asking: "What are Gaesser's main points? Do you agree or disagree?" One student summarized that: "Essentially what he was saying was it's not necessarily obesity that's the concern as much as it is health concerns prevalent in the obese population that are the concern. He says you don't necessarily need to lose weight to improve your health." Another student clarified with an example saying: "You can still lower your blood pressure, your cholesterol, and everything without losing weight."

Although students tended to understand Gaesser's main points, some were uncertain how they felt about the reading because of their preconceived notions regarding the relationship between health behaviors and weight loss. For instance, one student said he was "kind of on the fence because in all the examples [Gaesser] gave, like exercising and lowering blood pressure, these studies didn't include that there was associated weight loss. We think that people who exercise do lose weight." Another student held tightly to the notion that weight loss was a reasonable measurement of improved health:

> I felt the same way. I knew what he was trying to say … and I guess I might have a bias because I study public health but I feel like it's generally understood that it's not actually the act of

losing weight as much as it is the actions that everyone knows lead up to losing weight, such as diet and exercise, and losing weight is a measurable way to assess how well you're doing at those things. ... And especially because it's such a big concern and we talked about the *Let's Move!* campaign and we want Americans to take the initiative to improve their health. ... I think it's hard for them to do that at least without some kind of palpable goal, and also medical access is not as accessible as we would like especially in poorer populations. It's not like the standard person is going to know, "Oh, I've been dieting for 4 weeks now; I can feel my cholesterol is lower." It doesn't work like that. But they can say, "Oh I've lost 5 pounds."

We probed at this comment, asking,

Does that always happen though? Is body weight a good proxy for health? There seems to be a lot of uncertainty. However, when we see it presented in the media, it's dead certain. Does association equal causation? If you lose 5 pounds are you going to be less healthy than if you lose 20 or 30 pounds? What's the dose response?

One student said she definitely agreed that "you don't necessarily have to be lean to be fit." However, she argued Gaesser's argument may still have been a little flawed because he did not discuss whether health outcomes such as cholesterol levels and hypertension were different between individuals who had participated in the same level of physical activity but varied based on their weight status. She said, "People who were lean, I would guess, are healthier than people who were overweight."

Exploring How the Weight-Based Paradigm Is Mobilized in a Public Health Campaign

Next, we demonstrated how messages communicated throughout the *Let's Move!* website are underpinned by the three assumptions previously presented as being integral to the weight-based paradigm and how there is evidence that these assumptions may be misguided or inaccurate. For instance, messages such as "childhood obesity impacts health immediately and sets the stage for a number of health problems later in life" and "if we don't solve this problem, one third of all children born in 2000 or later will suffer from diabetes at some point in their lives"[1] speak to the idea that "obesity" directly contributes to health problems (assumption 1). To point out the potential inaccuracies in this claim, we illustrated the difference between association and causation by showing a hypothetical news story warning that "people with yellow teeth are more likely to die of lung cancer." We asked the students if they felt this was accurate, and they unanimously pointed out that it was *smoking* that would lead both to yellow teeth and lung cancer, and that yellow teeth themselves were not the cause of cancer. We used this example to talk about the role of confounding variables, with which the students were familiar already as this was previously covered in the course. We discussed potential confounding variables in the relationship between "obesity" and ill health. In critiquing the first assumption, we also pointed out that finding a relationship between weight and increased mortality does not confirm that weight *causes* ill health (Bacon & Aphramor, 2011) and that rather than a direct, linear relationship between weight and disease, there actually may be a more complex U-shaped relationship between weight and morbidity (Flegal, Carroll, Ogden, & Curtin, 2010) or mortality (Flegal & Graubard, 2009).

To illustrate how the *Let's Move!* campaign supports the notion that weight loss through measured food and activity choices will lead to better health (assumption 2), we presented quotes from the website such as "the ingredients [to reduce obesity] ... better food + more activity ... are clear."[2] To demonstrate how this assertion may be harmful, we shared research findings that reveal that negative messages such as "sugar and fat are bad" or the idea of "junk" food can contribute to a fear of food and weight gain (Shaw & Kemeny, 1989) and restricting eating can lead to weight-cycling, which also can lead to weight gain (Strohacker & McFarlin, 2010).

Finally, we provided examples of how, even though the *Let's Move!* campaign does urge families, schools, and communities to take action for improving children's health, the website also communicates the assertion that "obesity" is a question of individual control over lifestyle (assumption 3). We shared quotes such as "people who are successful at managing their weight track how much they eat every day" and "the good news is that by making just a few lifestyle changes, we can help our children lead healthier lives—and we already have the tools we need to do it. We just need the will."[3] We noted that an emphasis on lifestyle change often takes attention away from the social and environmental determinants of bodies and health (Evans & Rich, 2011), an idea that we had already spent a significant portion of the course exploring. We asked: "What are some factors that might keep someone from being able to participate in physical activity?" The students provided a variety of responses, including: "age; as you get older, certain mechanisms may change"; "SES [socioeconomic], resources, having safe places to play"; and "accessibility, for people who are handicapped or disabled."

Case Studies Demonstrating How the Weight-Based Paradigm Shapes Subjectivities

We began this part of class discussion by sharing some of the known unintended effects of the weight-based paradigm, including that it can result in fat children being bullied at school (Puhl, Leudicke, & Heuer, 2011), avoiding health care practitioners (Drury & Louis, 2002), engaging in disordered eating (Evans, Rich, Davies, & Allwood, 2008), and avoiding exercise (Puhl & Leudicke, 2012). We talked about how weight stigma itself may actually be at the root of some of the health effects thought to be caused by "excess" weight, such as cardiovascular disease (Farrell, 2011).

To further demonstrate how young people interact with the weight-based paradigm, we presented findings from our own research. Krishna discussed a research project, *Children's Constructions of Health and Healthy Bodies*, in which she interviewed nine children ranging from kindergarten to third grade about their constructions of health and "obesity" and integration of health practices in everyday life. She explained how, in comparison with the younger children, the older (third grade) children she spoke with (a) associated health with particular physical abilities and body size (e.g., "being healthy means you're thin"); (b) made stronger connections between the "right" body size and balance, perfection, individual behaviors, and health outcomes (e.g., when asked to point to a "healthy" figure from a range of body types and justify why they chose a particular silhouette, some children said "because she's perfect" and "because he exercised every day for at least 60 minutes"); and (c) reported more frequently that they received messages from their parents, teachers, and the media regarding the associations between health, behavior, and body size (e.g., one child said she learned from the media that "people start to lose weight because they exercise about 60 minutes long" and another said her parents told her that she should "only eat portions of food … [and] you only get fast food once a week"). The findings from this study imply that as children get older, the weight-based paradigm is more evident in their understandings, and is reinforced through their social networks and the media.

Shannon talked about a study, *Urban Native American Female Youths' Understandings of Health and Physical Activity* (ages 12 to 17). She explained that a major theme that emerged in these interviews was a paradox of "normal" body size and health: the girls felt that "health" was eating well and getting exercise, being skinny, or having "normal" body size, but they also recognized that concern with body size can paradoxically lead to ill health and several shared their own experiences and observations of bullying related to body size as well as extreme weight loss attempts to try to have a "normal" body.

This segment of the module was more didactic and did not present many opportunities for student interaction. In planning future modules, we will incorporate more discussion. We did leave some time for questions at the end, and one student asked a question that probed at the gendered nature of ideas about body weight: "Did you interview boys of the same age?" Since only Krishna was able to include three boys in her small sample, we were not able to delve into gender differences in these particular research projects. This comment suggests that these students acknowledge that boys and girls may interact differently with the weight-based paradigm and that they are interested in learning more about this phenomenon.

Evaluation

At the end of class, we gave students about 10 minutes to complete an anonymous, paper-and-pencil questionnaire that including the following prompts: "How has your understanding of 'obesity' changed after today's lecture, if at all? How has your viewpoint of 'obesity' interventions such as *Let's Move!* changed, if at all? What teaching tools/methods used in today's lecture were most compelling? The least compelling?" We collected a total of 30 questionnaires.

In responding to how their understanding of "obesity" may have changed, many students said that they now believe that losing weight is not necessary for health and that "obesity" as a measurement of health may be inaccurate and overstated. One student added: "although it seems to be the only thing that matters in the media and other societal influences." A few students indicated that although their understanding may not have changed much, they gained a new perspective, including the "anti-obesity" agenda's effect on young people, "obesity's" various determinants, and the stigma associated with "obesity." A couple of students wrote that their views regarding "obesity" had been reaffirmed. Finally, several students indicated that their views of "obesity" had not changed, but this may be because they were already aware of some of the arguments in the material we presented. For instance, one student said: "We've been taught as kinesiology majors that weight and BMI aren't great health indicators."

In their responses regarding their viewpoint towards interventions such as *Let's Move!*, many students wrote that they now felt that these campaigns should shift their focus away from weight and individual level factors and instead focus more on overall health and social factors. Some students also commented on the psychological consequences of focusing on "obesity." A few students indicated that their views regarding the campaign had not really changed, and that they feel that the campaign is better than nothing at all, that they still support it, or that they already had a similar viewpoint to what was presented during the module.

Finally, in responding to what teaching tools or methods used were most and least compelling, the majority of students commented that they thought the findings from our own research were most interesting and helpful. Other aspects that students enjoyed included the discussion questions, screenshots from the *Let's Move!* campaign, and the fact that we took turns presenting material. Less appealing to some students was the reading they had to complete prior to arriving to class and they recommended that there be even more discussion but less text in our presentation. A couple of students wrote that they did not think that the yellow teeth and lung cancer news story example was effective. Some students asked for additional resources.

Chewing the Fat: Reflections on Our "Intervention"

In this module, we aimed to bring students' attention to the harm being caused by the assumptions inherent in the weight-based paradigm. We challenged them to think critically by illustrating the existence of contradictory research on "obesity" and health, demonstrating how the assumptions of the weight-based paradigm are seamlessly folded into popular health campaigns, such as the *Let's Move!* campaign, and employing research to show evidence of the potential impacts of the weight-based paradigm on young people. Our goal was to challenge mainstream "obesity" discourse and, in doing so, also to provide the students with an alternative paradigm as they go forward in their careers as public health practitioners so that they won't further perpetuate the weight-based paradigm in their professional practice. It was also our hope that the ideas we shared might change the way they viewed their own health and their own bodies.

Based on our class discussions and results from the student evaluations, we have a few recommendations for designing pedagogical approaches dedicated to disrupting the weight-based paradigm in fields such as kinesiology. First, instructors should consider sharing recent, relevant, and "real life" examples and research to garner interest and foster discussion regarding the weight-based paradigm and its implications. An additional strategy might be to have students bring in an "obesity" artifact from their daily lives (e.g., food label, dietary advertisement) that could be analyzed and used to illustrate the way that knowledge, language, and power are written into, and function through, the products that they see and possibly use every day. We also recommend assigning readings or facilitating discussion that deconstructs healthist discourse more generally and addresses how the weight-based paradigm sustains specific relations of power. Comparative research evaluating the effectiveness of a similar module with students who are or are not as familiar with public health or kinesiology concepts would be illuminating. Finally, our module may have been even more effective had it been part of a longer, ongoing discussion over the entirety of the course or positioned within a course that incorporated insights from fat studies. One benefit of offering our module as one component of a traditional kinesiology course focused more broadly on health disparities was that it allowed the students to critically engage with questions around health inequity and stigmatization of different types of bodies, not only fat bodies, and perhaps reached students who might have been resistant to an entire course focused on "obesity" and problematizing the weight-based paradigm.

In closing, while we feel our lesson went some way towards our goal of disrupting students' unconditional acceptance of the weight-based paradigm, we fear that the pervasiveness of dominant obesity discourse, especially in the realm of public health, means that the shift towards a more critical understanding of "obesity" displayed by some of the students is likely temporary, and possibly forgotten once they walk down the hallway to other classes in which the weight-based paradigm is taught without question. Modules such as ours must be part of broader, sustained, and critical efforts in public health courses to disrupt the weight-based paradigm.

References

Bacon, L. (2010). *Health At Every Size: The surprising truth about your weight*. Dallas, TX: BenBella Books.

Bacon, L., & Aphramor, L. (2011). Weight science: Evaluating the evidence for a paradigm shift. *Nutrition Journal, 10*, 1–13.

Braveman, P., Kumanyika, S., Fielding, J., Laveist, T., Borrell, L. N., Manderscheid, R., & Troutman, A. (2011). Health disparities and health equity: The issue is justice. *American Journal of Public Health, 101*, 149–155.

Daníelsdóttir, S., Burgard, D., & Oliver-Pyatt, W. (2009). *Guidelines for childhood obesity prevention programs*. Retrieved from http://www.aedweb.org/web/index.php/23-get-involved/position-statements/90-aed-statement-on-body-shaming-and-weight-prejudice-in-public-endeavors-to-reduce-obesity-4

Drury, C., & Louis, M. (2002). Exploring the association between body weight, stigma of obesity and health care avoidance. *Journal of the American Academy of Nurse Practitioners, 14*, 554–561.

Evans, J., & Rich, E. (2011). Body policies and body pedagogies: Every child matters in totally pedagogised schools? *Journal of Education Policy, 26*, 361–379.

Evans, J., Rich, E., Davies, B., & Allwood, R. (2008). *Education, disordered eating and obesity discourse: Fat fabrications*. London, England: Routledge.

Farrell, A. E. (2011). *Fat shame: Stigma and the fat body in American culture*. New York, NY: New York University Press.

Flegal, K. M., Carroll, M. D., Ogden, C. L., & Curtin, L. R. (2010). Prevalence and trends in obesity among U.S. adults, 1999–2008. *Journal of the American Medical Association, 303*, 235–241.

Flegal, K. M., & Graubard, B. I. (2009). Estimates of excess deaths associated with Body Mass Index and other anthropometric variables. *American Journal of Clinical Nutrition, 89*, 1213–1219.

Gaesser, G. (2003). Is it necessary to be thin to be healthy? *Harvard Health Policy Review, 4*, 40–47.

Neumark-Sztainer, D. (2009). Preventing obesity and eating disorders in adolescents: What can health care providers do? *Journal of Adolescent Health, 44*, 206–213.

O'Reilly, C., & Sixsmith, J. (2012). From theory to policy: Reducing harms associated with the weight-centered health paradigm. *Fat Studies, 1*, 97–113.

Puhl, R., & Luedicke, J. (2012). Weight-based victimization among adolescents in the school setting: Emotional reactions and coping behaviors. *Journal of Youth and Adolescence, 41*, 27–40.

Puhl, R., Leudicke, M., & Heuer, C. (2011). Weight-based victimization toward overweight adolescents: Observations and reactions to peers. *Journal of School Health, 81*, 696–703.

Rail, G. (2002). Postmodernism and sport studies. In J. Maguire & K. Young (Eds.), *Perspectives in the sociology of sport* (pp. 179–207). London, England: Elsevier.

Rail, G. (2009). Canadian youth's discursive constructions of health in the context of obesity discourse. In J. Wright & V. Harwood (Eds.), *Biopolitics and the "obesity epidemic": Governing bodies* (pp. 141–156). New York, NY: Routledge.

Shaw, S., & Kemeny, L. (1989). Fitness promotion for adolescent girls: The impact and effectiveness of promotional material which emphasizes the slim ideal. *Adolescence, 24*, 677–687.

Strohacker, K., & McFarlin, B. (2010). Influence of obesity, physical inactivity, and weight cycling on chronic inflammation. *Frontiers in Bioscience, 1*, 98–104.

Weedon, C. (1997). *Feminist practice and poststructuralist theory*. London, England: Blackwell.

Wright, J. (2001). Gender reform in physical education: A poststructuralist perspective. *Journal of Physical Education New Zealand, 34*, 15–25.

Notes

1 http://www.letsmove.gov/learn-facts/epidemic-childhood-obesity
2 http://www.letsmove.gov/sites/letsmove.gov/files/pdfs/LetsMovePledge.pdf
3 http://www.letsmove.gov/sites/letsmove.gov/files/MyPlateCommunityToolkit.pdf

NINETEEN

Mitigating Weight Stigma Through Health Professional Education

Caitlin O'Reilly

Research has illustrated that weight stigma and weight-based discrimination are prevalent through-out society, including in education, media, and employment sectors (Brownell, Puhl, Schwartz, & Rudd, 2005; Puhl & Heuer, 2009). It also is manifested in and through health care. In a survey-based study, Gary Foster and colleagues (2003) found that 50 percent of doctors perceived fat patients as unattractive and non-compliant and one-third viewed them as lazy and weak-willed. Similarly, others have found that health care providers' attitudes towards heavier patients include stereotypes of laziness (Bocquier et al., 2005) and poor willpower (Brown, Stride, Psarou, Brewins, & Thompson, 2007). The experience of weight stigma can result in consequences such as emo-tional eating, lowered physical activity, body image disturbances, disordered eating (Puhl & Heuer, 2009), and avoidance of health care (Olson, Shumaker, & Yawn, 1994).

Interventions are thus urgently needed to shift weight-biased attitudes and practices, includ-ing amongst those working in health care. Currently, however, little is known about how to reduce weight bias in health care professionals. As Sigrún Daníelsdóttir, Kerry O'Brien, and Anna Ciao (2010) illustrate in a systematic review of published studies on weight stigma reduction, most extant weight bias reduction interventions have been tested on youths or with university students. Although some of this work has occurred with pre-service health students, little is known about how to address the problem among health care providers already in the field (Provincial Health Services Authority [PHSA], 2013). In this chapter, then, I theorize how to address weight bias through continuing health professional education based on a case study of a government-funded, anti–weight stigma initiative in the province of British Columbia (BC), Canada.

The Case Study

In 2011, a health agency in BC received money over three years to develop, pilot, implement, and evaluate an educational resource on weight stigma for health care professionals. The aim of the project was to reduce weight bias and stigma among health care practitioners in BC, including front-line medical, mental health, allied health care, and public health professionals.

Early on, two committees were formed to help guide the work: (1) a steering committee of health researchers and professionals with expertise in related topics (e.g., eating disorders, public health) (N=13); and (2) an advisory committee of health care providers in the province (e.g., doctors, dieticians) (N=8). These committees were used both to vet curriculum content and to think about how to achieve buy-in from the wider health care professional community. The first activity in the project was to conduct a literature review and interview professionals, academics, and patients to discover their ideas about promising practices to address weight stigma. The second step was to determine the format the resource would take, and it was decided it would be an online course. The third step was to decide on course content and how to best deliver it, which involved much back-and-forth between the various stakeholders and committees. The development phase lasted more than two years and the course is now in the process of being piloted. Future steps will involve making changes based on qualitative and quantitative pilot findings and ensuring the resource is widely available to health care providers in BC.

My role in this work has been multipronged. I began as a member of the steering committee and from there was invited to take on the role of research partner. I am also now one of two contracted evaluators of the project. During the development phase of the training, I observed and participated in the regular advisory and steering committee meetings, analyzed meeting minutes, and conducted interviews with some of the committee members involved in course development. Throughout the whole process, I kept a reflexive, autoethnographic[1] research journal to document my evolving feelings and thoughts about weight stigma reduction. This journal was particularly helpful in encouraging me to reflect on how various health care providers on the advisory and steering committees related to the many iterations of course content in the development phase.

Grounded in my learning from the collaborative development and vetting of this course with the steering and advisory committees, in this chapter I discuss important considerations when striving to address weight stigma through continuing health professional education. First, I theorize the need for complex solutions to what is a multifaceted problem. Second, I articulate the importance of developing a critical pedagogy about weight science and weight stigma and provide insight on what this could look like when working with health professionals, particularly suggestions for addressing challenges that may be encountered in addressing the medicalization of weight. Third, I discuss how to create a safe learning environment within which a critical pedagogy focused on weight stigma can flourish.

Complex Solutions for Complex Problems

Weight stigma is a complex social issue. Its roots in Western culture are deep and multifaceted. In relatively recent history, fatness has been devalued for religious, class, gender, and racial reasons. Amy Farrell (2011), for example, shows how an influx of immigrants in postindustrial America led to a cultural shift whereby fat was no longer associated with white-ness and affluence as it had been previously, and instead began to be associated with racialized, immigrant bodies constructed as "uncivilized." Although meanings ascribed to fat bodies have varied across time and place, at various points in history the thin body has been touted as the most virtuous: for example, through denial of the bodily requirement to eat, the thin soul was viewed as closer to God (Braziel & LeBesco, 2001). Although religious influence has decreased in the last century, related ideas about fatness as indicative of poor willpower and laziness con-tinue to be pervasive (Puhl & Heuer, 2009). Today, social constructions of thin bodies as the most beautiful are rampant in print, visual, and social media, affecting women in particular. The dominant anti-obesity "fat as unhealthy" rhetoric legitimized through medical institu-tions has also contributed to a devaluing of the fat body in contemporary society (McMichael, 2013). These are but a few aspects of the complex phenomenon of weight stigma. Given the various contributing factors to weight stigma, it follows that educational interventions to ad-dress the problem be designed with the complexity of the problem in mind.

A key learning from the literature review, initial interviews with experts (PHSA, 2013), and early committee meetings was that whatever was developed had to respond to this complexity and target multiple aspects of the problem to be effective. This is consistent with Daníelsdóttir et al.'s (2010) contention that educational initiatives using multiple tactics to reduce weight prejudice are the most promising. With this in mind, we incorporated four main stigma reduc-tion strategies into the curriculum: (a) addressing controllability beliefs; (b) evoking empathy; (c) engaging professional voices; and (d) encouraging self-reflection. All these strategies were viewed favorably by committee members.

First, to reduce stigma we drew upon attribution theory that suggests that stigma exists because of perceptions that the stigmatized condition is a matter of choice. Weight stigma re-duction thus necessitates providing information that challenges the idea that weight is entirely within an individual's control (Puhl & Brownell, 2003). For this, we provided extensive infor-mation about the challenges of controlling weight, including the complex factors leading to higher weights such as genetics, disease, and environment. The committee members responded favorably to this information, particularly when it was supported by corresponding scientific evidence and reinforced by well-respected health professionals.

Second, we drew from the literature on empathy approaches to stigma reduction that highlights the challenges of living with a stigmatized condition. To do so, we featured "patient voices" in a series of videos in which people shared their stories of experiencing weight bias in health care settings. Based on their own learning in the early steps of the process, the steering committee agreed that, in the words of one member, hearing "personal stories is an effective way to start to shift attitudes." The group cautioned, however, that we needed to be careful that empathy approaches promoted compassion for the challenges of living in a weight-biased *society*, rather than only highlight the challenges of living *in a fat body*.

Third, we also attempted to reduce stigma by engaging well-respected health professionals in the fight against weight stigma. This strategy is based on social consensus theory, a stigma reduction theory that suggests stigma can be mitigated through norms established by power-ful, influential "in-group" individuals (Puhl, Schwartz, & Brownell, 2005). We incorporated this through "professional voices" videos, in which we had several health care providers speak about the need to avoid biased care. In our own curriculum development and vetting process, the inclusion of influential health care providers at the table seemed to be effective in positively influencing our own group norms. One interviewee, for example, stated that she felt that the presence of two very influential and particularly "unbiased" health care providers at the table was key in challenging members of the group on some of their beliefs. In her view, hearing stories from peers about moving past their own stigmatizing attitudes helped "reassure learners who may hold weight bias that others have gone through similar experiences and have been able to effect change in their practice."

Lastly, we employed a tool to encourage critical self-reflection about one's values, attitudes, and/or behaviors. We hoped that such a tool might reduce stigma by fostering cognitive dissonance, a process by which individuals realize their attitudes or behaviors are not consistent with their overarching values. The discomfort of cognitive dissonance is theorized to increase the likelihood that individuals will modify their attitudes and behaviors to suit their value systems (PHSA, 2013). In the various committee meetings, it was acknowledged that this emotional discomfort and a subsequent period of reflexivity were essential to committee members' "unlearning" weight stigma. We thus chose to maximize the opportunity for reflective dialogue in the team's future meetings as well as in the online course itself by using scripted reflections whereby participants would be given specific prompts for writing about their experiences. We also used the online Implicit Associations Test (IAT) to encourage reflection, which is a pattern-matching exercise that is supposed to reveal implicit biases (Greenwald, Nosek, & Sriram, 2006). It was suggested by interviewees and committee members that it would be a useful starting point to gently help health care providers acknowledge their own biases about weight.

A key strategy for weight stigma reduction that the team identified early on in curriculum development was the need to "challenge the myths about weight and health." Next I discuss the rationale for wanting to include this, the challenges we faced in attempting to do so, and some suggestions for moving past such difficulties through cultivating a critical pedagogy.

Contemplating a Critical Pedagogy About Weight Science and Weight Stigma

A common refrain of fat activists and scholars is that designating "overweight" and "obesity" as diseased is inherently harmful and can lead to stigma (McMichael, 2013; Wann, 2009) as well as related consequences such as disordered eating and weight cycling (O'Reilly & Sixsmith, 2012). As Marilyn Wann (2009) articulates:

> "Overweight" is inherently anti-fat. It implies an extreme goal: instead of a bell curve distribution of human weights, it calls for a lone, towering, unlikely bar graph with everyone occupying the same (thin) weights. If a word like "overweight" is acceptable and even preferable, then weight stigma becomes accepted and preferred. (p. xii)

She also asserts: "If you believe that being fat is a disease and that fat people cannot possibly enjoy good health or long life … your approach is aligned with 'obesity' researchers, bariatric surgeons, public health officials who declare 'war on obesity'" (p. ix). I too have reflected on the consequences of considering "overweight" and "obesity" as medical problems and argue in other work (O'Reilly & Sixsmith, 2012) that the dominant weight-centered health paradigm advocated for in the medical tradition sets people up for disordered eating and weight cycling.

This issue is compounded by the uncertainty of the relationship between weight and health. As Linda Bacon and Lucy Aphramor (2011) contend in their review article on weight and health, the assumption that adiposity poses mortality risk is not grounded in strong evidence. They point out that many epidemiological studies show that people who are "overweight" or moderately "obese" live as long as, if not longer than, people in the so-called "normal" weight range. They suggest that the studies that do find a positive relationship between increasing weight and mortality risk have methodological shortcomings that call the findings into question. They point to the failure of many weight science studies to control for factors known to confound the data such as diet, fitness, socioeconomic status, and weight cycling (see also Campos, Saguy, Ernsberger, Oliver, & Gaesser, 2006). Bacon and Aphramor (2011) further argue that there is very little long-term evidence that suggests that people who try to lose weight will actually improve their health. Rather, most people regain the weight and this process of weight cycling detracts from rather than contributes to physiological health. In light of the harms of weight cycling and the increased risk that the pursuit of weight loss will lead to disordered eating, I have argued that weight-centered approaches to health should be considered systemic discrimination (O'Reilly & Sixsmith, 2012).

When we began to develop the anti–weight stigma course, we based much of our initial work on the ideas that medical frames of weight might be inaccurate, stigmatizing, and come with iatrogenic harms. We thus began with the premise that an essential part of unlearning weight stigma for health care providers should involve exposure to what we termed "the myths about weight and health." Indeed, challenging these myths was a key finding from the initial literature review as well as interviews with both patients and weight stigma experts on how best to address weight stigma through health professional education. We thus proceeded to develop course content based around this. Of the five modules, one was heavily dedicated to challenging mainstream ideas about weight and health. This curriculum was then extensively vetted through many meetings with the advisory and steering committees prior to the formal pilot test.

Unfortunately and interestingly, this proposed content did not go over well with some of the health professionals involved. Indeed, feedback from some health care providers was decidedly negative. Some, for example, believed the information we presented challenging the relationship between Body Mass Index (BMI) and health outcomes to be "factually incorrect." A few were so strongly opposed to the content we proposed that they wanted to stop the implementation of the course altogether should we proceed with this approach. Others on the committees working within the health sector felt unfairly targeted and hurt, saying that our strong position made them feel like they were being accused of engaging in stigmatization given their beliefs about weight and health despite them sitting at the table wanting to address weight bias with no intention to cause harm. They reported that their instinctive reaction was to disengage and warned us that if we proceeded as intended we would probably find our course ineffective due to attrition. As one interviewee shared: "Our worry was that if we do create those reactions where people are feeling offended, and … are just completely dismissing the resource because this conflicts so much with their existing belief system, that they just can't even start to be open to it."

Experiencing this resistance, I felt quite emotionally triggered. My first response was to staunchly defend my initial anti-medicalization stance. Through reflection and much dialogue, however, I came to reflect more critically on my original positioning. I realized that attempting to counter "myths about weight" with the "facts" employs the same strategy as mainstream weight science: framing one's research findings as the truth. Indeed, this mirrors the kind of absolutism and essentialism often present in dominant weight science. As a strategy for bias reduction, it can therefore only succeed if it can be proved as "true" or at least remain largely uncontested. It is therefore not as likely to create change among those who can locate alternative evidence. As Audre Lorde (1984) once argued, "the master's tools will never dismantle the master's house. They may allow us temporarily to beat him at his own game, but they will never enable us to bring about genuine change" (p. 2).

This is not to suggest that I no longer believe that medicalization does not relate to weight stigma. Abigail Saguy (2013) shows that individuals exposed to medical frames about weight are more likely to score as weight biased on attitudinal measures. Lonie McMichael (2013) also convincingly argues that the "fat is bad for you" argument justifies and promotes weight prejudice. However, rather than addressing medicalization through debunking the myths about weight and health—a strategy which, as I learned, can backfire—I suggest that instead what is needed is a critical pedagogy of weight science and weight stigma.

What can or should this critical pedagogy look like? Henry Giroux (2007) defines critical pedagogy as the process of encouraging and enabling students to "actively question and negotiate the relationships between theory and practice, critical analysis and common sense, and learning and social change" (p. 1). He emphasizes the importance of democracy of knowledge, whereby learners have an "unconditional freedom to question and assert" (p. 1). Giroux also argues that critical pedagogy requires a healthy skepticism about sources of authority and power and that cultivating this skepticism requires that learners be provided with the skills to question authority and power structures.

In the development of the weight stigma course, after extensive debate among committee members, the group opted to present a *balanced* perspective on the medicalization of weight. This meant offering evidence from *all* sides of the debate on weight, health, medicalization, and stigma in the course—including both those who support and those who critique medicalization—and encouraging participants to critically appraise the various perspectives for themselves. This strategy for curriculum development aligns with Giroux's (2007) notion of democratization of knowledge. Rather than prioritizing the voices of only those of us who believed medicalization was inherently negative, which led to an adverse reaction and significant resistance, we instead validated the voices of *all* of those at the table helping to develop the course. At the very least, this allowed for the course to continue without getting shut down (and there was a real threat that might happen), but it also created space for deeper learning for all of us.

Giroux (2007) also emphasizes providing learners with "the skills and knowledge necessary for them to expand their capacities to both question deep-seated assumptions and myths that legitimate the most archaic and disempowering social practices" (p. 2). What skills or knowledge might help learners undertake a transformation in how they think about weight and health if simply challenging the "myths about weight and health" is not a viable strategy? One skill set important to cultivate in learners is the ability to critically appraise the weight science literature. Interviewees agreed: "I think it's very important. I think it's always important to critically evaluate the literature." Jacquineau Azétsop and Tisha Joy (2011) argue that weight bias results in part from a cultural tendency to prioritize "common sense" thinking over intellectual, critical thought. This suggests that providing information on things such as the shortcomings of the BMI, as we have done in the project, may be helpful in addressing weight-biased beliefs. Other useful skills and knowledge we identified included understanding the difference between correlation and causation and the influence of the pharmaceutical industry on weight science research.

Giroux (2007) also recommends encouraging learners to connect theory and practice. Connecting evidence in the literature with practice implications was quite helpful in this case. As an interviewee involved in developing and vetting the content shared, "people want to see the evidence ... there's no reason to change my practice unless I see otherwise." This interviewee elaborated that health care providers are concerned about avoiding harm in clinical practice. She thus emphasized that one way of encouraging a learning shift is to provide knowledge about how weight-focused health approaches can lead to inadvertent harms:

> I think they—when they stick to their beliefs about a certain way of kind of approaching weight related issues—it's 'cause they believe that that's the best way and they really do believe that [being heavy] can't be healthy for their patients. So when you talk about some of these potential harms of ... like, eating disorders and weight cycling and, you know, some of the mental health effects ... that speaks to health care professionals because they get that. They don't want to cause any of those things in their patients and they can accept that there might be consequences of weight bias and stigma.

Dialogue and information provision on the possible harms of asserting a relationship between weight loss and health improvement seemed to be readily accepted by the team and influenced the health care professional committee members. Interestingly, this was particularly so when the information came from well-respected "in-group" members on the committees, such as the health care providers with well-established careers in relevant areas.

Cultivating a Safe Environment for Learning About Emotionally Charged Issues

Stigma is a topic that evokes strong emotions. An oft-heard refrain in the committee meetings during the curriculum development phase was that we needed to be cautious in how we presented information, lest people become so emotionally triggered that they disengage. One way we tried to create a safe learning environment was to avoid taking a blaming approach towards health care providers. This non-blaming approach was cultivated through an acknowledgment that weight bias is something deeply ingrained in our culture that most of us, at various points and to varying extents, internalize. As one interviewee shared:

> I think acknowledging that this is something that we all are coping with and dealing with and we are embedded within this culture [and] have common issues ... so even if, you know, a health care professional feels like, "Oh my gosh, I am being weight stigmatizing," not to, to encourage them not to, feel guilty about that but just to reflect ... not a blaming approach because ... I think if someone feels blamed they might turn away and turn off.

In the online course, we used the Implicit Attitudes Test (IAT) as one way of encouraging awareness of implicit weight bias without finger-pointing. We also strove to focus on areas of agreement, such as the harms of weight bias (e.g., eating disorders and weight cycling) rather than on points of contention (e.g., the exact relationship between weight and health). This minimized the level of emotional intensity at our various meetings. Interviewees shared that the presence of skilled facilitators at the table also helped mediate conversations and diminish upset.

While minimizing emotional intensity and blame can help create a viable learning space, a safe, democratic learning environment nonetheless must take care not to fail to provide room for marginalized voices to be heard. In this case, that meant including the contentions of fat activists who argue that the "war on obesity" feels like a war against fat people (Wann, 2009). Providing this perspective will inevitably trigger emotions among some and may sometimes result in an uncomfortable learning environment. Facing these emotions, however challenging, is nonetheless essential, as one committee member shared. How to manage these emotionally fraught conversations about medicalization is thus an area in which further exploration is required and we can perhaps learn from broader critical pedagogy efforts (e.g., see Sensoy & DiAngelo, 2011, on education about racism). Learning how to manage these challenging conversations is particularly important in the context of working with health professionals who are embedded within a medicalized tradition.

Conclusion

Based on lessons learned from developing and vetting an online educational resource for and with health care providers in BC, the importance of complex, multifaceted educational interventions to address weight stigma became clear. Health care providers on the committees involved in this case study seemed to be positively influenced by stigma reduction strategies based on attribution theory, empathy, social consensus, and self-reflection. However, since weight bias is legitimized through beliefs about fat as unhealthy (McMichael, 2013), these strategies also need to be infused with a more critical component so that we can consider how medicalized beliefs about weight may contribute to stigma and harm for heavier patients. How best to approach the medicalization of weight within stigma reduction, however, is an area in which further research is needed. Despite clear assertions by fat studies scholars that medicalization is stigmatizing (McMichael, 2013; Wann, 2009), we have little solid evidence about how to best translate this into educational interventions. The approach used in the case study was to present both sides of the debate on medicalization and to focus on common ground such as the health risks associated with an overemphasis on weight in health care. This helped create buy-in and a safe learning environment for committee members. Further research is required, however, to consider how else the medicalization of weight may be addressed within stigma reduction education, in health care and beyond. We also need more theoretical and empirical work on the relationship between weight stigma and medicalization if we are to get to a point where there is more widespread understanding and acceptance of this relationship.

As we advance knowledge concerning what works to reduce weight stigma through education, the importance of evaluation cannot be understated. Here I presented insights from qualitative research into the experiences of two committees of health care professionals involved in developing curriculum on weight stigma. More research, including that from the quantitative tradition, is still needed. For example, Daníelsdóttir et al. (2010) argue that in order to best understand how to reduce weight bias, studies should include some form of pre-and post-test survey measurement. Study design should also allow for the researcher to ascertain which aspects of a multimethod intervention were most effective. Future work in BC and elsewhere should incorporate these insights.

References

Azétsop, J., & Joy, T. R. (2011). Epistemological and ethical assessment of obesity bias in industrialized countries. *Philosophy, Ethics, and Humanities in Medicine, 6*(1), 1–16.

Bacon, L., & Aphramor, L. (2011). Weight regulation: A review of the evidence for a paradigm shift. *Nutrition Journal, 10*(9), 2–13.

Bocquier, A., Verger, P., Basdevant, A., Andreotti, G., Baretge, J., Villani, P., & Paraponaris, A. (2005). Overweight and obesity: Knowledge, attitudes, and practices of general practitioners in France. *Obesity Research, 13*, 787–795.

Braziel, J. E., & LeBesco, K. (2001). *Bodies out of bounds: Fatness and transgression.* Los Angeles, CA: University of California Press.

Brown, I., Stride, C., Psarou, A., Brewins, L., & Thompson, J. (2007). Management of obesity in primary care: Nurses' practices, beliefs, and attitudes. *Journal of Advanced Nursing, 59*, 329–341.

Brownell, K., Puhl, R., Schwartz, M., & Rudd, L. (2005). *Weight bias: Nature, consequences, and remedies.* New York, NY: Guilford.

Campos, P., Saguy, A., Ernsberger, P., Oliver, E., & Gaesser, G. (2006). The epidemiology of overweight and obesity: Public health crisis or moral panic? *International Journal of Epidemiology, 35*, 55–60.

Daníelsdóttir, S., O'Brien, K. S., & Ciao, A. (2010). Anti-fat prejudice reduction: A review of published studies. *Obesity Facts, 3*(1), 47–58.

Farrell, A. (2011). *Fat shame: Stigma and the fat body in American culture.* New York, NY: New York University Press.

Foster, G. D., Wadden, T. A., Makris, A. P., Davidson, D., Sanderson, R. S., Allison, D. B., & Kessler, A. (2003). Primary care physicians' attitudes about obesity and its treatment. *Obesity Research, 11*, 1168–1177.

Gingras, J. (2009). *Longing for recognition: The joys, complexities and contradictions of practicing dietetics.* York, England: Raw Nerve Books.

Giroux, H. (2007). Introduction: Democracy, education, and the politics of critical pedagogy. In P. McLaren & J. Kinchloe (Eds.), *Critical pedagogy: Where are we now?* (pp. 1–5). New York, NY: Peter Lang.

Greenwald, A., Nosek, B., & Sriram, N. (2006). Consequential validity of the implicit association test: Comment on Blanton and Jaccard. *American Psychologist, 61*(1), 56–71.

Lorde, A. (1984). *Sister outsider: Essays and speeches.* Berkeley, CA: Crossing Press.

McMichael, L. (2013). *Acceptable prejudice? Fat, rhetoric and social justice.* Nashville, TN: Pearlsong.

Olson, C. L., Shumaker, H. D., & Yawn, B. P. (1994). Overweight women delay medical care. *Archives of Family Medicine, 3*, 888–892.

O'Reilly, C., & Sixsmith, J. (2012). From theory to policy: Reducing harms associated with the weight-centered health paradigm. *Fat Studies, 1*(1), 97–113.

Provincial Health Services Authority (PHSA). (2013). *Reducing weight stigma and bias in the BC healthcare system: Findings from a critical review of the literature and environmental scan.* Vancouver, BC, Canada: BC Mental Health and Substance Use Services.

Puhl, R. M., & Brownell, K. D. (2003). Psychosocial origins of obesity stigma: Toward changing a powerful and pervasive bias. *Obesity Reviews, 4*(4), 213–227.

Puhl, R. M., & Heuer, C. A. (2009). The stigma of obesity: A review and update. *Obesity, 17*, 941–964.

Puhl, R. M., Schwartz, M. B., & Brownell, K. D. (2005). Impact of perceived consensus on stereotypes about obese people: A new approach for reducing bias. *Health Psychology, 24*, 517–525.

Saguy, A. (2013). *What's wrong with fat? The war on obesity and its collateral damage.* Oxford, England: Oxford University Press.

Sensoy, O., & DiAngelo, R. (2011). *Is everyone really equal? An introduction to key concepts in social justice education.* New York, NY: Teachers College Press.

Wann, M. (2009). Foreword: Fat studies: An invitation to revolution. In E. Rothblum & S. Solovay (Eds.), *The fat studies reader* (pp. ix–xxv). New York, NY: New York University Press.

Notes

1   Autoethnography is a method of self-reflection that helps bridge a researcher's personal experiences with broader social contexts (e.g., Gingras, 2009).

PART FOUR

Expanding Fat Pedagogies

TWENTY

Fat Studies in the Field of Higher Education: Developing a Theoretical Framework and Its Implications for Research and Practice

Heather Brown

Scholars, activists, and activist-scholars have been working for many years to develop fat studies as an academic field that draws on other disciplines, yet stands on its own: "In the tradition of critical race studies, queer studies, and women's studies, fat studies is an interdisciplinary field of scholarship marked by an aggressive, consistent, rigorous critique of the negative assumptions, stereotypes, and stigma placed on fat and the fat body" (Solovay & Rothblum, 2009, p. 2). While fat studies as an identifiable academic paradigm is becoming more commonplace in areas such as literature and sociology, other fields such as higher education (which includes the study of postsecondary student learning outcomes, student affairs, curricular elements, evaluation, administrative processes, and more) are in the nascent stages of exploring these issues. Instead, the relationship between weight and postsecondary academic achievement is most often framed and analyzed by scholars who utilize dominant obesity discourse where fatness is perceived as problematic and dangerous. For example, framing "obesity" as a medical or developmental problem for learners is commonplace in the literature (e.g., Kobayashi, 2009).

Here, I explore how four core components of fat studies as identified in other disciplinary areas are being translated into a fat studies framework designed for the field of higher education. I identify and describe how these key concepts are applicable to the research and practice of higher education: attentiveness to issues of language; challenging discrimination in higher educational practice and research; problematizing specious connections between weight, health, and academic performance; and placing the lived experience of the fat learner at the center of research on fat learners. I argue that using a fat studies approach in higher education scholarship and teaching can allow researchers and practitioners to consider the story of postsecondary fat learners' academic achievement from multiple perspectives and, by honoring participants' understandings of their own experiences, uncover new data that can help these students be successful without further stigmatizing or harming them.

Defining a Theoretical Framework

Fat studies scholars have been working to develop a theoretical framework, an ongoing and sometimes challenging process. The first challenge is that while many scholars identify themselves as working in the field of fat studies, very few talk about what it means to think of fat studies in a theoretical sense. As a result, working within a fat studies paradigm can become more about doing fat studies than interrogating and advancing the field theoretically. As a result, fat studies is defined not so much by what its theoretical foundations are, but by what it fights against: "As a new, interdisciplinary field of intellectual inquiry, fat studies is defined in part by what it is not" (Wann, 2009, p. ix). Marilyn Wann (2009) delineates a list of things you cannot do if you are "doing" fat studies, such as advocating weight loss and constructing fat as a disease.

Another challenge to the development of a fat studies theoretical framework is that fat studies is interdisciplinary (Harjunen, 2009) and intersectional (Watkins, Farrell, & Doyle Hugmeyer, 2012). Scholars who identify themselves as associated with fat studies come from a wide variety of disciplines including English, communication and rhetoric, sociology, politics, food science, nutrition, medicine, legal studies, education, and women's studies, to name a few. Each of these disciplines comes with its own set of assumptions and theoretical frameworks (Harjunen, 2009). In addition, fat studies scholars must also contend with the complexities associated with intersectionality. This plurality of backgrounds and the challenges the field faces in making sense of how they all fit (or do not fit) together are topics still being explored by fat studies scholars. Charlotte Cooper (2010), for example, writes, "Fat Studies currently makes use of a number of theoretical underpinnings which have given rise to as yet unexamined tensions arising from the differences between these theoretical approaches" (p. 1028). She highlights social stigma theory, Foucauldian analysis, poststructuralism, and Arendt's web of relations as only a few of the theoretical frameworks used by fat studies scholars. Despite these challenges, four core concepts that appear to delineate a fat studies theoretical perspective can be identified in the work of fat studies scholars no matter their home discipline.

Four Core Concepts

Lesleigh Owens (2008) argues that while there is no single definition of fat studies, researchers working in the field have shared sensibilities, including the centering of fat experience at the heart of research and discourse. Looking at the work of fat studies scholars, the following core characteristics can be identified as shared sensibilities: the importance of activism and the challenging of oppression of and discrimination against fat individuals; attentiveness to issues of language; problematizing fatness as a medical issue; and placing the actual experiences of fat individuals at the center of research, both in practice and in analysis.

Importance of activism

For Cooper (2010), activism and relationships between activism and scholarship are fundamental to a fat studies theoretical framework. Fat studies "provides a platform for identifying, building and developing fat culture as well as extending alliances between activism and the academy" (p. 1021). A poet with a doctorate in sociology, Owens (2008) also situates fat studies in its activist past, noting that "fat studies is political. Like cultural studies, feminist studies, African American studies, and others, fat studies emerged from a political movement devoted to pursuing the rights of an oppressed group" (p. 31). Similarly, Patricia Boling (2011) infuses her teaching around fat bodies with a feminist perspective grounded in social justice. This emphasis on social justice leads many fat studies scholars to focus their work on issues of weight bias and discrimination and advocate for basic human rights for fat individuals (Solovay, 2000).

Although working on behalf of social justice is an important cornerstone of fat studies, embracing social justice as a key component of a theoretical framework is not without its own challenges. One debated topic is whether or not one must be fat in order to do fat studies. Cooper (2010) suggests in her review of the literature that there are obvious distinctions between much of the scholarship of individuals who are themselves fat and those who are not. Specifically, in some research done by non-fat scholars, she argues that fat individuals "are abstract presences within it, a nebulous blob of people sometimes known as 'the obese,' which echoes contested approaches to fat people within more traditional medicalised obesity discourses" (p. 1024). Yet, fat activism and social justice are not limited by physical body size; thin people can be, and are, allies in fat activism and fat studies (Boling, 2011; Paullet, 2015). Wann (2009) argues that no one—fat or thin—doing fat studies can escape the effects of weight bias and prejudice: "Every person who lives in a fat-hating culture inevitably absorbs anti-fat beliefs, assumptions, and stereotypes, and also inevitably comes to occupy a position in relation to power arrangements that are based on weight" (p. xi). As an antidote, fat studies scholars argue for activism, both within oneself and a fat-hating culture, that "acknowledges the confines of a particular situation while simultaneously working to break through them" (Smith, 2015, p. 151).

Attentiveness to issues of language

Fat studies scholars pay a significant amount of attention to language, particularly language that constructs fatness as a medical issue and only a medical issue. This focus on language is a result of fat scholars' attempts to challenge dominant obesity discourse. For example, Erin Cameron (2015) noted in her analysis of fat studies courses that they often challenge mainstream "obesity" language and rhetoric. As Wann (2009) suggests, "Word choice is a good place to begin to examine assumptions" (p. xii). Cooper (1998) and Hannele Harjunen (2009) argue that words such as "obesity" and "overweight" are highly problematic because they are correlated with incorrect preconceptions of what it means to be fat. If "overweight" is a linguistic symbol of a socially normative category, who has the power to define that category and what does it mean to individuals who are stigmatized by the category and yet had no say in its creation?

Fat studies scholars thus rarely use terms such as "obese" or "overweight" without benefit of quotation marks. Instead, they prefer to use language they suggest is more purely descriptive. Use of the word "fat" is a form of social justice work for fat studies scholars: "using it is about reclaiming a word which has been used to hurt, and substituting its destructive power for a more positive and descriptive meaning" (Cooper, 1998, p. 9). Using "fat" instead of "obese" or "overweight" is an open challenge to dominant obesity discourse. As Wann (2009) writes: "Currently, in mainstream U.S. society, the O-words, 'overweight' and 'obese,' are considered more acceptable, even more polite, than the F-word, 'fat.' In the field of fat studies, there is agreement that the O-words are neither neutral or benign" (p. xii). Using language in this critical way helps "carry out the revolution that replaces the spoiled identity (in Goffman's sense) of fatness—so powerful that even fat people abhor their own bodies with a more inhabitable subject position" (LeBesco, 2004, p. 3).

Problematizing fatness as a medical issue

A third core component of fat studies is that the dominant discourse establishing "obesity" as a medical problem or a disease must be problematized. Fat studies scholars suggest the need to "expand the understanding of fatness beyond the narrow confines of medicalisation or pathology" (Cooper, 2010, p. 1020). For fat studies researchers, weight is never just a medical issue to be addressed using medical solutions; it is more complex than that: "The field of fat studies requires skepticism about weight-related beliefs that are popular, powerful, and prejudicial" (Wann, 2009, p. x).

Defining weight as a medical condition is of concern to the fat studies researcher because issues of health and disease are often conflated with issues of morality: "When we define fatness as a disease we are acting within powerful social boundaries which control what we believe to be right and appropriate, or shameful and abnormal" (Cooper, 1998, p. 71). This is especially true when fatness is presented as a temporary, fixable "problem" that is wholly under the control of the individual. With such framing, the fat individual becomes a pariah, responsible for all the hate and bias aimed at her or him, issues that would go away if only the fat person would just lose weight. As Wann (2009) suggests, "Belief in a 'cure' also masks that hatred. It is not possible to hate a group of people for our own good. Medicalization actually helps categorize fat people as social untouchables" (p. xiv). As social untouchables responsible for their own stigmatization, fat individuals become unworthy of the rights of "normal" citizens: "Fat people exist at a juncture where 'unhealthy' equals 'bad'. Our demands for rights and social acceptance are assumed to be invalidated by our unhealthiness, a condition for which we are responsible" (Cooper, 1998, p. 76).

Placing the individual at the center of research

Fat studies retains the feminist focus on centering research on the lived experiences of the individual. This practice is a hallmark of work done using a fat studies theoretical framework (Solovay & Rothblum, 2009). Just as feminist scholars "became increasingly aware of glaring contradictions between their lived experiences as women and mainstream research models, studies, and findings" (Brooks & Hesse-Biber, 2007, p. 5), so too have fat studies scholars shown that the experiences of fat individuals do not mirror what studies in dominant obesity paradigms suggest they should be.

Unlike earlier feminist scholars, however, fat studies scholars do not have to invent from whole cloth new methods that address shortcomings in traditional scholarship. Rather, they can borrow critical methodologies from feminist, queer, and other critical scholarship. Which methodologies best center the lives of fat individuals at the heart of knowledge building remains open for discussion, however. *The Fat Studies Reader*, for example, includes methods such as quantitative analysis, participatory action research, historical methods, literary criticism, ethnography, and legal analysis.

Developing a Fat Studies Theoretical Framework for Higher Education

There is a growing literature on the ways in which fat studies is being taken up in formal education, whether elementary, secondary, or postsecondary. While far from a complete list, examples include the work of Mary Renck Jalongo (1999) and Christina Fisanick (2006), both of whom used a fat activist perspective to explore the experiences of the fat professor. In her article exploring identity formation, Carla Rice (2007) analyzed how the hidden curriculum works in primary and secondary schools to teach fat girls that they are defined negatively, and only as, fat. As well, five chapters related to formal education were published in *The Fat Studies Reader*. Maho Isono, Patti Lou Watkins, and Lee Ee Lian (2009) conducted a qualitative study of the long-term effects of the "Trim and Fit" weight loss program for fat elementary school children in Singapore, while Ashley Hetrick and Derek Attig (2009) used participatory action research to explore college students' relationships with classroom furniture. Susan Koppelman (2009) investigated whether texts featuring fat individuals are included in postsecondary curricula and in what contexts those texts are used with students. As well, Julie Guthman (2009) and Yofi Tirosh (2006) reported on their own experiences teaching postsecondary courses using a fat studies perspective.

More recently, Ragen Chastain's (2015) anthology, *The Politics of Size: Perspectives From the Fat Acceptance Movement,* included an entire section of chapters focused on school and the workplace. Some focused on the academic experience like Ameerah Mattar's (2015) exploration of anti-fat interventions with school children around the world, Brittany Lockard's (2015) analysis of how weight bias affects fat scholars in the workplace, and my (2015) work on how family disapproval impacts fat daughters' sense of themselves as capable learners.

The previous summary is certainly not an exhaustive account of writing related to fat pedagogy nor of the growing literature on the experiences of teaching postsecondary fat studies courses (e.g., Cameron, 2015; Watkins, Farrell, & Doyle Hugmeyer, 2012). Nonetheless, there still remains a significant lack of research on fat pedagogy, including at the postsecondary level (Brown, 2012; Cameron, 2015). It is possible, however, through extrapolation to further develop theoretical frameworks useful to fat pedagogy in higher education. Moreover, it is critical to do so. In the following section, I explain how the core components of a fat studies theoretical perspective may lead to a useful framework for fat pedagogy in higher education.

Using language

Fat studies scholars who study higher education ask whether the language used in research treats fat learners as individuals worthy of respect and dignity or, instead, demonstrates bias and discrimination against fat learners. If a researcher uses fat-biased language, it raises questions about how it will lead to educational practices that will improve academic outcomes for fat learners rather than perpetuate discrimination. One example I found of language in educational research that I worried could lead to discrimination against fat learners is that by Sangeeta Singh and Shari McMahan (2006). They ground the introduction to their study of weight and learning in literature that compares the dangers of being "overweight" or "obese" with "the threats of bio-terrorism and small pox" (p. 207). Certainly, being the victim of a terrorist attack (biological or otherwise) or contracting a virulent disease would affect an individual's ability to learn. Do Singh and McMahan truly believe, and does their evidence show, that possessing plenty of adipose tissue affects the ability of the individual to learn in the same way? If not, why have they chosen to use such hyperbolic language?

Another example I found was in Futoshi Kobayashi's (2009) study of weight and academic achievement. He begins his article by stating, "it is very common these days to encounter 'super-sized' students on the campuses of many colleges and universities in the USA" (p. 555). While the term "super-sized" may have been used in a humorous attempt to describe weight in the American population, it would be perceived as hurtful and disrespectful by fat individuals since it is commonly used as a taunt. Scholars using a fat studies theoretical framework should avoid using terms or phrases that could be considered mocking of the fat learner or that suggest a connection between fatness and an individual's learning ability without benefit of evidence. As is done in this *Fat Pedagogy Reader*, they can also use scare quotes around terms such as "obese" and "overweight" to disrupt dominant obesity discourse. As noted earlier, many fat studies scholars prefer to use terms such as "fat" as a descriptive rather than a pejorative word (Cooper, 1998, 2010; Wann, 2009).

Challenging discrimination in educational practice and research

Given its genesis in the activism of the fat acceptance and fat rights movements, fat studies in higher education should honor that heritage by challenging discrimination against fat individuals both in practice and research. In practice, a postsecondary educator working within a fat studies frame would consider issues in the physical environment, such as one-piece chair-desk sets that might serve as a barrier to fat learners and work to eliminate these barriers in a fashion that does not further establish the fat individual as an Other (Brown, 2012, 2015; Hetrick & Attig, 2009).

Those working in fat studies would also champion the efforts of fat learners to succeed and protest any decisions by educational institutions that are based on assumptions of inability by fat students. An example of this type of activism can be seen in the case of *Sharon Russell v. Salve Regina* (Weiler & Helms, 1993). A fat student in the nursing program at Salve Regina, Russell was dismissed from the program one year prior to graduation not because she was performing badly in either her practicum or her classroom work, but because she failed to lose a certain number of pounds per week. When news of the case became public, Russell was recruited by another college's nursing program and not only went on to earn her degree but also to sue Salve Regina in a case that went all the way to the U.S. Supreme Court, which upheld a court's earlier decision to award her monetary damages for wrongful dismissal, intentional infliction of emotional distress, and discrimination.

Working from a fat studies theoretical framework in higher education also demands vigilance around learning materials that have the potential to be discriminatory against fat learners or in which the fat learner is ignored entirely. For example, "in recent decades, adult educators have become increasingly interested in previously unexplored aspects of adult learning, including somatic, emotional, and spiritual dimensions" (Kasworm, Rose, & Ross-Gordon, 2010, p. 442). However, for the fat learner, the very concept of somatic learning (or learning through the body) can be fraught with difficulty because it is hard to trust the body as an instrument of learning in a society that constantly tells the learner that her or his body is wrong. For example, Constance Russell discusses how challenging ecofeminist texts were for her in her early graduate student years since they often called for embodied knowing, yet she herself "was not so keen to reclaim this particular [fat] body" (Russell, Cameron, Socha, & McNinch, 2013,

p. 30). This is not to say that professors teaching or researching from a fat studies perspective avoid embodied knowing; indeed, I would argue quite the opposite. But they need to be sensitive to the unique experiences of fat learners even as they encourage reflective student inquiry and research on body size and learning.

Health and academic performance

Practice and research that frame weight as a medical or developmental problem for fat learners must be approached with a sense of skepticism (Cooper, 2010; Wann, 2009). While there may be legitimate connections between physical fitness and academic achievement, fat studies research makes clear that the connections between fatness and physical fitness are more complex than portrayed by the dominant obesity paradigm popular in "obesity" research and in mainstream media (Solovay & Rothblum, 2009; Wann, 2009). An example of this dominant paradigm can be found in a situation that occurred at Lincoln University. In 2006, the university decided to mandate that all students who were defined as "obese" according to the Body Mass Index (BMI) take an extra course called Fitness for Life (Hoover, 2009, para. 2). Failure to take and pass the class meant that these students would not be allowed to graduate (para. 7). Eventually, the Fitness for Life requirement was dropped in the interest of fairness (Seaton & Lockley, 2009, para. 1). Cameron et al. (2014) describe a similar situation in Quebec, Canada, and conclude that "[a]lthough schools are mandated to treat all children equally and with dignity, discrimination based on weight is reinforced, not challenged, by 'schooled healthy body' discourses and regimes of discipline" (p. 688).

A fat studies perspective makes clear that forcing one group of students to take a special class simply because of their weight is certainly unfair. It establishes fat students as deviant and deficient and could set them up for bullying, harassment, and other types of persecution. Also at issue is why other students are assumed to be fit simply because of their body weight, even though one can certainly be thin and unfit. It ought to be the case that all humans deserve to have the opportunity to learn how to be healthy and fit throughout their lives; singling out fat students is hardly the way to do so.

Centrality of fat experience to educational practice and research

Fat individuals, as a group, are still struggling for the right to define their own subjectivity. As Harjunen (2009) argues, "It is notable this stigmatized status of fat people is assigned from outside and usually explored as such" (p. 50). Moreover, as a group, fat individuals are often not seen by others nor, in many cases, even by themselves as "deserving sympathy, support, understanding, acceptance, or even tolerance in their surroundings" (p. 51). As a result, fat people's understandings of their own experiences are often not considered at all in either educational practice or research. There is a growing body of research that explores the experiences of fat people in their own words, including in educational settings. As one example, Hannah McNinch (2014) examined the experiences of girls who had been bullied in elementary and secondary school (as she had been herself as a student) and built on these to make recommendations for teacher education. In the way that McNinch did, a fat studies theoretical perspective calls for research to keep a focus on the lived experiences of fat learners at all stages of the research process, from the first stages of research design all the way through data analysis and dissemination. My own work (2012) focusing on practice calls on colleges to work with a wide variety of student populations, including fat students, to learn more about students' needs as they understand them before designing and building new buildings or renovating old structures—rather than assuming a "father knows best" approach to designing the physical environment.

Conclusion

Fat studies is becoming more common in disciplines from women's studies to nutrition to sociology. It is starting to grow as well in the field of higher education. Four core concepts from fat studies can inform a theoretical framework for research and practice in higher education. For fat learners in postsecondary settings, adoption of a fat studies theoretical framework cannot come soon enough if they are to have equitable access to educational opportunities that enable academic success in a stigma-free learning environment.

References

Boling, P. (2011). On learning to teach fat feminism. *Feminist Teacher, 21*(2), 110–123.

Brooks, A., & Hesse-Biber, S. N. (2007). An invitation to feminist research. In S. N. Hesse-Biber & P. L. Leavy (Eds.), *Feminist research practice: A primer* (pp. 1–24). Thousand Oaks, CA: Sage.

Brown, H. (2012). *Fashioning a self from which to thrive: Negotiating size privilege as a fat woman learner at a small liberal arts college in the Midwest* (Doctoral dissertation). Northern Illinois University, DeKalb, IL.

Brown, H. (2015). Never delivering the whole package: Family influence on fat daughters' college experiences. In R. Chastain (Ed.), *The politics of size: Perspectives from the fat acceptance movement* (Vol. 2, pp. 189–202). Santa Barbara, CA: Praeger.

Cameron, E. (2015). Toward a fat pedagogy: A study of pedagogical approaches aimed at challenging obesity discourse in post-secondary education. *Fat Studies, 4*(1), 28–45.

Cameron, E., Oakley, J., Walton, G., Russell, C., Chambers, L., & Socha, T. (2014). Moving beyond the injustices of the schooled healthy body. In I. Bogotch & C. Shields (Eds.), *International handbook of educational leadership and social (in)justice* (pp. 687–704). New York, NY: Springer.

Chastain, R. (2015). *The politics of size: Perspectives from the fat acceptance movement* (Vols. 1 & 2). Santa Barbara, CA: Praeger.

Cooper, C. (1998). *Fat and proud: The politics of size*. London, England: The Women's Press.

Cooper, C. (2010). Fat studies: Mapping the field. *Sociology Compass, 4*(12), 1020–1034.

Fisanick, C. (2006). Evaluating the absent presence: The professor's body at tenure and promotion. *Review of Education, Pedagogy, and Cultural Studies, 28,* 325–338.

Guthman, J. (2009). Teaching the politics of obesity: Insights into neoliberal embodiment and contemporary biopolitics. *Antipode, 4*(5), 1110–1133.

Harjunen, H. (2009). *Women and fat: Approaches to the social study of fatness* (Doctoral dissertation). University of Jyväskylä, Jyväskylä, Finland.

Hetrick, A., & Attig, D. (2009). Sitting pretty: Fat bodies, classroom desks, and academic excess. In E. Rothblum & S. Solovay (Eds.), *The fat studies reader* (pp. 197–204). New York, NY: New York University Press.

Hoover, E. (2009, November 19). Lincoln U. requires its students to step on the scale. *Chronicle of Higher Education.* Retrieved from http://chronicle.com/section/Home/5

Isono, M., Watkins, P. L., & Lian, L. E. (2009). Bon bon fatty girl: A qualitative exploration of weight bias in Singapore. In E. Rothblum & S. Solovay (Eds.), *The fat studies reader* (pp. 127–138). New York, NY: New York University Press.

Jalongo, M. R. (1999). Matters of size: Obesity as a diversity issue in the field of early childhood. *Early Childhood Education Journal, 27*(2), 95–103.

Kasworm, C. E., Rose, A. D., & Ross-Gordon, J. M. (2010). Conclusion: Looking back, looking forward. In C. E. Kasworm, A. D. Rose, & J. M. Ross-Gordon (Eds.), *Handbook of adult and continuing education* (pp. 441–451). Thousand Oaks, CA: Sage.

Kobayashi, F. (2009). Academic achievement, BMI, and fast food intake of American and Japanese college students. *Nutrition and Food Science, 39*(5), 555–566.

Koppelman, S. (2009). Fat stories in the classroom: What and how are they teaching about us? In E. Rothblum & S. Solovay (Eds.), *The fat studies reader* (pp. 197–204). New York, NY: New York University Press.

LeBesco, K. (2004). *Revolting bodies?: The struggle to redefine fat identity.* Amherst, MA: University of Massachusetts Press.

Lockard, B. (2015). The fat academy: Does being big keep you from getting big in scholarship? In R. Chastain (Ed.), *The politics of size: Perspectives from the fat acceptance movement* (Vol. 2, pp. 177–188). Santa Barbara, CA: Praeger.

Mattar, A. (2015). A "weigh" to go? Looking at school-based antifat interventions from a weight-based versus a health-based approach. In R. Chastain (Ed.), *The politics of size: Perspectives from the fat acceptance movement* (Vol. 2, pp. 159–176). Santa Barbara, CA: Praeger.

McNinch, H. (2014). *Fat bullying of girls in school: Implications for pre-service teacher education* (Master's thesis). Lakehead University, Thunder Bay, ON, Canada.

Owens, L. J. (2008). *Living large in a size medium world: Performing fat, stigmatized bodies and discourses* (Doctoral dissertation). University of California at Santa Cruz.

Paullet, M. (2015). Thin fat activism. In R. Chastain (Ed.), *The politics of size: Perspectives from the fat acceptance movement* (Vol. 1, pp. 119–130). Santa Barbara, CA: Praeger.

Rice, C. (2007). Becoming "the fat girl": Acquisition of an unfit identity. *Women's Studies International Forum, 30,* 158–174.

Russell, C., Cameron, E., Socha, T., & McNinch, H. (2013). "Fatties cause global warming": Fat pedagogy and environmental education. *Canadian Journal of Environmental Education, 18,* 27–45.

Seaton, J., & Lockley, N. (2009, December 5). University decides to drop BMI requirement. *The Lincolnian.* Retrieved from http://www.thelincolnianonline.com/

Singh, S., & McMahan, S. (2006). An evaluation of the relationship between academic performance and physical fitness measures in California schools. *Californian Journal of Health Promotion, 4*(2), 207–214.

Smith, E. (2015). The pragmatic attitude in fat activism: Race and rhetoric in the fat acceptance movement. In R. Chastain (Ed.), *The politics of size: Perspectives from the fat acceptance movement* (Vol. 1, pp. 151–162). Santa Barbara, CA: Praeger.

Solovay, S. (2000). *Tipping the scales of justice: Fighting weight-based discrimination.* Amherst, NY: Prometheus.

Solovay, S., & Rothblum, E. (2009). Introduction. In E. Rothblum & S. Solovay (Eds.), *The fat studies reader* (pp. 1–7). New York, NY: New York University Press.

Tirosh, Y. (2006). Weighty speech: Addressing body size in the classroom. *Review of Education, Pedagogy, and Cultural Studies, 28,* 267–279.

Wann, M. (2009). Foreword: Fat studies: An invitation to revolution. In E. Rothblum & S. Solovay (Eds.), *The fat studies reader* (pp. ix–xxv). New York, NY: New York University Press.

Watkins, P. L., Farrell, A. E., & Doyle Hugmeyer, A. (2012). Teaching fat studies: From conception to reception. *Fat Studies, 1*(2), 180–194.

Weiler, K., & Helms, L. B. (1993). Responsibilities of nursing education: The lessons of *Russell v Salve Regina. Journal of Professional Nursing, 9,* 131–138.

TWENTY ONE

We Take "Cow" as a Compliment: Fattening Humane, Environmental, and Social Justice Education

Constance Russell and Keri Semenko

"Fat cow!" How many women have had that insult hurled at them? Fat, thin, or somewhere in between, we imagine many readers have had that experience themselves or witnessed it. Some may have even directed it at another person at some point in their lives. There is much to unpack in this insult given its roots in fat hatred, sexism, and speciesism; in this chapter, we use this insult as a springboard for describing some of the ways in which we have "fattened" our own pedagogical praxis, particularly through intersectional analyses. While we both work in higher education, we are confident that our analysis and pedagogical attempts have applicability in other educational contexts.

We come to our work as two straight, abled, white, Anglophone Canadian, cisgender women who do not conform to ideal beauty standards of mainstream Western culture. One of us is fat, the other robust and athletic, and neither of us would be considered feminine in the traditional sense; we both grew up as working-class "tomboys," one on a farm, the other in a city known for auto manufacturing. We share these various identities not only to help readers situate our remarks, but also to make clear that while we have both experienced fat and class oppression, we are privileged in important ways (e.g., species, race, sexuality, ability). Now, as professors, we are committed to spending the privilege that we do have, including in our teaching.

Both of us have been on the receiving end of "fat cow" and over the years also have found ourselves unfavorably compared to pigs, hippos, elephants, and whales. We also have overheard students tossing these words at each other, sometimes playfully and sometimes with clear intent to hurt or marginalize; either way, we are particularly disheartened to see our young female students using language that serves to police not only the bodies and actions of other women but also their own. Further, they are reinforcing the dominant social view of other animals as lesser. Alas, we are not surprised by any of this. As other chapters in *The Fat Pedagogy Reader* demonstrate, we are marinated in a culture rife with fat phobia and sexism. Perhaps less obvious to readers is that most of us also are living in profoundly anthropocentric cultures wherein humans are viewed as the center of the universe and inherently superior to, and rightly dominant over, all other species. Anthropocentrism is understood as an underpinning of our exploitation of other life (Fawcett, 2013), so intersectional analyses that go beyond the human are key to our approach to fat pedagogy.

Framing Our Pedagogy

Animal referents used to stigmatize fat people, particularly women, are everywhere once you start looking for them. As Kathleen LeBesco (2004) notes, "It takes little imagination to conjure up 'pig' or 'cow' as a popular term of insult for fat people" (p. 86). Amy Farrell (2011), in her history of fat stigma in American culture, illustrates how fatness became a sign "of inferior, primitive bodies, a sure indicator of one's low position on the evolutionary scale" (p. 83) with the result that "fat people are often treated as *not quite human*" (p. 6, emphasis in original). Irene López Rodriguez (2009), in her analysis of English and Spanish animal words used to describe women, notes how "cow/vaca" and "heifer/vaquilla" imply both "fat and ugly" and how pig "and its female counterpart *sow/cerda* are metaphorically used as terms of opprobrium for a woman, implying fatness, dirtiness, ugliness and even promiscuity" (p. 88). These scholars, however, do not grapple with the underlying anthropocentrism that serves to make such associations so powerful.

Conversely, other writers interrogate the links between sexism and speciesism, but fail to address fat phobia. Ecofeminists have done important work outlining how the domination of women and animals intersect in ways that profoundly impact both, but some reproduce "obesity" discourse, especially in discussions of veganism (e.g., Gaard, 2013). Carol Adams (2014) offers a trenchant analysis of an image of a female pig reclining like a nude pin-up model in the satirical magazine *Playboar: The Pig Farmer's Playboy.* (And, yes, such a magazine existed. Connie remembers it well from her childhood.) Adding insights from fat studies, we argue, would make Adams' analysis even more powerful. Lorna Stevens, Matthew Kearney, and Pauline Maclaran (2013) examine representations of cows in advertising such as the Laughing Cow and Borden's Elsie, noting how these cows with their "exaggeratedly feminine features" are portrayed as "happy" cows who serve to erase the horrors of contemporary dairy production (p. 161). No mention is made of fatness in their analysis either and this too feels like a missed opportunity.

In fact, there are very few scholars who bring gender, fat, and animality together in their work.[1] Kristen Hardy (2014) is one exception. In her article "Cows, Pigs, Whales: Nonhuman Animals, Antifat Bias, and Exceptionalist Logics," she describes an advertisement for a weight loss spa that depicts a woman "evolving" from a cow (see Figure 21.1) alongside similar ads featuring a pig and a whale.[2] Using these ads to illustrate the dehumanization or, more precisely, the "animalization" of fat people, she asserts, "To be rendered as 'animal' is, in the context of a deeply anthropocentric system, to be marginalized in the most fundamental of ways" (p. 195). Such animalization has had profound material impacts. As Maneesha Deckha (2012) makes clear, slavery and the treatment of Indigenous peoples are "but a sampling of the array of international instances by which violence was enacted against colonized human beings through the differentiating logic of animalization, racialization, and dehumanization" (p. 539).

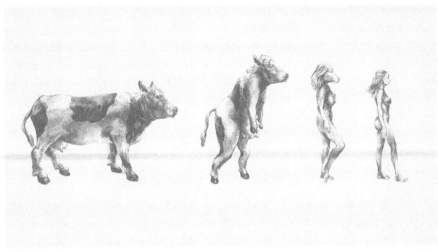

Figure 21.1. Weight loss spa advertisement. Retrieved from http://adsoftheworld.com/media/print/del_mar_cow. Reprinted with permission of Propaganda Advertising, Romania.

The animalization of women also has had horrifying consequences. As Joan Dunayer (1995) summarizes: "Applying images of denigrated nonhuman species to women labels women inferior and available for abuse" (p. 11). This may be particularly so for fat women. Consider the bumper sticker that reads "harpoon fat chicks" (Jones & Hughes-Decatur, 2012, p. 56). Or ponder the phenomenon of "hogging" wherein groups of young men competitively seek out fat women for sex (Prohaska & Gailey, 2010). While Ariane Prohaska and Jeannine Gailey suggest that participation in hogging might serve as a cover for some men who are embarrassed to admit that they find fat women attractive, when one takes into account the common practice of using alcohol to break down resistance to sex and the denigration of the targeted women, they argue that hogging should be called what it is: rape. Certainly, we do not think it is a coincidence that peppered throughout the interview excerpts shared by Prohaska and Gailey are words and phrases like "hog," "porker," "disgusting pigs," "road beef," "rodeo," "fat bitch," and "dog's night out."

For us, then, we see much pedagogical potential in intersectional analyses that include both fat and species. Ecofeminism served as our own introduction to what has come to be called intersectionality. Although ecofeminism fell out of favor in some circles because of the essentialist positions some of its advocates took (see Adams & Gruen, 2014) and its contributions are often erased in histories of intersectionality, we nonetheless continue to find ecofeminism helpful because it does insist on going beyond the human. We also see promise in the words of Sumi Cho, Kimberlé Crenshaw, and Leslie McCall (2013) who laud the "widening scope of intersectional scholarship" and view the emerging field of intersectionality studies as "a gathering place for open-ended investigations of the overlapping and conflicting dynamics" of various inequalities (p. 788). They further assert, "It is important to consider the intersectional project a communal one, one undertaken not in academic silos but in conjunction with fellow travelers with shared insights, approaches, and commitments, guiding critique and collaboration for communal gain" (p. 804). While neither fat nor animality is mentioned in Cho, Crenshaw, and McCall's article, it is clear that they are seeking solidarity with others committed to tackling oppression in all its complexity. So too are many fat studies scholars (e.g., Pausé, 2014). We turn now to the ways in which we apply such ideas to our teaching.

Fattening Our Pedagogy

Most of our pedagogical efforts are focused in postsecondary education, although we do make forays into other contexts such as elementary and secondary schools and work with nongovernmental organizations. Connie teaches BEd and graduate courses in social justice education and environmental education in a faculty of education. Keri is based in a community college where much of her work has a humane education[3] bent as she instructs students seeking positions in frontline animal care including as veterinarian assistants, zookeepers, and animal protection workers. Even though our students are on different professional pathways, our pedagogies overlap in substantial ways given that our intersectional approach makes clear the connections between humane, environmental, and social justice education. We must admit that it has been only in the past 10 or so years that we have incorporated fatness into our teaching, despite our own embodiment. Prior to our engagement with fat studies, we were mostly embarrassed by our bodies and avoided the topic. Below we share descriptions of a few ways in which we have attempted to fatten our pedagogy. Like Erin Cameron (2015b), we are not offering these as recipes but as illustrations.

Embodiment, Autobiography, and Thin Privilege

To begin, we recognize that even before we open our mouths on the first day of class, our bodies are already teaching (Cameron, 2015a; Jones & Hughes-Decatur, 2012). Connie's fat body, for example, is far from the "hard body" of the stereotypical environmental and outdoor educator (see Russell, Cameron, Socha, & McNinch, 2013). And Keri suspects her body calms some of her heavier students who, having accepted the false equivalency of thinness and fitness, worry that their bodies may not be up to the physically demanding work of animal care; this may be especially true for the young women who want to work with "exotic" animals given the often sexualized undertones of that work (Semenko, 2000). Determined to bring our embodiment out of the depths of the hidden curriculum to the explicit curriculum, we share our own experiences of being heavier in our respective professions and beyond. Students have responded positively to our frank stories and some have reported that hearing these felt empowering to them.[4]

We also use our own narratives as part of our teaching about privilege. Peggy McIntosh (1998), in her landmark essay, "White Privilege: Unpacking the Invisible Knapsack," illustrated the ways in which unearned privilege gives some people unfair advantages personally and professionally. More often than not, given that many believe in the myth that we live in a meritocracy, these privileges are unconscious despite having profound impacts on educational outcomes and much more (Sensoy & DiAngelo, 2011). Building on written autobiographical assignments that students complete at the beginning of our courses, we help students examine their own, often quite complicated, knapsacks. One activity useful for this is a variation of the "Power Flower" (Arnold, Burke, James, Martin, & Thomas, 1991) wherein students create "petals" that represent their positioning on various hierarchical dualisms (e.g., thin/fat, male/female, human/non-human). We take great care in facilitating this activity given that emotions such as guilt and anger can run high and we do not want to unwittingly marginalize any students, reproduce oppression, or reify the very dualisms we are trying to problematize. For us, the point is to demonstrate the complex interplay of identities and the structural underpinnings of oppression as well as to catalyze discussions of how students might address privilege in their own future work. What makes our variation of the Power Flower unusual, and of most relevance to this chapter, is that we include both thin privilege and species privilege in the mix.

In fat pedagogy, we certainly are not alone in wanting to address embodiment and thin privilege (e.g., Boling, 2011; Cameron, 2015a, 2015b; Jones & Hugh-Decatur, 2012; Watkins, Farrell, & Hugmeyer, 2012). Nor are we alone in wanting students to go beyond the individual and make connections to broader structural forces at play. One activity we have found helpful for doing that is the "Hegemony Treasure Hunt" (Fawcett, Bell, & Russell, 2002) wherein students seek out examples of oppression built into our campuses. The "treasures" they return with include photographs or descriptions of buildings that are next to impossible to navigate in a wheelchair, portraits of university presidents who are all white men, classrooms with chairs bolted to the floor pointing to a stage that assumes the use of lecture-based pedagogies, and signs that say "no animals allowed." They also take note of classroom furniture that does not accommodate fat bodies (see Hetrick & Attig, 2009), fat-phobic and sexist advertising plastered on the walls, and the limited food choices available in vending machines and cafeterias.

Media Activities

Another way we help our students to link the individual to the systemic is through media analysis and production. Given the attention to body image in much media literacy work in Ontario elementary and secondary schools, most of our students seem to have little problem identifying fat phobia in traditional and social media. What they are sometimes less good at is making connections between fat phobia and other oppressions. One activity to help us do that is called "Alien Spy." We bring to class a collection of magazines and ask students to imagine that they are spies from another planet whose only source of information on Earth's inhabitants is a small archive of magazines. One group might have fashion magazines while others have outdoorsy, health, and animal-focused magazines. After responding to a series of questions that seek physical descriptions of Earthlings alongside speculation about behaviors and beliefs (e.g., "What do they eat? What makes them happy? What do they worship?"), they are asked to depict a typical Earthling through collage or drawing. The results are often humouros (e.g., one group decided that the most powerful creatures on Earth must be dogs since their magazines featured ads showing humans following dogs around with "pooper scoopers"), but mostly they are poignant as they demonstrate the ways in which certain bodies are marginalized or erased.

Other times we select particular images to analyze to help them make specific connections. For example, to demonstrate the ways in which fat people are demonized in the environmental movement (Russell et al., 2013), we show a newspaper front page with a headline that blared that "Fatties Cause Global Warming" and a cartoon of a fat woman sitting on the planet. We can also readily find images that make clear the connection between fat phobia and sexism (e.g., Farrell, 2011) or that demonstrate the connections between sexism and speciesism (e.g., Adams, 2010). One image that we have found particularly powerful in demonstrating the intersection of sizeism, sexism, and speciesism is the People for the Ethical Treatment of Animals (PETA) billboard that depicts a cartoon image of a fat woman in a bikini on a beach with the tagline, "Save the Whales. Lose the Blubber: Go Vegetarian." This billboard generated a forceful negative response and PETA pulled it, but alas that does not mean that they learned much from the experience. Rather, PETA president Ingrid Newkirk (2009) responded to the controversy by citing "obesity" science, decrying the "coddling" of fat people who "shovel in food and haven't a clue," and asserting that "fat people need to have some discipline and remember that being fat means being a bad role model to our children" (para. 3). Given such statements, it should come as no surprise that PETA continues to use fat shaming in their campaigns. Reacting to another fat shaming billboard, Farrell (2011) insightfully observes, "PETA reduces their larger, and much more complicated, argument about animal ethics to an abhorrence of the fat body" (p. 15).

In her discussion of the billboard, Hardy (2014) applauded the work of an artist and blogger named Christie who created a parody ad in response: a photograph of herself in a bikini with the words, "I am vegetarian but I am still a whale" alongside contact information for PETA so that others could register complaints.[5] Similarly, we find it pedagogically useful to have students move beyond deconstruction to engage in media production themselves (McKenzie, Russell, Fawcett, & Timmerman, 2010). For example, we were inspired by Tema Sarick (2002), who brought together a group of friends to create a zine in response to heated debates about including transgender women at the Michigan Womyn's Festival. Using a collage of magazine cuttings, their own artwork, prose, and poetry, their zine problematized the various ways "nature" was used to police gender (see also Russell, Sarick, & Kennelly, 2002); they also disrupted fat phobia in creative ways throughout the entire zine. Cameron (2015b) describes similar media production activities being used in fat pedagogy in higher education, including the creation of videos and blogs.

Teaching About Other Animals' Lives
In her analysis of campaigns that use fat shaming, Farrell (2011) rightfully notes that PETA's "mockery of fat people is one of the more obvious examples of how those in the food activist movement use the motif of fatness to simplify, publicize, and garner support for their cause" (p. 15). She asserts, however, that

> food activists are aiming for one thing but have hit another. They want a complex overhaul of our food systems, but they aim at readers' waistlines … [and] the very diet-industrial system that food activists so abhor is strengthened, as fat denigration encourages people to turn to desperate measures to fight the stigma they experience. And, finally, by relying on the fat stigma motif, food activists alienate fat readers. (p. 17)

Hardy (2014), a fat vegan, also questions the fat-phobic tactics used in some campaigns for plant-based diets. Nonetheless, she recognizes how challenging it can be to discuss food choices such as meat eating within the fat acceptance movement given the damage caused by cultural obsessions with dieting. Hardy asserts, however, that these conversations need to happen: "personal dietary choices are inherently embedded with issues of power and privilege" and must be examined (p. 200; see also Dean, 2014). We agree and see much potential in a critical food education that attends to both fat phobia and speciesism.

For us, critical food education must include illuminating the horrifying conditions for both animals and human laborers in the factory farms and slaughterhouses responsible for much of the meat and dairy consumed by North Americans and elsewhere. While undoubtedly discomforting knowledge that many people would rather ignore (Corman & Vandrovcová, 2014; Kahn, 2011), understanding how food animals live and die is necessary for making informed decisions. Further, as Adams (2010) convincingly argues, feeling separate from, and above, certain animals enables our industrialized exploitation of them. For example, imagining a "fat cow" as a stupid and docile animal makes it easier to mistreat her in industrialized dairy production.

The two of us have firsthand experience with cows and pigs and we know that common characterizations of them are often inaccurate. We thus consider it vital that we bring the lives of other animals into our teaching. Keri is particularly fortunate to teach in a program that approaches animal care from both biological and sociological perspectives and this opens many avenues for her to resist dominant constructions of other animals. We both are committed to demonstrating the complexity of various animals' lives and making clear that they too are subjects of their own lives (Bell & Russell, 2000). Through learning more about, for example, the social dynamics of whales, the intelligence of pigs, and the complex emotional lives of cows (Armstrong & Botzler, 2008; Bell & Russell, 1999), it is our hope that students will come to appreciate these creatures' intrinsic value and begin to question the assumptions that undergird the insults they casually throw about. And this brings us back to where we began this chapter: animal insults.

Animal Insults

Analyzing insults can be very revealing. Adapting an activity called "Animal Adjectives" (Selby, 1995) that helps students deconstruct different ways other animals are represented, we narrow our focus to insults. We ask students to brainstorm insults that use animals as referents. With the classroom door shut so that they feel safer sharing insults that contain swear words or that they deem particularly offensive, we write the insults on the board. We then begin to group the insults together by target (e.g., women, men, racialized people, fat people) to unpack the associations that often have sexist, racist, homophobic, and ableist undertones. We also unpack the speciesist assumptions being made about the animals in question. Calvin Odhiambo (2012) describes a similar classroom activity that he calls the "Name Game." Focused on gender-based insults, he too finds a significant cluster of insults related to animals and adds fat to his analysis.

Insults like "fat cow" work, in part, because animal bodies, fat bodies, and female bodies are considered abject in much of contemporary Western culture, that is, they often evoke disgust. Writing about fat, Lesleigh Owen (2015) says:

> Fat bodies live. They breathe. They sneeze, sweat, menstruate, eat, talk, drink, urinate, vomit, belch, and defecate. In fact, many bodies do every one of these things, but fat, similar to other abject bodies, are more regularly linked to them. Fat bodies are regarded as disgusting in part

because they are considered more biological, more tied to their processes, their orifices. ... [F]at people are dirty, a word we tend to associate with coming into contact with bodies and nature. (p. 6)

Bringing together scholarship on abjection from gender studies, critical animal studies, and fat studies has much to add to this conversation (Leahy, 2009; Owen, 2015; Russell et al., 2013).

As a counterpoint, it is also important to make clear that there are always cracks in consent to hegemonic narratives (marino, 1997) that stigmatize. For example, Farrell (2011) describes Susan Stinson's poetry that challenges the stigma that comes with being labeled a fat whale: "The poems celebrate the beauty and sensuality of the whale slipping through the water. ... It is no surprise that Stinson draws on the idea and image of the whale, simultaneously rejecting the common insult and reclaiming the creature's beauty, finesse, and strength" (p. 154). In a similar vein, Anna Kirkland (2008) shares this quotation from a fat acceptance activist who liked to think of herself as a hippo: "I do a lot of swimming and I get in the water and I just feel like a total ballerina in the water. I'm very buoyant and graceful and amazing in the water. But then when I'm on land, I feel very clumsy and large and awkward. I feel just the opposite in the water" (p. 397). By challenging the speciesism underlying what are meant to be hurtful comparisons to whales and hippos, the power of these two insults is significantly diminished.

Reclaiming Fat Cow

To return to "fat cow" as we wrap up, can we problematize and reclaim this insult as part of the intersectional work we consider vital to fat pedagogy? As fat acceptance activists and fat studies scholars have argued, the word "fat" need not be considered an insult, but rather as a simple descriptor of a body. Further, in our personal experience with cows, we know them to be curious, highly social, gentle, and fiercely protective mothers. We appreciate their beautiful eyes, respect their strength, and enjoy their evocative mooing so long as they are not in distress. So, yes, we will take cow as a compliment.

References

Adams, C. (2014). Why a pig? A reclining nude reveals the intersections of race, sex, slavery, and species. In C. Adams & L. Gruen (Eds.), *Ecofeminism: Feminist intersections with other animals and the earth* (pp. 208–244). New York, NY: Bloomsbury.

Adams, C. J. (2010). *The sexual politics of meat: A feminist-vegetarian critical theory* (20th anniversary ed.). New York, NY: Continuum.

Adams, C., & Gruen, L. (2014). Groundwork. In C. Adams & L. Gruen (Eds.), *Ecofeminism: Feminist intersections with other animals and the earth* (pp. 7–36). New York, NY: Bloomsbury.

Armstrong, S. J., & Botzler, R. G. (2008). *The animal ethics reader* (2nd ed.). New York, NY: Routledge.

Arnold, R., Burke, B., James, C., Martin, D., & Thomas, B. (1991). *Educating for a change*. Toronto, ON, Canada: Between the Lines.

Bell, A., & Russell, C. (1999). Life ties: Disrupting anthropocentrism in language arts education. In J. Robertson (Ed.), *Teaching for a tolerant world: Grades K–6. Essays and resources* (pp. 68–89). Urbana, IL: National Council of Teachers of English.

Bell, A., & Russell, C. (2000). Beyond human, beyond words: Anthropocentrism, critical pedagogy, and the post-structuralist turn. *Canadian Journal of Education, 25*(3), 188–203.

Boling, P. (2011). On learning to teach fat feminism. *Feminist Teacher, 21*(2), 110–123.

Cameron, E. (2015a). Toward a fat pedagogy: A study of pedagogical approaches aimed at challenging obesity discourse in post-secondary education. *Fat Studies, 4*(1), 28–45.

Cameron, E. (2015b). Teaching resources for post-secondary educators who challenge dominant obesity discourse. *Fat Studies, 4*(2), 212–226.

Cho, S., Crenshaw, K. W., & McCall, L. (2013). Toward a field of intersectionality studies: Theory, applications, and praxis. *Signs, 38*(4), 785–810.

Corman, L., & Vandrovcová, T. (2014). Radical humility: Toward a more holistic critical animal studies pedagogy. In A. Nocella II, J. Sorenson, K. Socha, & A. Matsuoka (Eds.), *Defining critical animal studies: An introduction to an intersectional social justice approach to animal liberation* (pp. 135–157). New York, NY: Peter Lang.

Dean, M. A. (2014). You are how you eat? Femininity, normalization, and veganism as an ethical practice of freedom. *Societies, 4*(2), 127–147.

Deckha, M. (2012). Toward a postcolonial, posthumanist feminist theory: Centralizing race and culture in feminist work on nonhuman animals. *Hypatia, 27*(3), 527–545.

Dunayer, J. (1995). Sexist words, speciesist roots. In C. Adams & J. Donovan (Eds.), *Animals and women: Feminist theoretical explorations*. Durham, NC: Duke University Press.

Farrell, A. E. (2011). *Fat shame: Stigma and the fat body in American culture*. New York, NY: New York University Press.

Fawcett, L. (2013). Three degrees of separation: Accounting for naturecultures in environmental education research. In R. Stevenson, M. Brody, J. Dillon, & A. Wals (Eds.), *International handbook of research on environmental education* (pp. 409–423). New York, NY: Routledge.

Fawcett, L., Bell, A., & Russell, C. (2002). Guiding our environmental praxis: Teaching for social and environmental justice. In W. Filho (Ed.), *Teaching sustainability at universities: Towards curriculum greening* (pp. 223–238). New York, NY: Peter Lang.

Gaard, G. (2013). Toward a feminist postcolonial milk studies. *American Quarterly, 65*(3), 595–618.

Hardy, K. A. (2014). Cows, pigs, whales: Nonhuman animals, antifat bias, and exceptionalist logics. In R. Chastain (Ed.), *The politics of size: Perspectives from the fat acceptance movement* (Vol. 1, pp. 187–206). Santa Barbara, CA: Praeger.

Hetrick, A., & Attig, D. (2009). Sitting pretty: Fat bodies, classroom desks, and academic excess. In E. Rothblum & S. Solovay (Eds.), *The fat studies reader* (pp. 197–204). New York, NY: New York University Press.

Jones, S., & Hughes-Decatur, H. (2012). Speaking of bodies in justice-oriented, feminist teacher education. *Journal of Teacher Education, 63*(1), 51–61.

Kahn, R. (2011). Towards an animal standpoint: Vegan education and the epistemology of ignorance. In E. Malewski & N. Jaramillo (Eds.), *Epistemologies of ignorance in education* (pp. 53–70). Charlotte, NC: Information Age.

Kirkland, A. (2008). Think of the hippopotamus: Rights consciousness in the fat acceptance movement. *Law and Society Review, 42*(2), 397–431.

Leahy, D. (2009). Disgusting pedagogies. In J. Wright & V. Harwood (Eds.), *Biopolitics and the obesity epidemic: Governing bodies* (pp. 172–182). London, England: Routledge.

LeBesco, K. (2004). *Revolting bodies? The struggle to redefine fat identity*. Boston, MA: University of Massachusetts Press.

López Rodríguez, I. (2009). Of women, bitches, chickens and vixens: Animal metaphors for women in English and Spanish. *Cultura, lenguaje y representación, 7*, 77–100.

marino, d. (1997). *Wild garden: Art, education, and the culture of resistance*. Toronto, ON, Canada: Between the Lines.

McIntosh, P. (1998). White privilege: Unpacking the invisible knapsack. *Race, Class, and Gender in the United States: An Integrated Study, 4*, 165–169.

McKenzie, M., Russell, C., Fawcett, L., & Timmerman, N. (2010). Popular media, intersubjective learning, and cultural production. In R. Stevenson & J. Dillon (Eds.), *Environmental education: Learning, culture and agency* (pp. 147–164). Rotterdam, the Netherlands: Sense.

Newkirk, I. (2009, September 26). The skinny on our growing girth. *HuffPost Green*. Retrieved from http://www.huffingtonpost.com/ingrid-newkirk/the-skinny-on-our-growing_b_269353.html

Odhiambo, C. (2012). The name game: Using insults to illustrate the social construction of gender. *College Teaching, 60*(1), 25–30.

Owen, L. J. (2015). Monstrous freedom: Charting fat ambivalence. *Fat Studies, 4*(1), 1–13.

Pausé, C. (2014). X-static process: Intersectionality within fat studies. *Fat Studies, 3*(2), 80–85.

Prohaska, A., & Gailey, J. A. (2010). Achieving masculinity through sexual predation: The case of hogging. *Journal of Gender Studies, 19*(1), 13–25.

Russell, C., Cameron, E., Socha, T., & McNinch, H. (2013). "Fatties cause global warming": Fat pedagogy and environmental education. *Canadian Journal of Environmental Education, 18*, 27–45.

Russell, C. L., Sarick, T., & Kennelly, J. (2002). Queering environmental education. *Canadian Journal of Environmental Education, 7,* 54–66.

Sarick, T. (2002). *This zine is 100% naturally queer* (MES Major Project). York University, Toronto, ON, Canada.

Selby, D. (1995). *Earthkind: A teachers' handbook on humane education.* Oakhill, England: Trentham.

Semenko, K. (2000). *"Girly-girls need not apply": An ecofeminist analysis of gender and zoos* (MES Major Paper). York University, Toronto, ON, Canada.

Sensoy, Ö., & DiAngelo, R. (2011). *Is everyone really equal? An introduction to key concepts in social justice education.* New York, NY: Teachers College Press.

Stevens, L., Kearney, M., & Maclaran, P. (2013). Uddering the other: Androcentrism, ecofeminism, and the dark side of anthropomorphic marketing. *Journal of Marketing Management, 29*(1/2), 158–174.

Tirosh, Y. (2006). Weighty speech: Addressing body size in the classroom. *Review of Education, Pedagogy, and Cultural Studies, 28*(3/4), 267–279.

Watkins, P. L., Farrell, A. E., & Hugmeyer, A. D. (2012). Teaching fat studies: From conception to reception. *Fat Studies, 1*(2), 180–194.

White, F. R. (2013). "We're kind of devolving": Visual tropes of evolution in obesity discourse. *Critical Public Health, 23*(3), 320–330.

Notes

1   Other axes of oppression such as those based on race, class, sexuality, and ability also figure into the work of many of these scholars, as they do our own. For the purposes of this discussion, however, we focus mostly on gender, species, and body size.

2   For another discussion of visual evolutionary tropes in obesity discourse, notably of fat people "devolving" into pigs, see White, 2013.

3   Humane education refers to learning that enables compassion, kindness, respect, and responsibility towards other animals and grew out of a social movement concerned with both child welfare and animal protection (Selby, 1995). Similar work is being done under the auspices of environmental education that focuses on animality, ecopedagogy, critical animal pedagogy, and posthumanist education. Here, we are using humane education simply as a shorthand for learning that foregrounds other animals.

4   While there are debates in the field about instructors addressing their own or students' embodiment (e.g., Cameron, 2015a; Tirosh, 2006; Watkins, Farrell, & Hugmeyer, 2012), we prefer to do so given our theoretical and pedagogical commitments.

5   We planned to reprint the PETA billboard here, but they denied us permission to do so. It is easily found on the web by typing in the text and we recommend seeking it out since it is so pedagogically useful. To view both the original billboard and the parody, see: http://bastet2329.blogspot.ca/2009/08/petas-anti-fat-whale-campaign.html

TWENTY TWO

A Tale of Three Classrooms: Fat Studies and Its Intellectual Allies

Breanne Fahs

As an emerging field, fat studies has started the work of deconstructing and challenging notions of "obesity" and size normativity while also establishing itself as a powerful interrogator of stigma, oppression, and the haunting outcomes of teaching people to fear and dread fatness (Cooper, 2010; Hebl & Heatherton, 1998; Rothblum & Solovay, 2009). Notions of fat embodiment, fat resistance, and rebellions against fat shaming have cohered to form a new field of critical studies that is rapidly expanding within and outside of academia (Rothblum & Solovay, 2009). Further, with all of the work feminist scholars have done around bodies, embodiment, and the body as a site of resistance, fat studies is uniquely situated to have far greater prominence in years to come (Bobel & Kwan, 2011; Bordo, 1997; Rothblum & Solovay, 2009).

Although fatness as an identity category has received more and more attention in recent years, particularly related to stigma in the classroom (Hetrick & Attig, 2009) and prejudices and biases directed towards fat professors and fat students (Escalera, 2009; Fisanick, 2014; Koppelman, 2009), fat pedagogies—or how educators teach about fatness in formal classrooms, non-formal learning environments, and beyond—are still in their infancy. No universities offer fat studies majors or minors yet, although a few offer stand-alone fat studies courses (Cameron, 2015). Teaching fat studies is paramount to advancing social justice around issues of fatness. Charlotte Cooper (2010) argued that teaching about the cultural production of fat phobia enacts social change because fatness becomes a critical (and productive) site of analysis in comparison to only looking at the fat body. While some have started to integrate fat studies work into their core curricula, its presence within women and gender studies, for example, often lags behind other sites of critical body interrogation such as eating disorders, body hair, fashion and modeling, genital attitudes, trans studies, and so on. Fatness, it seems, is still far too often invisible and sidelined in feminist pedagogies of the body (Watkins, Farrell, & Doyle Hugmeyer, 2012).

In this chapter, I argue that fat pedagogies must draw heavily from the intellectual alliances and political "cousins" of fat studies—particularly queer studies, disability studies, gender studies, and the new and emerging freak studies—in order to advance its status within academia and activism. Drawing from clear pedagogical examples of teaching fat studies in three different undergraduate courses—a women and gender studies course on health and the body, a women and gender studies/social justice course on manifestos and radical writings, and a women and gender studies/social justice course on trash and freaks—I outline in this chapter the different intellectual, political, and personal stakes of framing fatness within these different rhetorical and political communities.

Seeing fat within the lens of health has far different consequences for students in comparison to seeing fatness within the context of rebellious social movements or "freak" bodies. Feminist health classes often critically examine constructions of the fat body as "sick," but positioning fatness as inherently rebellious occurs less often. For example, by situating fat studies as a discipline of resistance, fat empowerment, and body rebellion, professors can more easily situate fat studies texts into the context of manifestos and other radical responses to systematic forms of oppression; this helps students to frame fat studies not as a passive or health-related enterprise but as a field dedicated to outspoken resistance and flagrant fighting against oppression. When teaching about fat studies in the context of health and body studies, the stakes are quite different as students interrogate the fat body through the lens of public health discourses, medicalization, and "good body" frameworks. In these health and body studies classes, the drawing together of disability studies and fat studies can help dismantle assumptions about appropriate, good, and functional bodies while also provoking discussion about the limits of merging fatness into the framework of disability.

I conclude the chapter by reflecting on the powerful potential of teaching about fat studies in the context of the study of freaks, as the alliances formed between queer "freaks," fat "freaks," "freaks" of color, and women as "freaks" help students to understand and unpack the social conditions of the supposedly abject body present in these discourses. In doing so, the identity-based work of queer studies and gender studies (e.g., trans acceptance, the freak show) meets the critical body studies work of fat studies (e.g., fat shaming, fat manifestos) to help students better understand the critical intersections not only between emerging disciplines but also people's lived experiences.

Framing Fat Pedagogies

Critical fields such as women's studies/gender studies, ethnic studies, sexuality studies, religious studies, American studies, and Indigenous/First Nations studies have always faced numerous challenges when attempting to integrate themselves into the corporate university (Aronowitz, 2000). The relationship between critical fields (often with explicit goals to dismantle hierarchies, challenge power relations, give voice to the silenced, and upend disciplinary practices of exclusion) and the highly corporatized institutional practices of universities have often resulted in much contention (hooks, 2000; Rutherford, 2006). Even critical pedagogies suffer at times from replicating the very assumptions they seek to deconstruct and undermine; for example, Judith Butler (1997) has talked about the dangers of *producing* hate speech in an effort to understand and explore its meanings, just as Elizabeth Ellsworth (1989) has argued that critical fields still too often retain traditional notions of *who* can produce valid knowledge, thereby perpetuating relations of dominance in the classroom.

Fat studies scholars, fat professors, and fat activists also face a formidable uphill battle when seeking to combat fat shaming and fat phobia in the context of corporate/institutional universities. While other stigmatized identities can draw from progressive social movements (e.g., the women's movement, civil rights movement, queer movement), fat activists, even with the fat acceptance movement, do not have the advantages of a full-fledged progressive social movement. The mere mention of the word "fat" still elicits panic in some students. Because fatness is often seen as a symbol of self-indulgence, moral failing, and laziness, especially for women, fat bodies face stigma, assault, prejudice, and oppression in the classroom and elsewhere (Rothblum, 1992; Wray & Deery, 2008). Disgust about fatness and the dread of becoming fat permeates popular, medical, and psychological discourses, with several studies showing that women dieters were motivated more by their fear of fatness than by their desire for thinness (Dalley & Buunk, 2009, 2011; Vartanian, 2010). Fat women reported decrease in well-being as a result of fat prejudices, and more often divested themselves of sexuality and felt "uncultivated" and "uncared for" compared with thin women (Murray, 2004). While fat men felt more secure about their bodies than did fat women, these men also expressed more dislike of fat people than did fat women, suggesting that fatness impacts men and women differently (Aruguete, Yates, & Edman, 2006). In short, fat stigma permeates modern life throughout the United States, Canada, and much of the Western world, assaulting both men and women with clear messages about the "deviance" of fat and its various negative outcomes (Farrell, 2011; Rothblum & Solovay, 2009).

Within universities, fat shaming and fear of fatness may have particular salience, as college women routinely struggle with body image issues (Rudd & Lennon, 2000); specifically, sorority women reported especially strong fears of becoming fat along with more body dissatisfaction and more weight concern compared with other university women (Schulken, 1997). Fat students may withdraw and become invisible in light of the microaggressions they face on campuses and in their social spaces (Owen, 2012), as young women learn early on to conceptualize thinness as a requirement for feeling acceptable to themselves and others (Williamson, 1998). Even for groups historically protected from hatred of fatness such as African American and Latina women, studies have shown increasing bodily distress and fear of fatness within these groups (Lovejoy, 2001; Thompson, 1992; Williamson, 1998), even while white women reported the most body shame and fear of fatness (Abrams, Allen, & Gray, 1993; Rucker & Cash, 1992). College women clearly continue to struggle with body image and these struggles extend across identity groups (Harris, 1994; Lovejoy, 2001; Thompson, 1992), making a clear case for the urgency and necessity of critically understanding fatness and thinness.

Despite the clear evidence for the pervasive fear of, and hostility towards, fatness and the various impacts of fat phobia upon both women and men, few studies have interrogated fat pedagogies and how professors ultimately work to deconstruct and dismantle assumptions about thin and fat bodies (Escalera, 2009). When examining other critical fields that endorse and practice radical and critical pedagogies (e.g., women and gender studies, ethnic studies, American studies, queer studies), the relative blind spot around fat pedagogies, particularly for intersectional discourses, becomes even more glaring. With growing attention directed towards fat pedagogies, however, fat studies has presented itself as an emerging discipline wide open to new interpretations and conceptualization of its political allies (Boling, 2011; Cameron, 2015; Hopkins, 2011; Leahy, 2009; Sykes & McPhail, 2008).

Why, in an age when women learn to think about and demean their fat on a near daily basis, do universities rarely discuss or critically interrogate fatness? Why have medical and popular discourses failed to follow fat studies scholars in adjusting the cultural lexicon of fatness away from "obesity" and towards fatness? What does it mean when other modes of embodiment—gender identity, body hair, menstruation, dieting, fashion, body image, abortion, pregnancy, and so on—receive much attention in the classroom while fatness remains relatively unquestioned as an identity of "deviance"? Ultimately, because fat oppression has similar logics and practices compared with other forms of oppression such as racism, ableism, and misogyny, fat studies intuitively aligns with other subfields and disciplines that critically examine bodies and identities (van Amsterdam, 2013), just as fat phobia maps onto other forms of prejudice and discrimination (Perez-Lopez, Lewis, & Cash, 2001). In this chapter, I unravel how such alliances can usefully inform fat pedagogies both within and outside of the women's studies classroom.

Practicing Fat Pedagogies

As I teach several upper-division women and gender studies courses (some cross-listed with social justice and human rights) at a large, public southwestern university in the United States, I frame my observations about fat studies within that particular context. Students at my university come from a range of race, class, and sexual identity backgrounds and many students are outside of the traditional student age range (18 to 22). I typically also have approximately one-third male students and two-thirds female students in each course, along with at least one transgender or gender queer student each semester in my courses. During the semesters that I teach fat studies content, I typically introduce this material three to four weeks into the semester after students have been introduced to concepts in the theoretical foundations of the course.

Classroom 1: Gender, Bodies, and Health

Courses that critically examine bodies and medical/health discourses provide a solid framework for teaching critical material about fatness. In my course Gender, Bodies, and Health, I approach the critical examination of fatness through the study of food politics, medical discourses of mental and physical health, coming-of-age issues related to the development of body image and menstruation ideologies, and weight gain related to pregnancy and childbirth. More specifically, fat studies readings are wedged between discussions of how bodies are socially constructed and how bodies are subjected to forces of domination, control, and discipline by the culture at large. Eating and food, then, form the basis for such discussions, as the students and I link together food politics to discussions of how fatness gets constructed as "laziness" (Gregory, 2001; Hartley, 2001), how fatness connects to discourses of dieting and excess (Bordo, 1997; Hartley, 2001), and how our food system in general sabotages people into eating low-quality, low-nutrient food (Kaplan, 2012; Pollan, 2009). In this classroom, fatness relates to health, medicalization, and the politics of food.

Much of fat studies has sought to critically examine public health discourses that construct fatness as a mere health problem and thereby disguise the social control aspects of fat phobia within claims that "it's just healthier to be thinner." The largest body of fat studies work has sought to address the medicalization of fatness, and students can easily and readily access readings and ideas about these themes. Questioning whether one can be fat and healthy and examining how fatness and morality link together have both served as fruitful lines of discussion in this course. Further, thinking critically about food choices regardless of the students' size has brought about many vivid discussions on how food, morality, politics, the state, and the rhetoric of "personal choice" get tied together.

Teaching about fatness in a class on bodies and health also has allowed discussions of how fatness and disability studies can work together to dismantle notions of "good" bodies. By questioning ideas about functionality (e.g., must we all function similarly to be "normal"?), sexuality (e.g., whose bodies get sexualized and whose do not?), and morality (e.g., are "normal" bodies also "good" bodies, and if not, how can we challenge such links?), students interrogate fatness from the perspective of how bodies, ability, and desirability all work as social constructions. For some students, this is not only their introduction to thinking critically about fat shaming and fat phobia, but it also serves as their introduction to any critical body studies material. Some students have never critically examined notions of bodily control, media images around ideal bodies, family narratives of thinness as rewarded and fatness as discouraged, and beliefs that weight loss make people "good." This class most clearly links fat studies to disability studies and body studies, forming an intuitive alliance that facilitates larger discussions about gender, identity, and power. Still, by framing fatness under the umbrella of health and medical discourses, fat studies in this context faces limits to students being able to grasp its *political* potential and its fundamentally rebellious impulses, in part because the class may draw students more interested in health than in politics.

Classroom 2: Hate Speech, Manifestos, and Radical Writings

In contrast to the more intuitive and widely understood linkages between fat studies and bodies/health content, I have also taught fat studies in a course called Hate Speech, Manifestos, and Radical Writings. This course examines a range of radical and inflammatory writings that contextualize the fight against oppression within revolutionary and incendiary ideologies. More specifically, the class is designed to push progressive and liberal students to their logical endpoints in order to assess and critically examine the value of violence, open revolt, and dissent within contemporary and historical radical thought. We also work in this class to think about what constitutes hate speech and what hate speech *does* politically, socially, and legally (Butler, 1997).

Fat studies within this classroom, then, becomes situated as a form of resistance, fat empowerment, and bodily rebellion, as fat bodies conceptualized in this course are not passively awaiting acceptance or assimilation into mainstream society. Rather, fat studies is situated as a field that works towards explicit and unequivocal resistance, defiant rejection of contemporary body norms, and deep-seated unworking and unpacking of thin-centric ideologies. Students read *Big Fat Manifesto* (Vaught, 2008), a variety of anti-assimilationist queer/fat writings (Sycamore, 2008), and Amy Farrell's (2011) chapter "Refusing to Apologize" from her book *Fat Shame: Stigma and the Fat Body in American Culture*. In tandem with this, many students have chosen in previous semesters to write their own manifestos on fatness, often with blatant contempt for thin-centric discourse combined with a clear call for fat people (especially women) to take up space, declare war on fat phobia, and shamelessly exist as themselves. The fat studies content is presented alongside other outspoken body rebellion documents, including menstrual activist readings (e.g., Docherty, 2010) and body hair rebellions (Fahs, 2011). These pairings allow students to readily establish connections between fat shaming and other sorts of body shaming (e.g., menstrual shaming) directed towards women's bodies.

Notably, during class conversations, fat studies rarely elicits any talk of medicalizing fatness, and instead focuses on the expansive and radical potential for fat bodies to take up space, perform as excessive, and become purposefully and shamelessly "too much." Students critically interrogate fatness as a demarcation of power but rarely debate the health-related aspects of fat and thin bodies. They also engage with the emotional and affective components of fatness, particularly fat women's rage about being contained, humiliated, and controlled by mainstream society. Subtly, students identify fatness as one of many other forms of identity-based oppression that gets written onto the body, with many students making parallels between fatness, queerness, and other forms of embodied resistance (e.g., tattoos, body hair). By working with so many other forms of anti-assimilationist thought (e.g., black power, radical feminism), fat studies becomes shaped as an inherently rebellious force to be reckoned with.

Classroom 3: Trash, Freaks, and SCUM

As my newest iteration of bringing fat studies into the classroom, I have recently developed a course called Trash, Freaks, and SCUM, which takes as its philosophical premise the idea that knowledge should be produced and gleaned from the gutter. Working through texts such as Valerie Solanas' (1968) *SCUM Manifesto*, Edward Hume's (2013) *Garbology*, and Rachel Adams' (2001) *Sideshow U.S.A.*, students consider trash both literally (how much trash do we produce and what can we do about this?), and metaphorically (whose bodies are constructed as "trashy"?). As an offshoot of the emerging new field of freak studies, which seeks to unpack the idea of the abject Othered body embodied in the so-called "freak," fat studies in this classroom works on representations of extreme fatness and extreme "Otherness" to understand and unwork contemporary ideologies of fatness as morally sinful and ultimately abject.

The class focuses specifically on the production of the fat body as freak, alongside discussions of early anthropological efforts to cage and contain African men, Susan Stryker's (1994) compelling exposé on the plight of trans people as virtual Frankensteins, and Rachel Adams' (2001) analysis of freak photography. We read Amy Farrell's (2009) piece on fat women in tourist postcards and JuliaGrace Jester's (2009) analysis of fat burlesque. In this way, the fat "freak" becomes clearly aligned (politically and historically) with freaks of color, queer freaks, trans freaks, and women as freaks. The cartoon-like caricatures of fat women link up with the overtly racist and hateful portrayals of native Africans as "backward" and "primitive," the intensely self-loathing conditions of the trans existence (Stryker, 1994), and the overwhelming difficulty of circus performers with extreme bodies (Adams, 2001). Ultimately, these links work to situate fatness as one of many identities subjected to "freak" status by dominant (white, male, middle- and upper-class, heterosexual, thin, able-bodied) culture.

The Pedagogical Potential of Fatness

I present these three frameworks for teaching about fatness for several reasons, the most important of which is that fat studies, I believe, has not yet tapped into its full potential as a critical discipline or pedagogical tool. While there is definite utility in teaching about fatness in relation to discourses of medicalization (what is healthy?) and assimilation (how can fat people gain the social acceptance of thin and average-sized people?), my own pedagogical experiences have shown the tremendous possibilities inherent to teaching about fatness in more overtly political and even radical contexts.

Fat studies has a variety of important political allies, each of which can help fat studies reach wider audiences, gain relevance in university classrooms, and enter national and international discussions about hierarchies, power, social statuses, and political oppression. By linking up with disability studies, fat studies can unpack ideas around appropriate bodies, bodily excess, (de)sexualization, and functionality. How people take up space, and how people imagine the goals of bodies that are "out of bounds"—for example, should we work to assimilate disabled and fat bodies into able-bodied and thin models of being, or should we encourage and allow them to exist as is?—is something students can readily address when linking disability studies and fat studies together.

Similarly, connections between queer studies, fat studies, and critical race studies can also yield compelling classroom discussions and scholarly linkages (Perez-Lopez, Lewis, & Cash, 2001). If students learn that fat bodies are subjected to similar rhetoric and constraints as queer and black bodies, these connections work to establish clear intersectional and overlapping connective tissue between these fields (and people's lived experiences within these identities). Understanding the extreme mistreatment of fat bodies in tourist postcards, for example, seems easier to understand and examine when seeing the postcards in tandem with African men held at the Bronx zoo for "viewing" in 1906 (Adams, 2001). Ultimately, as each of these examples shows, the university classroom (especially in critical fields such as women and gender studies, critical race studies, and sexuality studies) is an important battleground in the fat studies revolution.

Situating Radical Fatness?

I want this chapter to serve both as an example of the pedagogical potential of fat studies and as a clear call to the fat studies field to embrace, encourage, and promote ideas of *radical fatness*. What would it look like if fat studies rejected notions of assimilation, mere "fat acceptance," and tepid criticisms of health discourse in favor of situating fat bodies as inherently rebellious and tools of *anti-assimilation*? I have longed for a more clear vision of radical fat politics and radical fat studies, one where students, scholars, and activists alike can tap into the angry emotional energy of oppressed fat people and use that energy to transform our understanding of the boundaries of the body and society. While some critical fields have embraced their more radical potential—particularly queer/trans studies and critical race studies—fat studies has a long way to go before it can fully embrace and realize its radical potential. Nevertheless, its radical potential is certainly there, bubbling underneath the surface, waiting to be utilized. The fat body is, I think, inherently dangerous, disruptive, and confrontational; fat pedagogies must showcase this potential.

To accomplish the goal of radicalizing fat studies and fat pedagogies, recognition of the deep connection between fat studies and its intellectual allies is necessary, particularly as fat studies embraces revolt and rebellion. Fat studies has the potential to lead the struggle for scholarly and activist work on bodily resistance and rebellion. I conclude here by asking: first, how can fat studies access its politically radical potential, especially by using notions of "excessiveness" as an advantageous, rebellious, and revolutionary force? Second, how can fatness in the classroom serve not only to illuminate the experiences of oppressed people but also to further map the body as the terrain upon which social inequalities are enacted? I want fat scholars, professors, students, and activists to move fat studies out of the more liberal terrain of assimilation and mere "acceptance" into the more provocative space of confrontational, in-your-face radical upheavals engendered by contemporary body politics.

References

Abrams, K. K., Allen, L. R., & Gray, J. J. (1993). Disordered eating attitudes and behaviors, psychological adjustment, and ethnic identity: A comparison of black and white female college students. *International Journal of Eating Disorders, 14*(1), 49–57.

Adams, R. (2001). *Sideshow U.S.A.: Freaks and the cultural imagination.* Chicago, IL: University of Chicago Press.

Aronowitz, S. (2000). *The knowledge factory: Dismantling the corporate university and creating true higher learning.* Boston, MA: Beacon Press.

Aruguete, M. S., Yates, A., & Edman, J. (2006). Gender differences in attitudes about fat. *North American Journal of Psychology, 8*(1), 183–192.

Bobel, C., & Kwan, S. (2011). *Embodied resistance: Challenging the norms, breaking the rules.* Nashville, TN: Vanderbilt University Press.

Boling, P. (2011). On learning to teach fat feminism. *Feminist Teacher, 21*(2), 110–123.

Bordo, S. (1997). Psychopathology as the crystallization of culture. In C. Counhan & P. Van Sterik (Eds.), *Food and culture: A reader* (pp. 226–250). Florence, KY: Psychology Press.

Butler, J. (1997). *Excitable speech: A politics of the performative.* New York, NY: Routledge.

Cameron, E. (2015). Toward a fat pedagogy: A study of pedagogical approaches aimed at challenging obesity discourse in post-secondary education. *Fat Studies, 4*(1), 28–45.

Cooper, C. (2010). Fat studies: Mapping the field. *Sociology Compass, 4*(12), 1020–1034.

Dalley, S. E., & Buunk, A. P. (2009). "Thinspiration" vs. "fear of fat": Using prototypes to predict frequent weight-loss dieting in females. *Appetite, 52*(1), 217–221.

Dalley, S. E., & Buunk, A. P. (2011). The motivation to diet in young women: Fear is stronger than hope. *European Journal of Social Psychology, 41*(5), 672–680.

Docherty, S. (2010). Smear it on your face, rub it on your body, it's time to start a menstrual party! *CTSJ: Critical Theory and Social Justice, 1*(1). Retrieved from http://scholar.oxy.edu/ctsj/vol1/iss1/12/

Ellsworth, E. (1989). Why doesn't this feel empowering? Working through the repressive myths of critical pedagogy. *Harvard Educational Review, 59*(3), 297–325.

Escalera, E. A. (2009). Stigma threat and the fat professor: Reducing student prejudice in the classroom. In E. Rothblum & S. Solovay (Eds.), *The fat studies reader* (pp. 205–212). New York, NY: New York University.

Fahs, B. (2011). Dreaded "Otherness": Heteronormative patrolling in women's body hair rebellions. *Gender & Society, 25*(4), 451–472.

Farrell, A. E. (2009). "The white man's burden": Female sexuality, tourist postcards, and the place of the fat woman in early 20th-century U.S. culture. In E. Rothblum & S. Solovay (Eds.), *The fat studies reader* (pp. 256–262). New York, NY: New York University.

Farrell, A. E. (2011). *Fat shame: Stigma and the fat body in American culture.* New York, NY: New York University Press.

Fisanick, C. (2014). Fat professors feel compelled to overperform. *Chronicle of Higher Education.* Retrieved from https://chroniclevitae.com/news/425-christina-fisanick-fat-professors-feel-compelled-to-overperform#sthash.EQn4lThq.dpuf

Gregory, D. (2001). Heavy judgment: A sister talks about the pain of "living large." In J. R. Johnston (Ed.), *The American body in context: An anthology* (pp. 311–318). Wilmington, DE: Scholarly Resources.

Harris, S. M. (1994). Racial differences in predictors of college women's body image attitudes. *Women & Health, 21*(4), 89–104.

Hartley, C. (2001). Letting ourselves go: Making room for the fat body in feminist scholarship. In J. E. Braziel & K. LeBesco (Eds.), *Bodies out of bounds: Fatness and transgression* (pp. 60–73). Berkeley, CA: University of California Press.

Hebl, M. R., & Heatherton, T. F. (1998). The stigma of obesity in women: The difference is black and white. *Personality and Social Psychology Bulletin, 24*(4), 417–426.

Hetrick, A., & Attig, D. (2009). Sitting pretty: Fat bodies, classroom desks, and academic excess. In E. Rothblum & S. Solovay (Eds.), *The fat studies reader* (pp. 197–204). New York, NY: New York University.

hooks, b. (2000). *Feminist theory: From margin to center.* London, England: Pluto Press.

Hopkins, P. (2011). Teaching and learning guide for: Critical geographies of body size. *Geography Compass, 5*(2), 106–111.

Hume, E. (2013). *Garbology: Our dirty love affair with trash.* New York, NY: Penguin.

Jester, J. (2009). Placing fat women on center stage. In E. Rothblum & S. Solovay (Eds.), *The fat studies reader* (pp. 249–253). New York, NY: New York University.

Kaplan, D. M. (2012). *The philosophy of food.* Berkeley, CA: University of California Press.

Koppelman, S. (2009). Fat stories in the classroom: What and how are they teaching about us? In E. Rothblum & S. Solovay (Eds.), *The fat studies reader* (pp. 213–222). New York, NY: New York University.

Leahy, D. (2009). Disgusting pedagogies. In J. Wright & V. Harwood (Eds.), *Biopolitics and the obesity epidemic: Governing bodies* (pp. 172–182). London, England: Routledge.

Lovejoy, M. (2001). Disturbances in the social body: Differences in body image and eating problems among African American and white women. *Gender & Society, 15*(2), 239–261.

Murray, S. (2004). Locating aesthetics: Sexing the fat women. *Social Semiotics, 14*(3), 237–247.

Owen, L. (2012). Living fat in a thin-centric world: Effects of spatial discrimination on fat bodies and selves. *Feminism & Psychology, 22*(3), 290–306.

Perez-Lopez, M. S., Lewis, R. J., & Cash, T. F. (2001). The relationship of antifat attitudes to other prejudicial and gender-related attitudes. *Journal of Applied Social Psychology, 31*(4), 683–697.

Pollan, M. (2009). *In defense of food: An eater's manifesto.* New York, NY: Penguin.

Rothblum, E. D. (1992). The stigma of women's weight: Social and economic realities. *Feminism & Psychology, 2*(1), 61–73.

Rothblum, E., & Solovay, S. (Eds.). (2009). *The fat studies reader.* New York, NY: New York University Press.

Rucker, C. E., & Cash, T. F. (1992). Body images, body-size perceptions, and eating behaviors among African-American and white college men. *International Journal of Eating Disorders, 12*(3), 291–299.

Rudd, N. A., & Lennon, S. J. (2000). Body image and appearance-management behaviors in college women. *Clothing and Textiles Research Journal, 18*(3), 152–162.

Rutherford, J. (2006). Cultural studies in the corporate university. *Cultural Studies, 19*(3), 297–317.

Schulken, E. D. (1997). Sorority women's body size perceptions and their weight-related attitudes and behaviors. *Journal of American College Health, 46*(2), 69–74.

Solanas, V. (1968). *SCUM manifesto.* New York, NY: Olympia Press.

Stryker, S. (1994). My words to Victor Frankenstein above the village of Chamounix: Performing transgender rage. *GLQ: A Journal of Gay and Lesbian Studies, 1*(3), 237–254.

Sycamore, M. (2008). *That's revolting: Queer strategies for resisting assimilation.* Berkeley, CA: Soft Skull Press.

Sykes, H., & McPhail, D. (2008). Unbearable lessons: Contesting fat phobia in physical education. *Sociology of Sport, 25*(1), 66–96.

Thompson, B. W. (1992). "A way outa no way": Eating problems among African-American, Latina, and White women. *Gender & Society, 6*(4), 546–561.

van Amsterdam, N. (2013). Big fat inequalities, thin privilege: An intersectional perspective on "body size." *European Journal of Women's Studies, 20*(2), 155–169.

Vartanian, L. R. (2010). Disgust and perceived control in attitudes toward obese people. *International Journal of Obesity, 34*(8), 1302–1307.

Vaught, S. (2008). *Big fat manifesto.* New York, NY: Bloomsbury.

Watkins, P. L., Farrell, A., & Doyle Hugmeyer, A. (2012). Teaching fat studies: From conception to reception. *Fat Studies, 1*(2), 180–194.

Williamson, L. (1998). Eating disorders and the cultural forces behind the drive for thinness. *Social Work in Health Care, 28*(1), 61–73.

Wray, S., & Deery, R. (2008). The medicalization of body size and women's healthcare. *Health Care for Women International, 29*(3), 227–243.

TWENTY THREE

A Public Pedagogy Approach
to Fat Pedagogy

Emma Rich

In this chapter I argue that the emerging academic field of "public pedagogy" has a great deal to offer fat pedagogy, in terms of its potential both to problematize and belie some of the taken-for-granted beliefs about fatness and to generate more critical and potentially more empowering and humanistic forms of knowledge and understandings about fat. I begin by exploring how the construct of public pedagogy (Sandlin, O'Malley, & Burdick, 2011) challenges the idea that pedagogical phenomena reside only in formal educational spaces. Public pedagogy recognizes that the spaces in which meanings are made, including those about fatness, weight, and the body, are contested and contingent. In this vein, a case is made for harnessing public pedagogical approaches for disrupting and troubling weight-based oppression.

My intention is not to present some kind of typology of fat pedagogies, but rather to offer a heuristic method through reflecting on various processes and practices of public pedagogy. Specifically, I ask, is there anything distinctive about public pedagogy that might help to challenge, trouble, or disrupt weight-based oppression? Throughout, I take up some of the challenges laid down by Jake Burdick, Jennifer Sandlin, and Michael O'Malley (2014) in their problematization of public pedagogy, to make clearer "its meaning, context or location" (p. 3). The chapter therefore considers the particular conditions of a range of "publics" and "sites" that might help to expand our collective knowledge of possibilities for articulating alternative ways of thinking about fat. These include, but are not limited to, arts, social media, community health, the activities of public intellectuals and public figures, and various sites of activism.

Learning About Fat: Adopting a Public Pedagogy Approach

In developing an account of "learning" about fatness beyond formal health education, it is necessary to start with a vision of education that recognizes how learning, including about one's body and health, often occurs in sites/contexts beyond formal education. A number of scholars have contributed to the field of "public pedagogy"[1] (e.g., Ellsworth, 2005; Giroux, 2003, 2004; Kellner, 1995; Sandlin et al., 2011) focusing on contemporary sites of learning beyond the boundaries of formal education sites. Public pedagogy theorizes learning as not only located in formal institutions (Sandlin, Schultz, & Burdick, 2010; Sandlin et al., 2011), but also operating across a range of sites, such as popular culture (Sandlin et al., 2010), social activism (Brady, 2006), the Internet, and museums (Sandlin et al., 2011), to name a few. From this perspective there is a broad range of "forms, processes and sites of education outside of formal schooling" (Sandlin et al., 2011, p. 338) through which claims about the consequences of "obesity" are constituted through an array of cultural and public settings.

If public pedagogy is characterized by how learning takes place outside of formal educational structures, then it follows that learning about fat occurs across a variety of different contexts and sites. A number of studies have already revealed the problematic and often limited ways in which the media frame fatness, particularly in terms of their representation of an "obesity epidemic." As Natalie Boero (2013) notes, "the media in its various forms is critical not only to how we learn about various social problems, but also to the very construction of these problems" (p. 371). In other words, the media play a crucial role in the public pedagogy of fat; they do not just reflect discourses on fat, they are active in constituting meaning and subject positions. Elsewhere, research has examined "makeover" shows (see Raisborough, 2014; Sender & Sullivan, 2008), reality television (Rich, 2011), and fictional media, revealing how fat people are usually "the objects of derision" (Sender & Sullivan, 2008, p. 573). Examining these media sites would certainly fall within a public pedagogy perspective, but thinking more broadly in terms of setting agendas for future research, there is a much greater range of noninstitutional spaces that warrant exploration of fat pedagogies.

Practicing Public Pedagogy: Disrupting Pedagogies

At this juncture, it is worth noting Glenn Savage's (2010) concern that the field of public pedagogy has been somewhat plagued by an "enveloping negativity" (p. 109). Partly in response to this, next I consider how public pedagogy might aid in developing what Stephanie Jones and Hilary Hughes-Decatur (2012) describe as "a theory of a critical body pedagogy that can contribute to a larger justice-oriented project" (p. 51).

So, just what are the possibilities for creating alternative pedagogies of fat? Given the contemporary climate of neoliberal thinking about the body, we might ask what potential there is for a more critical public pedagogy (Sandlin & Milam, 2008), not just for scholars, but also for teachers, researchers, cultural workers, practitioners, and activists. In other words, public pedagogy prompts us to consider "what informal and non-institutional sites of education might offer in terms of differing forms, articulations, enactments and traces of pedagogy" (Burdick & Sandlin, 2013, p. 143) to mobilize counterhegemonic learning. Public pedagogy recognizes that the spaces in which meanings are made, including those about fatness, weight, and the body, are contested and contingent. This may provide opportunities for learning in which individuals can circumvent dominant knowledges of health and develop those with a more critical perspective. There are, already, examples of these pedagogies emerging across different sites and there are a number of approaches I could explore in this chapter. Below I make reference to some of the intersecting sites and approaches that have particularly captured my interest lately; these are not meant to be exhaustive but rather point towards the potential purpose, process, and practices of public fat pedagogy.

"Public" Scholarship

I begin first with some observations about what public pedagogy might offer scholars contributing to critical perspectives on weight, "obesity," and fatness. Sam Beck (2011), in a "practice of critical public pedagogy," offers an autobiographical account of how public pedagogy developed out of his research experiences and teaching projects that seek to enhance justice and empowerment, which he described as being "more involved in the political engagement of people and communities under study" (p. 715). The idea that research ought to bridge the gap between academe and various "publics" is not particularly new, yet given the recognition that fat people are largely absent from research on "obesity," this is important (see Bombak, 2014). As Boero (2013) states, "[t]he omission of fat people's voices from research on obesity is of special concern when considering the increased media focus on particular groups of fat people" (p. 378). This is a significant omission, particularly given the focus on particular communities (related to gender, class, and ethnicity) in both the media framing and policy responses to the alleged "obesity epidemic."

Nonetheless, in any move towards public engagement through research, Beck (2011) warns us that we need be mindful of any "latent oppression" whereby we might "damage the population on which the work was carried out" (p. 718). Safeguarding against this might involve building research on everyday experience where there is also a strong engagement with those communities to actually improve the conditions of their lives. Or, it could mean campaigning against fat oppression in advancing perspectives such as public sociology and public education. Michael Burawoy (2005) suggests that "public sociology brings sociology into a conversation with publics, understood as people who are themselves involved in conversation" (p. 7). As scholars, in this regard, we might ask how engaging with particular movements and associations involved in alternative fat pedagogies might also help to shape our conceptual frameworks, to help us to ask different questions and inform theory as part of the public conversation about fat. Different forms of knowledge, truth, methodologies, and public engagement therefore potentially will lead to different public pedagogies such as the emergence of the Health At Every Size (HAES) movement.

Students as Publics

In developing this conversation, we might ask, just who are the publics beyond those individuals who are fat? Burawoy (2005) suggests that "students are our first and captive public" (p. 7) and in this regard it seems helpful to consider students as a "potential public." I concur with Beck (2011) that self-reflexivity can act as a "teaching/learning device" (p. 718) to explore one's positionality and to create learning environments that explore the socio-cultural aspects of everyday life. This approach orients us towards understanding the impact of a way of thinking about weight, fat, and the conditions through which individuals are positioned as particular subjects such as "healthy" or "fit" or "morally abject" "citizen."

Like others working on developing critical fat pedagogies (Cameron, 2015; Cameron et al., 2014; Guthman, 2009; Jones & Hughes-Decatur, 2012), next I reflect on some relevant teaching experiences within higher education (see also Cameron, 2015; Hopkins, 2011; Watkins, Farrell, & Hugmeyer, 2012). With colleagues (Silk, Francombe-Webb, Rich, & Merchant, in press), I have attempted to build some of these principles into a degree program centered on sport and social sciences to develop a more self-reflexive and democratic curriculum/pedagogy. In my context, in some respects students share a relatively homogenous background (white, young, able bodied) and so assignments and class activities are oriented towards understanding the experience of others as well as exploring "what they find significant in their lives" (Beck, 2011, p. 716). This means examining the pernicious thinking about the body that occupies so many cultural sites where the "physical" is given meaning and then moving towards a critical curriculum of the corporeal (see Francombe, 2013). In an advanced seminar class, one of the goals is to learn about diversity of the body and so the class includes an approach similar to Julie Guthman (2009) in exploring "the politics of obesity" and its impact on their own and others' subjectivity. Students in this seminar write a journal in which they reflect on the seminar discussion and readings, and relate this to contemporary cultural artifacts (e.g., commercial products, traditional media, social media). Doing so also provides a space for self-reflexive writing in which students write about their own experiences related to their bodies, weight, and health practices.

Additionally, in a group assignment students use the knowledge from public pedagogy and critical scholarship to design a way to publicly contextualize knowledge into shared community learning experiences. Students have designed public talks, body awareness road shows, workshops, social media campaigns, short films, and exhibitions to challenge dominant thinking about weight. For other ideas, a recent article by Erin Cameron (2015) offers a more comprehensive resource to "expand our knowledge base of classroom practices that help to problematize rather than promote dominant notions of fat" (p. 223). Building on this work, I can imagine future practices that involve providing opportunities for students to engage more with different populations and communities, where in the context of learning about their professions (health, sport, diet), they engage with a broader range of populations and publics to understand how health practices (Cohn, 2014) are contingent on and constrained by factors such as the unequal distribution of resources.

As Guthman (2009) reports, one of the challenges is the "considerable investment students had in their bodies as neoliberal subjects" (p. 1110). Many of the students I teach are athletes or enjoy physical activity, actively monitor their bodies, and are invested in the very discourses of health that I encourage them to critique. These include neoliberal discourses of governance as articulated through healthism (see Crawford, 1980) wherein it is assumed that one is responsible for one's own health (and in the case of "obesity," one's own weight). To this end, the healthy neoliberal subject is deemed one who can demonstrate self-control, self-improvement, and responsibility by making the correct choices to actively engage in health practices and avoid the risks of weight gain (Evans, Rich, Davies, & Allwood, 2008). In turn, "obesity" is read as a moral problem and thinness comes to represent the healthy neoliberal subject. In part, this is where a rationalist educational approach reveals its limitations. After reading some of the critical literature concerning "obesity," many students can articulate a rationale for critique but remain invested through their own embodiment. Many of them report a visceral response to fat bodies, reflecting what Elspeth Probyn (2004) describes as "the goose bump effect—that moment when a text sets off a frisson of feelings, remembrances, thoughts, and the bodily ac-tions that accompany them" (p. 29). Further work is needed to develop critical pedagogies that provide spaces for students to examine these visceral responses.

Towards Affective Pedagogies?

Another way in which we might engage a public pedagogy approach is to focus on affective responses to fat. One such way is to utilize contemporary visual spaces as pedagogies that pro-vide "visceral" experiences. As Sarah Brophy and Janice Hladki (2012) suggest, "contemporary visual culture generates unsettled forms of communication, empathy politics, thereby inviting ongoing contestation" (p. 76). As one example, in 2011, my research focused on the regulation and surveillance of young people's bodies in relation to fat (Evans et al., 2008; Rich, 2010) and was the subject of an exhibition, *Body Culture*, curated by artist Kerrie O'Connell. Artists cre-ated work seeking to unsettle, trouble, and challenge the normalcy of weightism and represent some of the more harmful effects this has on young people's subjectivity and health (Rich & O'Connell, 2012). The value of using art to prompt a visceral response is captured succinctly in the words of Probyn (2004), who argues that "affect amplification makes us care about things" (p. 26). For example, in Alexandra Unger's (2011) performance art at the exhibition, a provocative and affective response was created in a way that perhaps could not be achieved through words alone:

> I would like to do a performance, which has the provisional title "Fantasy to let go" in which I will allow myself to lose control and to be seen losing the control. I will interact with a block of gelatin, destroy its square shape, eat it but also soil myself and the floor around me. The sound of handled gelatin tends to be repulsive. I would like this eventually to turn into a sensual ex-perience where I am making peace with food and body, connecting the outside with the inside of it and make peace with this connection. (n.p.)

Alexandra's piece explored the regulation of the body and weight by bringing alive "the imbri-cation of bodies, intimacy, sensation, shame and ethical relations" (Brophy & Hladki, 2012, p. 77). In this way, as Jones and Hughes-Decatur (2012) suggest, "bodies are pedagogy" (p. 58). Such public pedagogies "privilege the intersection of the subject and object of pedagogy—the relational meanings that are generated via active, sensate, embodied interactions" (Burdick & Sandlin, 2013, p. 147). The performance produced powerful generative intensities in the for-mation of people's relations with loss of control, use of fluids, and food products to capture the complexities of control associated with weight and body culture. In this regard, visual forms such as those in the *Body Culture* exhibition can provide spaces where representation becomes a pedagogical site focused on relationally.

Fat Activism and Pedagogies of Reimagining

Counterhegemonic public pedagogies can also be clearly registered through the critical contri-butions of fat activism. Charlotte Cooper (2011) suggests that the earliest documented exam-ples of fat activism occurred between 1967 and 1989 and she considers Fat Power, the National Association to Advance Fat Acceptance (NAAFA), and the Fat Underground to be founding bodies for fat activism. The work of fat activists often uses transgressive and playful pedagogies to mobilize political and social discourses that are then re-imagined. The pedagogies attempt to disrupt knowledge about particular kinds of bodies that underpin forms of stigma and adopt pedagogical processes that attempt to subvert dominant discourses. As Burawoy (2005) suggests, "publics can be destroyed but they can also be created" (p. 7). Communities can be built from the ground up and be mobilized to make visible new publics. An example is the fat activist group the Chubsters (Cooper, 2014a).[2] Emerging communities and groups such as the Chubsters occupy "liminal spaces within the public sphere that manifest a pedagogical imperative" (O'Malley & Nelson, 2013, p. 41) to reimagine the fat subject in different ways.

Others perform the fat body as way of debunking the myths or critiquing the biomedical models that frame the capacities of the fat body in limited ways. This might also involve occupying public spaces in subversive ways, as captured in Josée Johnston and Judith Taylor's (2008) research on the Toronto-based grassroots fat activist organization Pretty, Porky, and Pissed Off (PPPO) that also targets feminine beauty ideals: "Frustrated with ill-fitting clothing options for plus-size women, a group of artists and activists from women's studies and queer activist communities formed PPPO in 1996. Their first event was a street protest in a trendy shopping district in which members handed out candy and questioned passersby about their attitudes toward fat" (p. 942).

Digital Activism and Public Pedagogy

With a colleague, I wrote, "In advancing a public pedagogy approach to theorising digital health, it is necessary to recognise how technology is inextricable from the manner in which people learn about health. Furthermore, these apparatus dictate conditions of self-tracking, collection of data, and monitoring, which have a bearing on what and how people learn about their bodies and health" (Rich & Miah, 2014, p. 301). In that article, we attempted to articulate how public pedagogies are evident in an increasing range of digital systems being used to predict, diagnose, treat, and monitor health, not just by health professionals, but increasingly by users themselves for purposes such as monitoring their weight loss. In these new territories of health engagement, there is a growing market in mobile health apps that relate to physical activity and lifestyle. Such apps allow users to track their exercise behavior, body weight, and food consumption. While concerns about the regulative and surveillant nature of these digital tools have been raised (Lupton, 2014), digital environments have also provided opportunities for subversive cultures. Digital spaces and cultures provide possibilities for resistance and for the democratization of knowledge as explored in Richard Freishtat and Jennifer Sandlin's (2010) work on Facebook. What people can learn across social media and whether this counts as social activism is still being debated. However, it is clear that Web 2.0 is increasingly being harnessed to produce pedagogies that challenge weight-based oppression as a kind of digital activism; fat blogs, e-zines, and other social media now feature centrally in the pedagogic practices of fat activists and critical weight scholars.

These digital spaces are often used in the critical pedagogic practices of public pedagogues advocating Health At Every Size (Aphramor, 2005; Robison, 2005), a perspective that challenges the weight-centered approach to health. HAES "evolved from the frustrations of actual clinical practice, by a cohort of health-care workers, fitness professionals, nutritionists, coaches and therapists" (Burgard, 2009, p. 50). Many within the HAES community have taken to the microblogging platform of Twitter to connect with others adopting this perspective. They have built a community and reached wider audiences through the hashtag #HAES, surely an act of public pedagogy. Another example is Golda Poretsky's (2013) Tedx Talk, "Why It's Okay to Be Fat." At the time of writing, this talk had received more than 202,047 views on YouTube and is still being circulated via Twitter. Twitter accounts and usernames among this community vary from the more self-reflexive autobiographical to those who are "practicing" such as @ HAEScoach to those who are advocating a particular perspective in their pedagogical intent such as @neverdietagain. In 2014, Cooper mobilized these international social media networks in her work, *No More Stitch-Ups! Developing Media Literacy Through Fat Activist Community Research.*[3]

That being said, given the dominance of healthism in contemporary society, many practicing HAES face resistance and contempt from those advocating weight loss strategies. One need only explore some of the debate on Twitter around the hashtag #fatacceptance to see how members of this community are publicly derided, for example, "#fatacceptance movement sounds like #Igaveup." The blurring of public and private spaces may leave individuals vulnerable to vociferous attacks and of course could intensify the expression of fat hatred and stigma witnessed in other social contexts. But from a public pedagogy perspective, it can also provide a counterinstitutional space for learning about weight, fat, and health and a way to circumvent the dominant biomedical narratives that often dominate public debate about weight. Digital activism enables the critical pedagogical work of these individuals and organizations to be brought into more public spaces.

Resisting Fat Stigma in Popular Culture

A final approach drawing from public pedagogy is to use "popular culture as cultural resistance," which can be seen "as a site where domination is fought against and [as] framing popular culture as a critical and emancipatory pedagogy" (Sandlin et al., 2011, p. 347). Critical possibilities are emerging through a counter-discourse in popular culture. For example, in 2013 the four-part documentary series *The Men Who Made Us Thin* was screened on the UK's BBC Two television channel; it attempted to decode, debunk, and interrupt some of the science behind the weight loss industry. As well, back in 2004, Dove launched its campaign for "real beauty" in what could be seen as "corporate appropriation of social movement ideals" by "using feminist critiques and concerns about beauty ideals to revitalize the Dove brand. Billboard, television, and magazine ads depicted women who were wrinkled, freckled, pregnant, had stretch marks, or might be seen as fat (at least compared with the average media representation of women)" (Johnston & Taylor, 2008, p. 942).

Conclusion

There is certainly a strong rationale for challenging weight-based oppression as part of a formal critical health education, both in schools and in the training of health professionals. Public pedagogy expands the potential for teaching and learning beyond the formal classroom and into everyday and public sites. Each of the cases described in this chapter can be recognized as a pedagogical context and each shares some key interrelated aspects of a public pedagogy, which I outline next.

First, they highlight the relationship between a range of sites in the production of knowledge about fat and possible ways of engaging with that knowledge. Public pedagogies that employ relational and affective practices can advance alternative readings of fat across intersecting spaces. These various sites can provide opportunities for learning about fat for a range of different publics. The pedagogical strategies outlined earlier can be found in media, social media, activist communities, organizations, protests, artwork, and in the pedagogical practices of academics. These emerging spaces might represent what Elizabeth Ellsworth (2005) describes as anomalous places of learning that are "peculiar, irregular, abnormal, or difficult to classify [as] pedagogical phenomena" (p. 5).

Second, many of the examples of public pedagogy outlined see knowledge as a thing that is constituted relationally rather than as "knowledge already made" (Ellsworth, 2005, p. 5) to be transmitted to another. If we are to provide spaces for alternative learning that can challenge these tacit knowledge forms, this means moving beyond a solely rational approach to pedagogy to one that engages with public pedagogy through relationality, affectivity, and embodiment (see Burdick, Sandlin, & O'Malley, 2014).

Third, while I have explored the potential for developing public pedagogies through research and teaching, it is clear that public pedagogy does not necessarily require the work of a public intellectual or an institution-based pedagogue. As many chapters in this book testify, there are many ways of engaging "the public" pedagogically to both open up and reimagine public spaces that position multiple citizens as potential educators.

Finally, in each of the cases here there are some attempts to "create structures and practices that are yet unimagined" (Brady, 2006, p. 59). There are intersecting and overlapping sites of learning about fat, both already existing and those being imagined; some reiterate dominant messages while others work in tension with one another such that the constitution of fat is in a process of always becoming. It is in these relationalities that we might develop alternative ways of imagining fat. In this sense, we need continued debate about what public pedagogy is and how it might evolve. Burdick et al. (2014) have begun to take up this challenge in their work on "problematizing public pedagogy" and I believe their work is particularly useful for those looking to engage further with possibilities for public fat pedagogies.

References

Aphramor, L. (2005). Is a weight-centred health framework salutogenic? Some thoughts on unhinging certain dietary ideologies. *Social Theory & Health, 3*(4), 315–340.

Beck, S. (2011). Public anthropology as public pedagogy: An autobiographical account. *Policy Futures in Education, 9*(6), 715–734.

Boero, N. (2013). Obesity in the media: Social science weighs in. *Critical Public Health, 23*(3), 371–380.

Bombak, A. E. (2014). The contribution of applied social sciences to obesity stigma-related public health approaches. *Journal of Obesity, 2014*, 267–286.

Brady, J. F. (2006). Public pedagogy and educational leadership: Politically engaged scholarly communities and possibilities for critical engagement. *Journal of Curriculum & Pedagogy, 3*(1), 57–60.

Brophy, S., & Hladki, J. (2012). Introduction: Pedagogy, image practices, and contested corporealities. *Review of Education, Pedagogy, and Cultural Studies, 34*, 3–4.

Burawoy, M. (2005). For public sociology. *American Sociological Review, 70*, 4–28.

Burdick, J., & Sandlin, J. A. (2013). Learning, becoming, and the unknowable: Conceptualizations, mechanisms, and process in public pedagogy literature. *Curriculum Inquiry, 43*, 142–177.

Burdick, J., Sandlin, J., & O'Malley, M. P. (2014). *Problematizing public pedagogy*. New York, NY: Routledge.

Burgard, D. (2009). What is "Health At Every Size"? In E. Rothblum & S. Solovay (Eds.), *The fat studies reader* (pp. 42–53). New York, NY: New York University Press.

Cameron, E. (2015). Teaching resources for post-secondary educators who challenge dominant obesity discourse. *Fat Studies, 4*(2), 212–226.

Cameron, E., Oakley, J., Walton, G., Russell, C., Chambers, L., & Socha, T. (2014). Moving beyond the injustices of the schooled healthy body. In I. Bogotch & C. Shields (Eds.), *International handbook of educational leadership and social (in)justice* (pp. 687–704). New York, NY: Springer.

Cohn, S. (2014). From health behaviours to health practices: An introduction. *Sociology of Health & Illness, 36*(2), 157–162.

Cooper, C. (2011). Fat lib: How activism expands the obesity debate. In E. Rich, L. Monaghan, & L. Aphramor (Eds.), *Debating obesity: Critical perspectives* (pp. 164–191). Basingstoke, England: Palgrave.

Cooper, C. (2014a). *Chubsters.* Retrieved from http://charlottecooper.net/b/chubsters/

Cooper, C. (2014b). No more stitch-ups! Developing media literacy through fat activist community research. In A. Wardop & D. Withers (Eds.), *The para-academic handbook: A toolkit for making-learning-creating-acting* (pp. 206–231). Bristol, England: Hammer On Press.

Crawford, R. (1980). Healthism and the medicalisation of everyday life. *International Journal of Health Services, 10*(3), 365–388.

Ellsworth, E. (2005). *Places of learning: Media, architecture, and pedagogy.* New York, NY: Routledge.

Evans, J., Rich, E., Davies, B., & Allwood, R. (2008). *Education, disordered eating and obesity discourse: Fat fabrications.* London, England: Routledge.

Francombe, J. (2013). Methods that move: A physical performative pedagogy of subjectivity. *Sociology of Sport Journal, 30*(3), 256–273.

Freishtat, R. L., & Sandlin, J. A. (2010). Shaping youth discourse about technology: Technological colonization, manifest destiny, and the frontier myth in Facebook's public pedagogy. *Educational Studies, 46,* 503–523.

Giroux, H. A. (2003). Public pedagogy and the politics of resistance: Notes on a critical theory of educational struggle. *Educational Philosophy and Theory, 35,* 5–16.

Giroux, H. A. (2004). *The terror of neoliberalism: Authoritarianism and the eclipse of democracy.* Boulder, CO: Paradigm.

Guthman, J. (2009). Teaching the politics of obesity: Insights into neoliberal embodiment and contemporary biopolitics. *Antipode, 4*(5), 1110–1133.

Hopkins, P. (2011). Teaching and learning guide for: Critical geographies of body size. *Geography Compass, 5*(2), 106–111.

Johnston, J., & Taylor, J. (2008). Feminist consumerism and fat activists: A comparative study of grassroots activism and the Dove Real Beauty campaign. *Signs, 33*(4), 941–966.

Jones, S., & Hughes-Decatur, H. (2012). Speaking of bodies in justice-oriented feminist teacher education. *Journal of Teacher Education, 63,* 51–61.

Kellner, D. (1995). *Media culture: Cultural studies, identity and politics between the modern and the postmodern.* New York, NY: Routledge.

Luke, C. (1996). *Feminisms and pedagogies of everyday life.* Albany, NY: SUNY Press.

Lupton, D. (2014). *Digital sociology.* New York, NY: Routledge.

O'Malley, P., & Nelson, S. (2013). The public pedagogy of student activists in Chile: What have we learned from the Penguins' Revolution. *Journal of Curriculum Theorizing, 29,* 41–56.

Poretsky, G. (2013, May 19). Why it's okay to be fat. Retrieved from https://www.youtube.com/watch?v=73SXX0w4eY8

Probyn, E. (2004). Teaching bodies: Affects in the classroom. *Body & Society, 10*(4), 21–43.

Raisborough, J. (2014). Why we should be watching more trash TV: Exploring the value of an analysis of the makeover show to fat studies scholars. *Fat Studies, 2*(2), 155–165.

Rich, E. (2010). Obesity assemblages and surveillance in schools. *International Journal of Qualitative Studies in Education, 23*(7), 803–821.

Rich, E. (2011). "I see her being obesed!": Public pedagogy, reality media and the obesity crisis. *Health, 15*(1), 3–21.

Rich, E., & Miah, A. (2014). Understanding digital health as public pedagogy: A critical framework. *Societies, 4,* 296–315.

Rich, E., & O'Connell, K. (2012). Visual methods in physical culture: Body culture exhibition. In M. Atkinson & K. Young (Eds.), *Qualitative research on sport and physical culture* (pp. 101–128). Bingley, England: Emerald Press.

Robison, J. (2005). Health At Every Size: Toward a new paradigm of weight and health. *Medscape General Medicine, 7*(3), 13.

Sandlin, J. A., & Milam, J. L. (2008). Mixing pop (culture) and politics: Cultural resistance, culture jamming and anti-consumption activism as critical public pedagogy. *Curriculum Inquiry, 38,* 323–350.

Sandlin, J. A., O'Malley, M. P., & Burdick, J. (2011). Mapping the complexity of public pedagogy scholarship. 1894–2010. *Review of Educational Research, 81*(3), 338–375.

Sandlin, J., Schultz, B., & Burdick, J. (2010). *Handbook of public pedagogy: Education and learning beyond schooling.* New York, NY: Routledge.

Savage, G. (2010). Problematizing "public pedagogy" in educational research. In J. A. Sandlin, B. D. Schultz, & J. Burdick (Eds.), *Handbook of public pedagogy: Education and learning beyond schooling* (pp. 103–115). New York, NY: Routledge.

Sender, K., & Sullivan, M. (2008). Epidemics of will, failures of self-esteem: Responding to fat bodies in "The Biggest Loser" and "What Not to Wear." *Continuum: Journal of Media & Cultural Studies, 22*(4), 573–584.

Silk, M., Francombe-Webb, J., Rich, E., & Merchant, S. (in press). On the transgressive possibilities of physical pedagogic practices. *Qualitative Inquiry.*

Unger, A. (2011). *"Body Culture" art exhibit* (Proposal for the Social Body & Art Exhibition). Retrieved from http://body-culture-art.tumblr.com/

Watkins, P. L., Farrell, A., & Hugmeyer, A. (2012). Teaching fat studies: From conception to reception. *Fat Studies, 1*(2), 180–194.

Notes

1   Burdick, Sandlin, and O'Malley (2014) offer an instructive trajectory for public pedagogy based on an architecture of three key areas: "*framing*, exploring the problematics of public pedagogy's definition, the organization and historicity; *studying*, emphasizing the ways in which our research simultaneously illuminates and obfuscates the object of inquiry; and *enacting*, taking up the ways in which we view and engage with our own pedagogical acts outside of institutional spaces" (p. 3, emphasis in original). The focus on popular culture and everyday life as a context for learning was addressed in the feminist work of scholars such as Carmen Luke (1996) who explored "pedagogies of everyday life." The field has continued to develop, although not without contestation and debate given that it is located at the intersection of a range of disciplines, including but not limited to education, sociology, and cultural studies. While there are differences among scholars in terms of theoretical predilections, there is some general consensus within the field that it comprises a focus on the kind of learning that takes place *outside* of formal schooling.

2   Fat studies scholar and activist Cooper (2014a) describes the Chubsters: "I started The Chubsters as an international girl gang, a fat girl gang, a fat and queer girl gang, actually, but Chubsters don't have to be queer, female or even fat to be a part of it. The Chubsters are vicious and belligerent, they will do anything to tear down Narrow Fucks, Chubster-speak for narrow-minded fatphobes, or anyone else who gets in their way, and they are always itching for a dirty fight. Chubsters embrace idiocy and aggression, they love to cause mayhem. … The Chubsters takes that shame-free queer or punk approach to life and applies it to fat. It expands our fat habitus and enables us to think beyond the usual expectations, it suggests: life does not have to be like this, there are other possibilities" (n.p.).

3   On her website, Cooper (2014b) describes this work: "It's research by and about fat people, by and about fat activism, and is a product of our international networks. It recognises and builds on fat community expertise. It's about fat people and our agency, about how we might help change some of the world's most powerful institutions. It's a valuable community resource. It is an example of how scholars might produce research beyond the usual academic boundaries. It's free and available to anyone who wants to read it or make use of it. It is released under a Creative Commons licence and can be republished non-commercially" (n.p.).

Twenty Four

Navigating Morality, Politics, and Reason: Towards Scientifically Literate and Intellectually Ethical Fat Pedagogies

Michael Gard

Having spent a great deal of my academic work arguing about fatness and obesity[1] research, it was probably inevitable that one of my faults as a teacher would be a tendency towards didacticism. I often begin by telling students that my intention is to stimulate their thinking and not, necessarily, to change their minds. Hand on heart, this is an ideal I am determined to uphold, and yet, as with most things, the reality is more complicated. For one thing, the systems designed to evaluate university teaching tell us—or at least me—that students *do* want to be entertained. They seem to appreciate people who are lively and "passionate" about their subject matter, a point that is tempting to interpret as meaning that our job is to advocate *for* something through our teaching. And if at least some students prefer certainty over gray circumspection, then maybe certainty is what I need to give them. But is this actually my job?

On the other hand, *not* pushing one's agendas through one's teaching is, in my experience, a hard thing to do. The material I select to teach is not only shaped by my opinions but also is the subject matter with which I feel myself to be most comfortable. In fact, these two things—my opinions and my expertise—could, in reality, be one and the same thing. And then there is the tendency of students to make statements and ask questions. How should my responses and strategies differ according to whether or not the thinking of the student appears to accord with my own? I want to help broaden their knowledge but how much the devil's advocate am I prepared to be when I approve of their views?

My sense is that some academics approach this problem by saying "what problem?" I have regularly been advised that my concern with a distinction between teaching and advocacy is not only old fashioned but also a false dichotomy; if all positions are political, the argument goes, then we might as well prosecute a politics that we believe in. To my mind, this is an over-simplification. In particular, I am inclined to take seriously the proposition that as the teacher I am still and always a learner. What right do I have visiting my own intellectual commitments on students if my own journey is unfinished?

Taking this point a little further, a recent study published in the *Proceedings of the National Academy of Sciences* (Fiske & Dupree, 2014) considered the degree to which a variety of different professions, including researchers, scientists, and university professors, are trusted and liked by the public. The study's general finding that people are more likely to distrust professors and scientists if they are perceived to be pushing a premeditated agenda strikes me as important. In other words, there is a fine but important distinction between informing and persuading. The authors write: "Rather than persuading, we and our audiences are better served by discussing, teaching, and sharing information, to convey trustworthy intentions" (Fiske & Dupree, 2014, p. 13596). In short, if our goal is to teach then we need to avoid preaching.

My goal in this chapter is to explore the moral, political, and intellectual complexities we face when teaching about fatness. To some extent, my suggestions cut against the position taken by other fat studies scholars including, perhaps, some of the authors in this volume. For this reason, I propose to briefly unpack my thinking before moving on to some more concrete suggestions for fat pedagogy.

Advocacy and the Birth of Fat Studies

Partly because of its historical connections with fat activism, the scholarly field of fat studies is in many respects a form of advocacy. Its birth shortly after the turn of the current century was a direct and appropriate response to biomedical and popular rhetoric about an "obesity epidemic." As I have argued elsewhere (Gard, 2011; Gard & Wright, 2005), the clear intention of many academic and media commentators in the early years of the "obesity epidemic" was to attract attention, cause alarm, and provoke action. In this context it was inevitable that, even with the best of intentions, much of what was written and said would be hyperbolic, lazy, inaccurate, and counterproductive. The situation demanded a response and fat studies was part of this response.

As they began to find their voice, dissenters largely fell back on familiar ideas about social and cultural difference and the ideological dimensions of science. After all, the case *for* a looming obesity crisis was usually prosecuted via contestable statistics and scientific techniques—such as the Body Mass Index—and unsupported throw-away predictions—such as the claim that rising obesity levels would lead to declines in life expectancy. In short, the idea of an "obesity epidemic" reeked of naïve scientism and fit neatly into existing feminist, post-structuralist, and broadly social constructionist critiques of science.

From this starting point, dominant obesity discourses could then be criticized for the way they "positioned" or "individualized" or "stigmatized" certain kinds of people, particularly women, ethnic minorities, and the poor. It was then easy to construct biomedical obesity discourses as either explicitly or implicitly evil, mean-spirited, or misguided. This established an understandably reactive but ultimately limiting dynamic in which the "obesity epidemic" was seen as a phenomenon that was being *done* to particular groups of people by other groups of people.

And yet there were at least two important weaknesses to these essentially morally driven critiques. First, they struggled to articulate a credible understanding of the health implications of body weight. Second, they tended to ignore questions of human agency, responsibility, and culpability. This is not to insist that health risk and personal responsibility need always be foregrounded above all other concerns. Equally, though, if one's intention is to increase and potentially shift people's understanding of obesity as a social issue, it is probably preferable that we find ways of talking about health risk and personal responsibility rather than being completely silent about them (for a discussion about health risk within a feminist pedagogical context, see Boling, 2011).

To suggest that fat studies has been populated by people inclined to pursue specific moral and social agendas is to say nothing that is not true of any other scholarly enterprise. Scholars must begin their work from *somewhere*. Likewise, there will always be many more interesting and important things to study than any of us have the time to actually pursue. But having registered this point, I think there is value in stepping back and at least attempting to view one's subject matter with a more disinterested eye.

For example, in the years I have been studying them, I have seen rising obesity levels blamed on a very long list of culprits that incudes but is by no means exhausted by the following: cars, televisions, computers, fast food, fizzy drinks, shopping centers, urban planning, crime rates, working mothers, lax parenting, gay marriage, declining religious observance, snacking, disrupted sleep patterns, affluence, poverty, capitalism, liberalism, individualism, feminism, Western culture, non-Western cultures, psychology, the weight loss industry, schools, dietary fat, carbohydrates, protein, and genetics. But the same is true on the other side of the fence. Unconvinced that obesity is quite the public health crisis it is claimed to be, sceptics have attributed the intensification of anti-obesity rhetoric on an equally dizzying and, in some cases, overlapping cast of players and cultural forces: the medical "establishment," science, the enemies of science, dietetics, Western culture, the New Age movement, the weight loss industry, the fashion industry, the fast food industry, the enemies of the fast food industry, misogyny, racism, elitism, capitalism, socialism, liberalism, neoliberalism, individualism, conservatism, neo-conservatism, psychology, and a pervasive hatred of fat people. The question I would pose to readers is this: if our task is to teach students about fatness, what should our attitude to this cacophony of voices be? Do we just add our own voice and advocate via our own political commitments?

I realize that the terms "sceptics" and "fat studies" are not interchangeable. It would be foolish also not to acknowledge that the many different contexts in which we might find ourselves teaching about fatness call for different pedagogies. But again, drawing on my own experience, I have seen many impassioned conference presentations and undergraduate lectures given by well-meaning fat studies scholars (including me) fall flat or provoke unnecessary hostility. Invariably the problem has been a failure to deliver a calibrated message, to treat one's audience with respect, and to take seriously the fact that one's own knowledge is partial. I have squirmed uneasily while listening to speakers claim that the obesity epidemic is a "myth," or that there is "no evidence" that a higher body weight is bad for one's health, or that public health campaigns against fatness are "oppressive to women" or a form of social prejudice like racism. It is one thing to pursue the legitimate task of teasing out the different discursive threads that make up a social phenomenon like the "obesity epidemic." It is quite another to communicate with—or teach—people who may take for granted dominant biomedical narratives about fatness and who will certainly hear what we say through *their own* political, ideological, and theoretical commitments. To return to the words quoted earlier, "Rather than persuading, we and our audiences are better served by discussing, teaching, and sharing information" (Fiske & Dupree, 2014, p. 13596).

Let me make this point slightly more concrete with a brief example. I have very much enjoyed Julie Guthman's thoughtful writing on fat pedagogy, and yet I invite readers to consider her 2009 paper in which she argues that it was her students' investment in neoliberal biopolitics that explained their, at times, extreme hostility to non-mainstream ideas about fatness. While the undergraduate course she describes began by problematizing scientific concepts like the Body Mass Index, the overwhelming focus, as Guthman herself says, was deconstructive. Students received presentations from a fat activist and were asked to see the "obesity epidemic" as a historical and social instantiation of power relations and political economy. These are perfectly reasonable strategies, but Guthman's quite strident criticism of her students seems unfair to me, primarily because she asked them to move so far so quickly without an opportunity to work through the scientific claims that constitute the *very discursive substance* of the "obesity epidemic" itself. While Guthman argues that they were hopelessly blinded by society's anti-fat biases, her students' comments show that some felt "preached at" and on the receiving end of someone else's personal and political agendas. Guthman seems unable to hear this criticism, preferring instead to blame her students and their corporeal privilege. Why are some critical pedagogues so fast to demonize their students and why are they so determined to change their students' attitudes? Why do they see this as their task? My argument is not that a more slavishly scientific approach to fat pedagogy will rid the world of fat oppression. My argument is that the credible, skillful, and strategic use of obesity science by critical pedagogues is an important ingredient in helping students to question their assumptions as well as leaving them feeling better informed and less manipulated.

So far I have said a lot about what one should *not* do when teaching about fatness. On a more positive note, the approach I advocate *for* is one which attempts to move backwards and forwards between the work of scholars from across the academic and non-academic spectrum; to make unexpected and, I think, subversive links between knowledge claims, statistics, and ideas that are not normally linked. No doubt some readers will sniff hypocrisy and point out that there is nothing particularly "neutral" or "objective" about this kind of fat pedagogy. True enough, although my response is that neutrality or objectivity is not my goal. Rather, my commitment is to the labyrinthine complexities of knowledge production per se. And while leaving students in a state of confusion is not something I would ever endorse, I also think that respecting one's audience/students/listeners includes resisting neat conclusions or premature clarity. The fact that the study of body weight produces so many bizarre, counterintuitive, and contradictory knowledge claims is not, ultimately, a sign that the people making these claims are especially flawed. They aren't. The reason is that secure knowledge about most things is elusive, and if there is a truth that teachers owe their allegiance to, it is this.

Life, Death, and Fat Pedagogy

Like their teachers, one of the most obvious challenges that students face is moving beyond the intense security of righteous conviction. As a physical education teacher educator, I have worked with many students for whom the war on obesity is central to their personal and professional identities (see Sykes & McPhail, 2008, for a discussion of fat bodies within physical education). Whatever else they might be prepared to compromise on, their thinking returns as if magnetically drawn to the same place: "But we've got to do something about obesity!" It is difficult to blame them; the claim that rising obesity rates will lead to a significant decline in life expectancy is repeated in the scholarly literature and popular media so often that few will not have been exposed to it.

I do not pretend that there is a fail-safe next move in the pedagogical dialogue I might now want to have with students. One playfully sadistic choice, however, is to ask students to locate the evidence. This is a sadistic choice because there is very little to be found. Students will easily locate thousands of instances where the claim is repeated but very few in which it is substantiated. For some students, this can be a stimulating or troubling finding. At the very least, many will quickly see that assertions about obesity and life expectancy have rebounded around the world as if contained within a giant echo chamber where the original source is impossible to locate.

Some students, however, will find Jay Olshansky and colleagues' 2005 *New England Journal of Medicine* paper, "A Potential Decline in Life Expectancy in the United States in the 21st Century." Whether found by students or teacher, the paper is worthy of close analysis because it is by far the most regularly cited study—more than 2,000 Google citations last time I checked—with any relevance to the life expectancy implications of obesity.

What this highly cited paper does and does not say will startle many students. To begin with, it deals only with U.S. data and so its relevance to other countries where obesity levels are lower—which is most of the world—is questionable. It is also worth considering what a complex task calculating the mortality implications of overweight and obesity is. People die for many reasons and it is rarely clear what role body weight has played. Just because a clinically obese man suffers a fatal heart attack does not necessarily mean his body weight caused his heart attack. Faced with this problem, Olshansky and colleagues (2005) simply assumed that if a person with a Body Mass Index above 30 dies, then their body weight *must* have been the cause. Ergo, whether they were eaten by a shark or had lung cancer, they would not have died if they weren't obese. In my experience, although a somewhat technical point, a discernable quiet sometimes descends on the room when students begin to digest the implications of this obviously flawed assumption.

But even with this assumption built into their calculations, Olshansky and colleagues (2005) found that, based on year 2000 statistics, obesity's effect on life expectancy in the United States was likely to be only a fraction of a year. This too will surprise some students because they will know that this paper is regularly used to support the prediction that obesity's effect on life expectancy will be measured in years, not months. Olshansky and colleagues conclude their paper by speculating about the future impact on life expectancy if obesity rates continue to rise, and it is here—and only here—that the prospect of more significant declines in life expectancy is raised.

This example is a reminder of people's tendency to interpret research findings in ways that confirm their existing biases. Olshansky and colleagues' (2005) paper does *not* demonstrate that obesity will lead to a significant decline in life expectancy and yet it is continually referenced to support this claim. The paper is also an example to students of the effect of sloppy referencing practices. In my own work I have shown how this claim has popped up all over the world in academic papers, government reports, on TV talk shows, and in newspapers.

At this point I like to ask students why the obesity/life expectancy claim has proved so promiscuously mobile. I think this is an important step in the pedagogical process that should not be rushed. Returning to my comments earlier, I have seen some teachers jump in and prematurely impose conclusions on students. For example, they will say that people are inclined to believe the claim because they are dazzled by science and statistics or because the claims confirm pre-existing biases against fat people. In my experience, given time to think students will generate a number of other possibilities, including the time pressures journalists work under, thus discouraging them from checking their facts, or the preference of politicians for simple sound-bite health messages. Some will talk about the tendency in Western societies for bad news to be big news, so the more startling the claim the more likely it is to be reported. A few might also reflect on the impossibility of checking the veracity of every single scientific claim that one is exposed to. Sometimes researchers preparing academic papers for publication or students writing last-minute essays make the all-too-human decision to rely on secondhand sources.

In short, given time to do so students will explain the spread of "obesity epidemic" rhetoric in ways that do not fall back on the moral failings, ideological agendas, or malicious intent of particular groups of people. The result, in my opinion, can be a sociologically richer picture of the world that students can, if they wish, use to take their thinking further.

Before leaving the matter of life expectancy, some students will be suspicious if discussions do not progress beyond a narrow focus on a single paper, such as the one by Olshansky and colleagues (2005). Teachers whose intention it is to wade critically into the science of fatness must do so with a credibly broad feel for the literature. When I make this point to colleagues, it is sometimes misinterpreted as meaning that teachers must have an encyclopaedic knowledge of the scientific literature. Far from it. My contention is that, for better or worse, many students will want to be reassured that their teacher speaks from a solid scientific foundation *before* they will entertain the more subversive ideas a teacher might put forward. Rather than science being all one needs, my point is merely that one's pedagogical job is harder without scientific foundations. To this end, I invite students to consult other studies that have considered the life expectancy impact of obesity. Although not numerous, the clear majority of these (such as Reynolds, Saito, & Crimmins, 2005; Stewart, Cutler, & Rosen, 2009) offer very little support for the more apocalyptic predictions about life expectancy that continue to circulate.

In a similar vein, we might ask students to consider the mainstream—as opposed to obesity focused—life expectancy literature where, perhaps not surprisingly, life expectancy in Western countries is generally expected to continue to increase (Christensen, Doblhammer, Rau, & Vaupel, 2009; Oeppen & Vaupel, 2002). This is a point of view totally at odds with much of what we read in the obesity literature. I am still surprised by how many students, colleagues, and friends are aware of utterly contradictory sets of predictions about life expectancy without stopping to consider the reasons for, or implications of, these differences. Once again, this strikes me as an important pedagogical opportunity; will increasing obesity cause a decline in human longevity or not? What reasons would different researchers, particularly those who specialize in the study of obesity, have for favoring different points of view? Are these differences a sign of healthy scientific debate or something else? Bias? Scientific error?

Perhaps these are unfair questions. I am certainly not confident I could definitively answer any of them but, as I have tried to stress, what matters here are the complexities of knowledge construction; how *exactly* have each of us come to believe certain things? In fact, even if they are posed only rhetorically, these questions still offer students intellectual room to pause and reflect on their own preconceptions in the light of competing knowledge claims.

Returning to my hypothetical students burning with the crusader's fervor to do something about obesity, it is noticeable how often they raise concerns about the "health budget" to frame the problem. This has always struck me as a strange connection to make, not least because of how little most people seem to be concerned about the more well-documented drivers of health care costs such as advancing technology. Nonetheless, having considered life expectancy, the obvious next question is whether predictions of falling life expectancy are consistent with a concern about increasing health expenditure. The answer to this question is probably no. Most researchers who have addressed the issue argue that it is *increasing* life expectancy, not the reverse, that leads to greater health costs (Lubitz, Cai, Kramarow, & Lentzner, 2003; Schneider & Guralnik, 1990). More troubling for our student crusaders, however, is the consistent research finding that winning the war on obesity will have little net effect on health budgets. As Pieter Van Baal et al. (2008) concluded:

> Although effective obesity prevention leads to a decrease in costs of obesity-related diseases, this decrease is offset by cost increases due to diseases unrelated to obesity in life-years gained. Obesity prevention may be an important and cost-effective way of improving public health, but it is not a cure for increasing health expenditures. (p. e29)

There are, of course, risks in teaching in this "myth busting" fashion. It is important for students not to feel they are being toyed with or that their teacher is being selectively mischievous. Tone is everything and, echoing Susan Fiske and Cydney Dupree (2014), if scientific findings are used in a way that appears designed to prove the teacher's superiority or the students' ignorance then they are less likely to engage with the message. My overriding point, though, is that rather than being the enemy of a critical fat pedagogy, as it is often portrayed, the mainstream obesity literature can be our ally.

Nothing Works?

Throughout this chapter I have emphasized the pedagogical need—for both teachers and students—to put certainty to one side and to grapple with the perverse uncertainties that the study of body weight produces. It should be obvious from this that I am placing a higher value on the educational journey—grappling with claim and counter-claim—rather than the destination—offering conclusions. Nonetheless, at some point students eventually ask for my point of view on the issues we have been discussing and my normal practice is to give it. However, I attempt to frame my "answers" by transparently weighing the available evidence. This is not easy because there is *always* contradictory evidence that one can potentially call upon. I conclude this chapter, then, by unpacking this point a little.

I have said that my students in physical education, exercise science, and the sociology of human movement tend towards a default position that values scientific knowledge above other knowledge traditions. However, it does not follow from this that they hold narrowly biomedical, individualistic, or judgmental opinions about fatness. Some do, but others are inclined to blame obesity on a lack of education, or economic disadvantage, or the aggressive marketing of fast food and soft drink companies, or the urban environments in which many people are forced to live. Indeed, the fat studies literature is full of scholars who appear to share these views.

There is a problem, however; finding compelling empirical evidence to refute each of these beliefs is disconcertingly easy. For example, Michael Daly, Christopher Boyce, and Alex Wood (2015) have recently found that a person's *relative* wealth may be more important to a person's health, including weight status, than the absolute level of wealth or poverty. Others have found that the association between weight status and socioeconomic status varies a great deal according to gender and ethnicity (Fradkin et al., 2015), and disappears altogether in some geographic areas (Lebel, Kestens, Clary, Bisset, & Subramanian, 2014). Likewise, a long list of studies have tried to prove the causal link between "junk food" and childhood obesity but produced data that show very little effect (for example, O'Neil, Nicklas, Liu, & Berenson, 2013).

I am not suggesting that these studies are the last word on any of the issues they purport to address. In fact, I am sure they are not. As a number of obesity researchers have pointed out, the tens of thousands of published research papers devoted to understanding the causes and cures of obesity have produced staggeringly few reliable and useful "truths." A recent paper by James Hebert and colleagues (2013) exploring this point is, I think, essential reading for fat studies teachers and students. It discusses how the biases, assumptions, and prejudices of obesity researchers have dogged obesity science, thus echoing the arguments that many of us in the fat studies social sciences have been making for some time. As such, this paper looks to me like a perfect jumping off point from which to introduce students to ideas about fatness that do not begin with positivistic biomedical assumptions.

The difficulties that obesity science has had producing generalizable knowledge also partly explains why so many obesity-focused public health interventions fail to work. But rather than using this point as a stick with which to beat obesity scientists, I take this as a sign that strident knowledge claims about body weight are a luxury few of us, including fat studies scholars, can afford, especially in our teaching. In my own teaching, I take as my starting point that one's role is to offer resources for understanding rather than recruiting students to particular points of view. Of course, pushing this line of thinking too hard courts the sin of naïve objectivism and, as I have tried to show, this is not my project. Rather, my concern is that educators make the limits of their political and moral motivations more transparent to themselves so that we might teach more credibly and, perhaps paradoxically, more rather than less subversively.

References

Boling, P. (2011). On learning to teach fat feminism. *Feminist Teacher, 21*(2), 110–123.
Christensen, K., Doblhammer, G., Rau, R., & Vaupel, J. W. (2009). Ageing populations: The challenges ahead. *The Lancet, 374*(9696), 1196–1208.
Daly, M., Boyce, C., & Wood, A. (2015). A social rank explanation of how money influences health. *Health Psychology, 34*(3), 222–230.
Fiske, S. T., & Dupree, C. (2014). Gaining trust as well as respect in communicating to motivated audiences about science topics. *Proceedings of the National Academy of Sciences, 111*(Suppl. 4), 13593–13597.
Fradkin, C., Wallander, J. L., Elliott, M. N., Tortolero, S., Cuccaro, P., & Schuster, M. A. (2015). Associations between socioeconomic status and obesity in diverse, young adolescents: Variation across race/ethnicity and gender. *Health Psychology, 34*(1), 1–9.
Gard, M. (2011). *The end of the obesity epidemic.* London, England: Routledge.
Gard, M., & Wright, J. (2005). *The obesity epidemic: Science, morality and ideology.* London, England: Routledge.
Guthman, J. (2009). Teaching the politics of obesity: Insights into neoliberal embodiment and contemporary biopolitics. *Antipode, 4*(5), 1110–1133.
Hebert, J. R., Allison, D. B., Archer, E., Lavie, C. J., & Blair, S. N. (2013). Scientific decision making, policy decisions, and the obesity pandemic. *Mayo Clinic Proceedings, 88*(6), 593–604.
Lebel, A., Kestens, Y., Clary, C., Bisset, S., & Subramanian, S. V. (2014). Geographic variability in the association between socioeconomic status and BMI in the USA and Canada. *PloS One, 9*(6), e99158.
Lubitz, J., Cai, L., Kramarow, E., & Lentzner, H. (2003). Health, life expectancy, and health care spending among the elderly. *New England Journal of Medicine, 349*(11), 1048–1055.

Oeppen, J., & Vaupel, J. W. (2002). Broken limits to life expectancy. *Science, 296*(5570), 1029–1031.

Olshansky, S. J., Passaro, D. J., Hershow, R. C., Layden, J., Carnes, B. A., Brody, J., … Ludwig, D. S. (2005). A potential decline in life expectancy in the United States in the 21st century. *New England Journal of Medicine, 352*(11), 1138–1145.

O'Neil, C. E., Nicklas, T. A., Liu, Y., & Berenson, G. S. (2013). Candy consumption in childhood is not predictive of weight, adiposity measures or cardiovascular risk factors in young adults: The Bogalusa Heart Study. *Journal of Human Nutrition and Dietetics, 28*(Suppl. 2), 59–69.

Reynolds, S. L., Saito, Y., & Crimmins, E. M. (2005). The impact of obesity on active life expectancy in older American men and women. *The Gerontologist, 45*(4), 438–444.

Schneider, E. L., & Guralnik, J. M. (1990). The aging of America: Impact on health care costs. *Journal of the American Medical Association, 263*(17), 2335–2340.

Stewart, S. T., Cutler, D. M., & Rosen, A. B. (2009). Forecasting the effects of obesity and smoking on US life expectancy. *New England Journal of Medicine, 361*(23), 2252–2260.

Sykes, H., & McPhail, D. (2008). Unbearable lessons: Contesting fat phobia in physical education. *Sociology of Sport, 25*(1), 66–96.

Van Baal, P. H., Polder, J. J., de Wit, G. A., Hoogenveen, R. T., Feenstra, T. L., Boshuizen, H. C., … Brouwer, W. B. (2008). Lifetime medical costs of obesity: Prevention no cure for increasing health expenditure. *PLoS Medicine, 5*(2), e29.

Notes

1   It has become something of a convention among some fat studies scholars to place the word obesity in quotation marks. I have deliberately chosen not to do this. In part, this is because of my concern in this chapter with the development of intellectual independence, both for my students and myself. To my mind, creating or following rules about how certain words should be used or written is surely antithetical to the job of the critical scholar or teacher. I would prefer to be bound neither by the orthodoxies of obesity science nor of fat studies scholars. *Of course* "obesity" is an unstable and contested term, and my acceptance of this point will become obvious to the reader soon enough. In general, I favor an approach in which the writer at least attempts to be clear about his or her usage of words such as "obesity" each time it is used. For example, when I talk about "obesity levels," I am referring to statistics about the prevalence of people technically classified as obese. When I talk generally about "obesity discourse" or obesity as a social issue, I am roughly equating obesity with a word like "fatness." That is, while it *can* mean many things, when I and my students talk about obesity we know that—if nothing else—we are referencing a broader public conversation about the amount of body fat people have.

Conclusion: A Fat Pedagogy Manifesto

Constance Russell and Erin Cameron

So here we are at the end of *The Fat Pedagogy Reader* and the two of us find ourselves feeling in the mood for a manifesto. We have been inspired by our fellow authors who have shared heartfelt stories of oppression, privilege, resistance, and action, fascinating descriptions of empirical research, confessional tales of pedagogical (mis)adventures, and diverse accounts of educational interventions that show promise. Taken together, they illuminate possibilities and pitfalls for fat pedagogy. While we are pleased with the contributions, by no means do we think this book is anywhere near being the final word on fat pedagogy. Far from it! Considering "fat pedagogy" entered the lexicon only a few years ago, we imagine that this book is but a glimmer of what is to come in addressing weight-based oppression in and through education.

When we first pitched the book, we envisioned it containing insights gleaned from a wide variety of educational sites, including elementary and secondary schools, colleges and universities, governmental and non-governmental organizations, and informal and social learning contexts. Yet it has unfolded as a decidedly academic book given who responded to the call. The vast majority of chapter authors are employed in postsecondary institutions, and many of these share descriptions of their own teaching experiences. Given we both are university professors and our own chapters are reflections on our own teaching practices, obviously we value such work. Still, we firmly believe that fat pedagogy must extend beyond the academy. In fact, it already does; as a number of chapter authors make clear, there are numerous examples of public pedagogies out there including art, blogs, demonstrations, films, and multimedia projects that reach wider audiences than do most books. We need to hear more about such work.

There are other obvious gaps in the book. The chapter authors hail from Australia, Canada, New Zealand, the United Kingdom, and the United States and all the chapters are written in English. There are far more female contributors to the book, which likely reflects the feminist roots of much fat scholarship and activism. While the contributors come in various shapes and sizes and seem somewhat diverse in terms of class origins and sexuality, as a group we appear fairly homogenous when it comes to race and ability. The two of us consider attending to the implications of the backgrounds of authors in this book to be important, including the ways in which our identities intersect in various contexts. We all must acknowledge, and work with, the complexity of the social contexts within which weight-based oppression and this emerging field of fat pedagogy occur, whether we are scholars, teachers, activists, or all of the above. Further, we imagine that contributions from an even more diverse group of scholars and activists would have enriched the book. It is our hope, then, that as the field of fat pedagogy grows, other voices and perspectives will flourish and be heard since this can only improve our praxis.

Another trend that became increasingly obvious to the two of us as we engaged in the process of lumping and splitting chapters into sections is which disciplines or interdisciplines were represented, and which were not. We have many chapters devoted to school-based education and numerous other chapters from authors working in various fields within education including adult education, critical pedagogy, environmental education, feminist pedagogy, health and physical education, higher education, humane education, public pedagogy, queer pedagogy, social justice education, and teacher education; given the book's focus on pedagogy, this does not come as a surprise. We also have chapters by authors working in American studies, animal care, counseling, health sciences, human movement, kinesiology, medicine, nursing, nutrition, public and community health, psychology, recreation, sociology, visual arts, and women's and gender studies. As one would expect, critical obesity studies, critical weight studies, and fat studies have inspired many of the authors and so too have other interdisciplinary fields such as critical animal studies, critical race studies, critical disability studies, cultural studies, environmental studies, feminist theory, freak studies, intersectionality studies, media studies, and queer studies. As well, authors are working in various research traditions and with diverse methodologies and methods. Still, it is clear that many disciplines are *not* well represented in the book including some that have obvious connections such as anthropology, biology, communications, economics, geography, history, law, languages, literature, political science, philosophy, and social work.

The previous caveats aside, we do believe that this book offers significant insights into the ways in which education might help address weight-based oppression. Authors use a variety of rhetorical styles, from memoir and confessional to description of practice and research report. Through these multifaceted approaches they build on a range of theoretical tools and research evidence. Such variety is important, we believe, since it is clear that there is no single right way of doing fat pedagogy. That means, however, that there are a number of tensions in the book. This is not unexpected given the authors' different backgrounds, contexts, disciplines, and theoretical commitments. It also reflects genuine debates in the field that will undoubtedly continue. These debates include the role of weight science, how or even whether to make pedagogical use of teachers' and learners' embodiment, and the role of advocacy in education (which is a tension present in all forms of education closely tied to social movements such as anti-racist education, environmental education, feminist pedagogy, humane education, Indigenous and decolonizing education, and queer pedagogy).

What all authors do agree on is that weight-based oppression is a serious problem and that education is an important form of intervention. As such, fat pedagogy is inherently radical; the status quo is not working and will not do. In this we echo Marilyn Wann (2009), who called the very existence of the field of fat studies an "invitation to revolution" (p. ix). Many revolutions, both big and small, often are kicked off with manifestos. It is telling, for example, that *The Fat Studies Reader* reproduced the 1973 "Fat Liberation Manifesto" at the end of the book (Freespirit & Aldebaran, 2009), making very clear the activist roots of the field. As Breanne Fahs illustrates well in her chapter in this book, there is much pedagogical potential in not only critically examining but also creating and sharing manifestos and other radical writing. Fahs has found fat-themed work such as Amy Farrell's (2011) chapter on the history of fat activism, "Refusing to Apologize," and Susan Vaught's (2008) teen fiction book, *Big Fat Manifesto*, helpful in her own teaching about manifestos and radical writing. Another piece of writing of this ilk that is regularly mentioned by those working in fat pedagogy is the "Basic Tenets of Size Acceptance" (see Cameron, 2015, p. 226).

The field of education is rife with manifestos. We did a Google search for "education manifesto" and more than 37,000,000 results popped up! There were manifestos by political parties setting out their educational platform, manifestos by faith groups, think tanks, and non-governmental organizations, manifestos written by and for art educators, educational technologists, geography educators, global educators, outdoor educators, science educators, librarians, and the list goes on. Some were rather apolitical policy statements, others were personal statements that the authors clearly hoped had broader implications, some attempted to establish a set of foundational principles for a field, and others were clearly grounded in radical politics with strong social change agendas.

One manifesto that did not make it to the top of that particular search but nonetheless stands out in Connie's memory was one that she read as she neared the end of her graduate studies and found so helpful that she used it in her social justice education courses for years afterwards: the chapter by Suzanne deCastell and Mary Bryson (1998) in the book *Queer Theory in Education*. They concluded their chapter with a section titled "Notes Towards a Queer Researcher's Manifesto" (p. 206) that consisted of seven points they used to guide their own practice as educational researchers. It included statements such as: "I will not sacrifice the chance to learn about how homophobia works in schools simply to be permitted to work in them" and "I will not engage in any educational intervention designed to promote heteronormativity in schools; on the contrary, any interventions in which I participate will be designed expressly to encourage and nurture difference" (p. 206). They ended their chapter with the following questions for readers: "Can you sign on? What will it mean for the future of your research if you do? What does it mean for the condition of your research if you do not?" (p. 206). Clearly, deCastell and Bryson's manifesto was written not just for those already working in queer pedagogy, but for all educational researchers. In much the same way, we hope that *The Fat Pedagogy Reader* reaches a wide audience, including educators who have not yet noticed that weight-based oppression exists. Perhaps having the word "manifesto" in the title of this concluding chapter will draw in a few readers who would not otherwise have the book on their radar. We can hope.

The two of us suspect that manifestos are best constructed in community through a participatory, democratic process. Ideally, then, we would have physically brought together the entire group of authors who contributed to *The Fat Pedagogy Reader* as well as the many other folks we know who are working in the area but for whom writing a chapter for the book at this moment was not possible. We imagine we may have had to stay up late as we engaged in playful and serious discussions and debates, and some of us likely would have found ourselves laughing, swearing, or crying, but in the end we may have emerged with one big, fat, messy manifesto. Alas, such a meeting remains in the realm of fantasy. So, the next best option for the two of us was to review all the chapters in search of emerging themes and key insights. Given this and our earlier discussion on the obvious gaps in the book, we recognize that what we offer is a highly situated and necessarily partial manifesto. Nonetheless, we wanted to give it a whirl, so here we humbly provide a list of some of the elements we consider important to fat pedagogy in the hope that we spark further reflection, discussion, and action.

- We are marinated in a culture rife with weight-based oppression. Fat or thin or somewhere in between, all of us are impacted by it in one way or another. Some of us feel the effects more keenly, however, and intersectional analyses can help clarify how various oppressions interact in complex ways. Fat pedagogy can and ought to help make weight bias, fat phobia, and fat hatred, in all their complexity, more visible. And fat pedagogy must, in the end, make a positive difference to fat people's lives.

- Fat pedagogy needs to be grounded in research and scholarship on weight-based oppression. Since different disciplines offer useful insights that become even more powerful when brought together, fat pedagogy is, and must be, an interdisciplinary, multidisciplinary, and transdisciplinary endeavor. Therefore engaging each other generously, attempting to communicate across our different discourse communities, and collaborating with one another can only serve to benefit this emerging field.

- Fat pedagogy scholars and practitioners need to seek one another out. This is a two-way street; scholars sharing findings in accessible ways and practitioners keeping abreast of research and scholarship in the field are both key. (Of course, many of the contributors to this book and many readers themselves are both scholars and practitioners, so we do not wish to imply that these two groups are necessarily as far apart as this statement implies.)

- Fat pedagogy needs to build on the lived experiences of those who have experienced weight-based oppression *and* of those who have grappled seriously with their thin privilege. As a fat person, Connie likes the phrase popularized by the disability rights movement: "nothing about us without us." It applies to the research we conduct, the teaching materials and resources we share, and who we invite to lead or participate in our pedagogical activities. As someone with thin privilege, Erin understands that thin people have much to learn through critical self-reflection and can spend their privilege in productive ways as thin allies.

- There is no "one size fits all" approach to fat pedagogy; the efficacy of different approaches will vary by geographical, cultural, linguistic, and sociopolitical contexts. In higher education, disciplinary traditions will likely influence what approaches best reach particular groups of students. Elementary and secondary school teachers and others working with children and youths need to ponder what is age appropriate and also would be wise to determine where administrative, policy, and other supports are to be found, especially when moving into territory deemed controversial by those in power. The built and physical environment also requires attention given that it can influence how welcoming a learning site will feel to fat learners.

- Regardless of learning context, it is vital that we start where learners are and not work from a deficit position that assumes learners, particularly those expressing fat phobia and demonstrating weight bias, are simply foolish and hateful. While this is standard fare in critical pedagogy and constructivist approaches to education, it may be less well understood in other disciplines. We do not need to reinvent the wheel in fat pedagogy but instead can glean insights from existing educational theory, research, and practice, particularly from those fields already deeply invested in and knowledgeable about tackling oppression. We want to be clear that starting where students are does not mean that we must tolerate fat hatred, but rather that we need to find ways of naming and disrupting it in ways that do not simply shut learners down and send them scurrying. We must challenge ignorance when we encounter it, but need to do so in compassionate ways that clearly acknowledge the systemic forces at play. Recalling our own journeys of learning and unlearning weight bias may be helpful in that regard.

- Fat pedagogy must raise awareness and encourage critical thinking. Learners may have heard little about weight bias and not know that counterhegemonic movements like fat activism and Health At Every Size even exist. Further, as the old cliché goes, education ought not be about teaching learners *what* to think, but *how* to think. Helping learners build skills so that they can critically assess dominant obesity discourse, be that in the media, the doctor's office, grocery stores, research reports, or classroom materials, is important. But we cannot stop there, as learners need to be able to turn a critical eye on *all* information they encounter, including that produced by scholars working within critical obesity studies, critical weight studies, fat studies, and, yes, fat pedagogy.

- Emotions can run high in fat pedagogy. The chapters in this book are peppered with stories of frustration, discomfort, anger, denial, guilt, curiosity, excitement, love, and hope. The "affective turn" that is occurring in many disciplines, including education, makes it increasingly clear that knowledge alone is insufficient in making change. Fat pedagogy would do well to remember this.

- Given the fat-phobic contexts within which most of us operate, unlearning weight bias is an ongoing process even for those who have been doing this work for years. Further, as the authors in this book demonstrate, working to address weight-based oppression through education can be very challenging. It behooves all of us engaged in fat pedagogy, then, to continue to push at the edges of our own knowledge and continually engage in thoughtful self-reflection. Many of the authors in this book did a fine job of modeling what this can look like as they shared both the challenges they have faced and successes they have enjoyed as teachers and learners.

Fat pedagogy is a nascent field, ripe with possibility. Still, it needs sustenance of various sorts in order for it to grow to a size where it can make more of a difference in the world. We need more scholarship of all sorts, including theoretical work and empirical research grounded in diverse methodologies, more accounts of practice from a wider variety of contexts, more resources for educators, and more professional development for those on the education frontlines. Let us make the most of this moment in time when there appears to be growing recognition of weight-based oppression and a desire among educators of all stripes to do something about it.

References

Cameron, E. (2015). Teaching resources for post-secondary educators who challenge dominant obesity discourse. *Fat Studies, 4*(2), 212–226.

deCastell, S., & Bryson, M. (1998). From the ridiculous to the sublime: On finding oneself in educational research. In W. Pinar (Ed.), *Queer theory in education* (pp. 203–207). Mahwah, NJ: Lawrence Erlbaum.

Farrell, A. E. (2011). Refusing to apologize. In *Fat shame: Stigma and the fat body in American culture* (pp. 137–171). New York, NY: New York University Press.

Freespirit, J., & Aldebaran. (2009). Fat liberation manifesto, November 1973. In E. Rothblum & S. Solovay (Eds.), *The fat studies reader* (pp. 341–342). New York, NY: New York University Press.

Vaught, S. (2008). *Big fat manifesto.* New York, NY: Bloomsbury.

Wann, M. (2009). Foreword: Fat studies: An invitation to revolution. In E. Rothblum & S. Solovay (Eds.), *The fat studies reader* (pp. ix–xxv). New York, NY: New York University Press.

The Fat Pedagogy Reader

Biographical Statements for Contributors

Editors

Erin Cameron is an Assistant Professor in the School of Human Kinetics and Recreation at Memorial University in St. John's, Newfoundland, Canada. As a retired professional athlete and public speaker on health and wellness, her research interests are interdisciplinary and span across the fields of sport development, health and physical education, health promotion, and critical pedagogy. Dr. Cameron's most recent research examines strategies to reduce weight bias and discrimination and promote positive body image in diverse settings such as sport, education, and health care. Relevant publications include "Toward a Fat Pedagogy: A Study of Pedagogical Approaches Aimed at Challenging Obesity Discourse in Post-Secondary Education" and "Teaching Resources for Post-Secondary Educators Who Challenge Dominant Obesity Discourse," both published in *Fat Studies: An Interdisciplinary Journal of Body Weight and Society*. Email: ecameron@mun.ca

Constance Russell is a Professor in the Faculty of Education, Lakehead University, Thunder Bay, Ontario, Canada, where she teaches courses in environmental education, social justice education, and proposal writing. She has long used intersectional analyses in her research, including the implications of feminism, ecofeminism, queer theory, critical animal studies, and fat studies for environmental, humane, and social justice education. Other research interests include fat pedagogy, interspecies relations, climate change education, and interdisciplinary and academic/activist collaboration. Dr. Russell is the author of numerous articles and book chapters, the editor of the *Canadian Journal of Environmental Education*, and co-editor of the Rethinking Environmental Education book series for Peter Lang. Email: crussell@lakeheadu.ca

Contributing Authors

Ellen S. Abell, EdD, is a Professor of Psychology and Women's and Gender Studies at Prescott College, Prescott, Arizona, teaching courses in feminist theory, counselor education, and critical psychology. Ellen's lived experiences as a fat teenage girl and adult woman have informed her perspective on the important role that sizeism plays in U.S. culture, and has sensitized her to the damaging effects that fat oppression can have on the social, emotional, and physical lives of fat people. She shares an excerpt from her memoir in *The Fat Pedagogy Reader* as a tribute to the strength and resilience of fat girls everywhere. Email: eabell@prescott.edu

Angela S. Alberga is a Banting CIHR Postdoctoral Fellow at the University of Calgary, Alberta, Canada, researching effective ways to reduce weight bias in education, health care, and public policy. As an exercise physiologist by training, her doctoral research focused on promoting physical activity for teenagers living in larger bodies. Dr. Alberga advocates for change in how physical activity and health is framed in educational settings and for promoting physical activity for overall health and well-being without a focus on body weight. Email: aalberga@ucalgary.ca

Lucy Aphramor, RD, PhD, is a co-founder of Critical Dietetics and pioneered the use of Health At Every Size (HAES) in the U.K. National Health Service. Her Well Now course teaches HAES from a liberatory pedagogy, bridging self-care and social justice. Dr. Aphramor is widely published, often collaboratively, and commitments to ethics, equity, embodiment, and compassion are hallmarks of her work. Her co-authored book, *Body Respect: What Conventional Textbooks Leave Out, Get Wrong or Just Plain Fail to Understand About Weight*, with physiologist Linda Bacon, rewrites weight science from a socially just perspective. Lucy is also a poet and uses the arts as a practitioner-activist. Email: lucy@well-founded.org.uk

Linda Bacon, an internationally recognized interpreter of Health At Every Size science, is a Professor teaching health and social justice at City College of San Francisco, an Associate Nutritionist at the University of California, Davis, and holds graduate degrees in physiology, psychology, and exercise metabolism. She has conducted federally funded health research, is well-published in top scientific journals, and is the author of *Health At Every Size* and co-author, with Lucy Aphramor, of *Body Respect*. Well-known for her skills at critical thought and her political and social commentary, Dr. Bacon has generated a large following on social media platforms and the international lecture circuit. Email: linda@lindabacon.org

Natalie Beausoleil, PhD, is a feminist critical obesity scholar and Associate Professor of Social Sciences and Health in the Division of Community Health and Humanities in the Faculty of Medicine at Memorial University of Newfoundland. Her research, teaching, and activism focus on the social production and experiences of the body and health. Relevant publications include "An Impossible Task? Preventing Disordered Eating in the Context of the Current Obesity Panic" in Wright and Harwood's edited book, *Biopolitics and the 'Obesity Epidemic'* (Routledge, 2009), and, with Pamela Ward, "Fat Panic in Canadian Public Health Policy" in *Radical Psychology: A Journal of Psychology, Politics, and Radicalism* (2010). Email: nbeausol@mun.ca

Krishna Bhagat is a doctoral candidate in the Department of Behavioral and Community Health at the University of Maryland School of Public Health. She has experience teaching courses in global health and research methods. Her dissertation project seeks to examine children's conceptualizations of health, healthy bodies, and health practices as well as how these conceptualizations compare with the dominant obesity discourse and children's functional, communicative, and critical health literacy. She and Shannon Jette recently published a piece in the journal *Sport, Education, and Society*: "Governing the Child Citizen: 'Let's Move!' as National Biopedagogy." Email: knbhagat@umd.edu

Heather Brown is Executive Director of the Women + Girls Research Alliance at the University of North Carolina, Charlotte. She earned her EdD in adult and higher education at Northern Illinois University. Her research focuses on the intersections between weight and learning in girls and women as well as on the ethics and practice of research with stigmatized populations. She is co-editor of the *Journal of Research and Practice for Adult Literacy, Secondary, and Basic Education* and provides peer review for *Adult Education Quarterly* and the *Journal of Diversity in Higher Education*. Email: dr.heather.a.brown@gmail.com

Lisette Burrows is a Professor in the School of Physical Education, Sport, and Exercise Sciences at the University of Otago, New Zealand. She has been researching and teaching health and physical education pedagogy for more than 20 years. Her research draws on poststructural theoretical tools and insights from the sociology of education, sociology of youth, curriculum studies, and cultural studies to explore the place and meaning of physical culture and health in young people's lives. She is keen to understand how socially critical perspectives on enduring issues such as 'obesity' and 'health' are taken up, or not, by tertiary students. Email: lisette.burrows@otago.ac.nz

Breanne Fahs is an Associate Professor of Women and Gender Studies at Arizona State University, where she specializes in studying women's sexuality, critical embodiment studies, radical feminism, and political activism. She has published widely in feminist, social science, and humanities journals and has authored four books: *Performing Sex* (SUNY Press, 2011), *The Moral Panics of Sexuality* (Palgrave, 2013), *Valerie Solanas* (Feminist Press, 2014), and *Out for Blood* (SUNY Press, forthcoming). She is the director of the Feminist Research on Gender and Sexuality Group at Arizona State University, and she also works as a private practice clinical psychologist specializing in sexuality and body image. Email: breanne.fahs@asu.edu

Amy E. Farrell is Executive Director of the Clarke Forum, Ann and John Curley Chair of Liberal Arts, and Professor of American Studies and Women's and Gender Studies at Dickinson College in Carlisle, Pennsylvania. She is the author of *Fat Shame: Stigma and the Fat Body in American Culture* and *Yours in Sisterhood: Ms. Magazine and the Promise of Popular Feminism*. She regularly teaches both fat studies and the history of American feminism as well as theory and writing courses within her fields. Email: farrell@dickinson.edu

Michael Gard is Associate Professor of Sport, Health, and Physical Education in the School of Human Movement and Nutrition Sciences at the University of Queensland, Australia. He teaches, researches, and writes about how the human body is and has been used, experienced, educated, and governed. He is the author of four books, including *The Obesity Epidemic: Science, Morality and Ideology* and *The End of the Obesity Epidemic*. His most recent major work, written with Carolyn Pluim, is *Schools and Public Health: Past, Present, Future* (Rowman & Littlefield). Email: michael.gard@scu.edu.au

Olga Heath, PhD, R. Psych, is an Associate Professor and Registered Psychologist at Memorial University of Newfoundland, Canada. Her principal areas of research/practice interest are eating disorders and teaching collaborative practice skills to health care students. These interests often intersect both in her interprofessional teaching and in her work leading a project designed to educate health care professionals about the continuum of care in eating disorders and how to work together to ensure the best possible treatment. Her experiences teaching health care students and professionals have highlighted the unconscious level of prejudice towards larger people existing in these groups and the need to sensitize and educate towards change. Email: oheath@mun.ca

Shannon Jette is an Assistant Professor in the Department of Kinesiology at the University of Maryland School of Public Health. She uses a range of qualitative research methods and social theory to examine the production, dissemination, and interpretation of knowledge about the active body. Much of her research focuses on the issue of prenatal exercise and gestational weight gain—from examinations of the production of medical knowledge around maternal exercise and weight gain to the ways that women of varying cultural backgrounds experience maternal weight gain and movement in their daily lives. She has published in such journals as *Sociology of Health & Illness* and *Health, Risk & Society*. Email: jette@umd.edu

Victoria Kannen, PhD, is an Assistant Professor in Communication Studies at Huntington University in Sudbury, Ontario, Canada. She has taught courses such as The Decorated Body as Communication, Media and Popular Culture, Introduction to Gender, and Gender, Globalization and Social Change. Her research has appeared in journals such as *Teaching in Higher Education*, *Journal of Gender Studies*, and *Gender, Place and Culture*. Email: vx_kannen@huntingtonu.ca

Deana Leahy is a Senior Lecturer in the Faculty of Education at Monash University, Australia. Her research interests are framed by a concern about the political and moral work that is 'done' under the guise of improving the health of children and young people in educational settings. Her research draws from Foucauldian and post-Foucauldian writings on governmentality to consider the various mentalities that are assembled together in policy and health education curriculum and how they are translated into key pedagogical spaces. Dr. Leahy is the co-author of the recently published book *School Health Education in Changing Times* (Routledge, 2015). Email: deana.leahy@monash.edu

Lori Don Levan is an Instructor for the School of Visual Arts at Pennsylvania State University. She holds an EdD in art education from Teachers College, Columbia University, New York City. She holds an MS in administration and supervision with a visual arts focus from Bank Street College of Education, New York City, and a Parson's School of Design certificate. Her BFA (with K–12 art teaching certification) is from Wilkes University, Wilkes-Barre,

Pennsylvania. Dr. Levan's teaching experience has covered a wide range of age groups from young children to adults. She is an active artist/researcher who explores issues concerning the fat female body, corporeality, and beauty. Email: ldl7@verizon.net

Hannah McNinch, BA, BEd, MEd, is a teacher with the Simcoe Muskoka Catholic District School Board, Ontario, Canada. Her interest in fat phobia fueled the development of her MEd thesis research on fat bullying of girls in elementary and secondary school. She co-authored "'Fatties Causing Global Warming': Fat Pedagogy and Environmental Education" for the *Canadian Journal of Environmental Education* (with Russell, Cameron, & Socha, 2013). She is very interested in fat pedagogy as a response to the prevalence of weight-based oppression in the Canadian education system. In her teaching, she works to challenge the fat-phobic discourse she witnesses being reproduced by children, teachers, and parents every day. Email: hmcninch@lakeheadu.ca

Moss Norman is in the Faculty of Kinesiology and Recreation Management at the University of Manitoba, Canada. He uses a qualitative lens to examine the relationship between physical culture, health, and embodiment. Currently, he is using a community-based research design to explore contemporary and historical Indigenous physical cultural masculinities in Fisher River Cree Nation, Manitoba. Dr. Norman also maintains secondary but active research interests in masculinity, fatness, and health; rural youth and recreation; and biomedicalized constructions of youth, health, and embodiment. He has numerous peer-reviewed publications, including in journals such as *Men and Masculinities, Gender, Place and Culture, Sport in Society, Sociology of Sport Journal,* and *The Journal of Rural Studies.* Email: Moss.Norman@umanitoba.ca

Caitlin O'Reilly is a PhD candidate in the School of Kinesiology at the University of British Columbia, Canada. Recent publications on weight stigma include an article with Judith Sixsmith, "From Theory to Policy: Reducing Harms Associated With the Weight-Centered Health Paradigm" in *Fat Studies* (2012), and an article with Erin Cameron, "Sizing Up Stigma: Weighing in on the Issues and Solutions to Diabetes and Obesity Stigma" in *Biochemistry & Cell Biology* (2015). Caitlin is currently involved in research on both weight stigma in health care and eating disorders and is deeply committed to research for social change. Email: caito@interchange.ubc.ca

Cat Pausé is the Lead Editor of *Queering Fat Embodiment* (2014, Ashgate). She is Senior Lecturer in Human Development and Fat Studies Researcher at Massey University, New Zealand, and her research focuses on the effects of spoiled identities on the health and well-being of fat individuals. She has published in top journals such as *Human Development, Feminist Review, HERDSA,* and *Narrative Inquiries in Bioethics.* Dr. Pausé hosted the Fat Studies: Reflective Intersections conference in 2012, and is gearing up for Fat Studies: Identity, Agency, and Embodiment in 2016. Her work has been featured on *Huffington Post*, Yahoo, NPR, and *20/20*. She also maintains a presence in the Fatosphere through Tumblr, YouTube, Twitter, podcasts, and the blog Friend of Marilyn. Email: c.pause@massey.ac.nz

LeAnne Petherick is on the Faculty of Kinesiology and Recreation Management at the University of Manitoba, Canada. She is a qualitative researcher who uses feminist poststructural approaches to disrupt dominant ways of thinking about the body in physical and health education. Focusing on the cycle of knowledge production, particularly in relation to school-based health promotion curricula, Dr. Petherick examines how these initiatives are taught and taken up in everyday life and how they shape how students and teachers alike come to think about health, the body, and human movement. Dr. Petherick has numerous peer-reviewed publications in journals such as *Sport, Education and Society*, *Critical Methodologies: Cultural Studies*, and *Canadian Journal of Education*. Email: leanne.petherick@umanitoba.ca

Darren Powell is a Lecturer of Health Education and Physical Education at the University of Auckland, New Zealand. Formerly an elementary school teacher, Darren's research focuses on the 'childhood obesity crisis' and the ways in which corporations (especially those of the food and drink industry) are reinventing themselves as 'part of the solution.' This includes an investigation of how schools, teachers, and children are drawn into the global war on obesity, and how corporations are using concerns about children's allegedly unhealthy lifestyles to promote themselves as healthy, philanthropic, and educational. Email: d.powell@auckland.ac.nz

Richard Pringle is Associate Professor of Socio-Cultural Studies of Sport and Physical Education at the University of Auckland, New Zealand. He is the co-author of *Foucault, Sport and Exercise: Power, Knowledge and Transforming the Self*, *Sport and the Social Significance of Pleasure*, and co-editor of *Examining Sport Histories: Power, Paradigms and Reflexivity*. His critical qualitative research draws on poststructural theories to predominantly examine issues associated with sport, exercise, gender, sexuality, health, and the body. Email: r.pringle@auckland.ac.nz

Emma Rich is a Reader in the Department for Health, University of Bath, United Kingdom. Over the past decade, Dr. Rich has been undertaking critical health research examining the recent changes in policies and practices geared towards tackling the perceived risks associated with obesity and the impact this has on young people's experiences of their bodies, weight, and health practices. Her recent work is focused on digital health and the relationships between learning, technologies, and health (e.g., exergaming, mobile health, social media). Her major books are *The Medicalization of Cyberspace* (2008, Routledge); *Education, Disordered Eating and Obesity Discourse: Fat Fabrications* (2008, Routledge); and *Debating Obesity: Critical Perspectives* (2011, Palgrave). Email: E.Rich@bath.ac.uk

Esther D. Rothblum, PhD, is Professor of Women's Studies at San Diego State University, California. Her research and writing have focused on the stigma of weight, and she has edited more than 20 books, including *Overcoming Fear of Fat* (with Laura Brown in 1989). Her most recent book, *The Fat Studies Reader* (with Sondra Solovay in 2009), was reviewed in *The New Yorker*, the *New York Times*, *Ms.* magazine, the *Chronicle of Higher Education*, and elsewhere. Dr. Rothblum is a member of the advisory board of the National Association to Advance Fat Acceptance and a founding co-chair of the Size Acceptance Caucus of the Association for Women in Psychology. Email: erothblu@mail.sdsu.edu

Tracy Royce is a fat feminist writer, poet, and sociology graduate student at the University of California, Santa Barbara. Her scholarly and/or creative work has appeared in various places, including *Affilia: Journal of Women and Social Work*, *Archives of Sexual Behavior*, *The Fat Studies*

Reader, Frogpond, Modern Haiku, and *Mother of Invention: How Our Mothers Influenced Us as Feminist Academics and Activists.* She lives in Los Angeles with animator Rob Renzetti and their naughty rabbit, Zigzag. Email: troyce@umail.ucsb.edu

Shelly Russell-Mayhew is a Registered Psychologist and Associate Professor in the Werklund School of Education, University of Calgary, Canada. Recently awarded the Werklund Research Professorship, her vision is to lead and transform prevention research about weight-related issues such as body image (perceptions, attitudes, and experiences about the body), disordered eating (e.g., unhealthy methods of weight change), weight-related disorders (e.g., obesity and eating disorders), and professional conversations and interactions about weight (e.g., weight bias). Dr. Russell-Mayhew believes that physical activity messages should be divorced from messages about weight and size and every*body* has a right to be physically active. Email: mkrussel@ucalgary.ca

Keri Semenko is a Professor in the Animal Care Program at Durham College in Oshawa, Ontario, Canada. She primarily teaches courses related to ethics and animal welfare law, wildlife science, and exotic animal care. Her passion for animal studies has guided her educational and personal journey and she brings years of frontline experience in animal sheltering work to her teaching. Her interest in fat pedagogy is connected to her desire to understand the intersectionality of oppressions faced by women and non-human animals, which began during her master's research related to women working in zoological parks. Email: keri.semenko@durhamcollege.ca

Marilyn Wann, MA, has been a fat activist since the mid-1990s when she published the print zine *FAT!SO?.* She is author of the book *FAT!SO? Because You Don't Have to Apologize for Your Size!* and is the creator of *Yay!Scales.* Email: marilyn@fatso.com

Pamela Ward, PhD, RN, is a Nurse Educator at the Centre for Nursing Studies and an Adjunct Professor with the Faculty of Medicine at Memorial University of Newfoundland, Canada. She utilizes qualitative and critical feminist approaches in her research with special attention to the social construction of the body in relation to health, fitness, and bodily norms. She is also the co-chair of the Body Image Network and has been involved in projects designed to enhance interprofessional practice in the promotion of positive body image and the prevention and treatment of eating disorders throughout the province of Newfoundland and Labrador. Email: pamela.ward@mun.ca

Patti Lou Watkins is an Associate Professor in Psychology at Oregon State University where she has developed and teaches the classes Women, Weight, and Body Image and Fat Studies. Her research has examined weight bias, body image, and physical activity, including evaluation of a weight-neutral program to facilitate exercise participation by larger women. She is currently on the editorial board of *Fat Studies: An Interdisciplinary Journal of Body Weight and Society* and has previously published in the area of fat studies pedagogy. She is also on the Education and Programming Committee for the Association for Size Diversity and Health. Email: pwatkins@oregonstate.edu

Jan Wright is a Professorial Fellow in the Faculty of Social Sciences at the University of Wollongong, Australia. Her most recent research draws on feminist and poststructuralist theory to critically engage issues associated with the relationship between embodiment, culture, and health. Dr. Wright's books include: *Biopolitics and the 'Obesity Epidemic': Governing Bodies* (Routledge 2009), co-edited with Valerie Harwood; *Young People, Physical Activity and the Everyday* (Routledge 2010), co-edited with Doune Macdonald; *The 'Obesity Epidemic': Science, Ideology and Morality* (Routledge 2005), co-authored with Michael Gard; and *School Health Education in Changing Times* (Routledge 2016), co-authored with Deana Leahy, Lisette Burrows, Louise McCuaig, and Dawn Penney. Email: jwright@uow.edu.au

Author Index

Y

Z

Subject Index

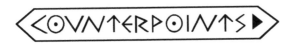

Studies in the Postmodern Theory of Education

General Editor
Shirley R. Steinberg

Counterpoints publishes the most compelling and imaginative books being written in education today. Grounded on the theoretical advances in criticalism, feminism, and postmodernism in the last two decades of the twentieth century, Counterpoints engages the meaning of these innovations in various forms of educational expression. Committed to the proposition that theoretical literature should be accessible to a variety of audiences, the series insists that its authors avoid esoteric and jargonistic languages that transform educational scholarship into an elite discourse for the initiated. Scholarly work matters only to the degree it affects consciousness and practice at multiple sites. Counterpoints' editorial policy is based on these principles and the ability of scholars to break new ground, to open new conversations, to go where educators have never gone before.

For additional information about this series or for the submission of manuscripts, please contact:

Shirley R. Steinberg
c/o Peter Lang Publishing, Inc.
29 Broadway, 18th floor
New York, New York 10006

To order other books in this series, please contact our Customer Service Department:

(800) 770-LANG (within the U.S.)
(212) 647-7706 (outside the U.S.)
(212) 647-7707 FAX

Or browse online by series:
www.peterlang.com

Lightning Source UK Ltd.
Milton Keynes UK
UKHW032119030522
402438UK00009B/2006